# *INSTRUCTOR'S MANUAL TO ACCOMPANY COPSTEAD:*

# *Perspectives on Pathophysiology*

*Jacquelyn Banasik, PhD, RN*
*Intercollegiate Center for Nursing Education*
*Spokane, Washington*

W. B. SAUNDERS COMPANY
*A Division of Harcourt Brace & Company*
Philadelphia London Toronto
Montreal Sydney Tokyo

W. B. SAUNDERS COMPANY
*A Division of Harcourt Brace & Company*
The Curtis Center
Independence Square West
Philadelphia, PA 19106

Instructor's Manual to Accompany Copstead: Perspectives on Pathophysiology

ISBN 0-7216-4754-5



Printed in the United States of America.

Last digit is the print number: 9 8 7 6 5 4 3 2 1

# *Preface*

Pathophysiology can be a daunting subject for students because of the large volumes of material to be learned. The textbook *Perspectives on Pathophysiology* has been written to help students focus on key pathophysiologic concepts. To help students identify what is most important among the many facts and details in the texbook, **KEY CONCEPTS** are identified regularly within the chapters and printed in an accent color in bulleted lists. A similar conceptual approach is used in this Instructor's Manual. **Key Questions, Case Examples,** and **Test Items** in this manual are reflective of the **KEY CONCEPTS** identified in each chapter of the textbook.

Instructional aids such as a **Sample Course Syllabus** and suggested **Teaching Strategies** are included for the beginning instructor. Seasoned instructors using *Perspectives on Pathophysiology* will find the Case Examples, Test Items with Answer Keys, and **Transparency Masters** useful. Approximately 500 test items are provided for the units; in addition, a **Sample Comprehensive Exam** containing 100 multiple choice questions is included.

The fourth section of this manual is a unique 140-page **Lecture Guide**, which can be used by instructors to organize content or can be photocopied for students by instructors who have adopted the book for classroom use. Students will find the Lecture Guide useful for notetaking during lectures and for review.

The promotion of critical thinking is a widespread goal. For example, the National League for Nursing accreditation criteria have placed heavy emphasis on the inclusion of critical thinking in nursing curricula. To help instructors meet these goals, supportive materials have been included. The Key Questions and Case Examples in Section Two of this Instructor's Manual are particularly helpful in providing practice with critical thinking about pathophysiology. Many of the Key Questions included in the manual are not easy to answer, nor do they necessarily have only one answer. They go beyond recall of factual information from the text and are designed to enhance students' thinking skills.

Teaching pathophysiology can be a challenging undertaking, and our aim in *Perspectives on Pathophysiology* and in this Instructor's Manual has been to help both instructors and students in their mutual endeavor.

## *Contents*

# List of Transparency Masters

| Transparency Number | Textbook Figure Number | Description |
|---|---|---|
| 1. | 1-18 | Etiologic Classification of Disease |
| 2. | 2-2 | Structure of Cell Membrane |
| 3. | 2-16 | Mitochondrial Electron Transport Chain |
| 4. | 2-17 | Schematic of ATP Synthetase |
| 5. | 2-20 | Membrane Channels and Carriers |
| 6. | 2-23 | The Sodium-Potassium Ion Pump |
| 7. | 2-24 | Membrane Calcium Ion Pumps |
| 8. | 2-27 | Effect of Potassium Concentration on Resting Membrane Potential |
| 9. | 2-29 | Ion Conductance During Action Potential |
| 10. | 2-31 | Action Potential in Ventricular Myocardium |
| 11. | 2-33 | Receptor Mechanisms |
| 12. | 3-4 | Cellular Responses to Injury |
| 13. | 5-1 | Chromosome Nondisjunction |
| 14. | 5-9 | Autosomal Dominant Inheritance Patterns |
| 15. | 5-11 | Autosomal Recessive Inheritance Patterns |
| 16. | 5-13 | Periods of Fetal Vulnerability |
| 17. | 6-4 | Mechanisms of Oncogene Activation |
| 18. | 6-6 | Mechanisms of Altered Growth Control |
| 19. | 7-1 | Sympathetic Alarm Reaction |
| 20. | 7-7 | Organs of the Immune System |
| 21. | 7-12 | Potential Stress Reactions |
| 22. | 8-4 | Factors Affecting Infectious Processes |
| 23. | 9-1 | Hematopoietic Cells |
| 24. | 9-11 | Typical Immunoglobulin Structure |
| 25. | 10-10 | HIV Structure |
| 26. | 10-11 | Sequence of HIV Infection |
| 27. | 13-1 | The Clotting Cascade |
| 28. | 14-13 | Factors Affecting Transcapillary Filtration |
| 29. | 16-12 | Sarcomere Structure |
| 30. | 16-15 | Proteins of the Thin Filament |
| 31. | 16-18 | The Role of Calcium Ion in Crossbridge Formation |
| 32. | 16-19 | Mechanisms of Calcium Ion Removal from the Sarcoplasm |
| 33. | 16-22 | Conduction System of the Heart |
| 34. | 17-2 | Subendocardial (A) and Transmural (B) Infarct |
| 35. | 17-6 | Mitral Stenosis |
| 36. | 17-7 | Mitral Regurgitation |
| 37. | 17-10 | Aortic Stenosis |
| 38. | 17-15 | Fetal Circulation |
| 39. | 18-1 | Compensatory Mechanisms in Heart Failure |
| 40. | 18-4 | Pathophysiology of Left Heart Failure |
| 41. | 18-5 | Manifestations of Left Heart Failure |
| 42. | 18-6 | Pathophysiology of Right Heart Failure |
| 43. | 18-7 | Manifestations of Right Heart Failure |
| 44. | 19-5 | Pulmonary Alveoli |
| 45. | 19-8 | Lobes and Segments of the Lungs |

# SECTION ONE

## *Teaching Strategies: Getting Started*

- *Approaches to Teaching Pathophysiology*
- *Sample Course Syllabus*

# *Approaches to Teaching Pathophysiology*

Pathophysiology concepts frequently are taught using the lecture format. This approach allows coverage of large volumes of material, but it may not stimulate students to think about and internalize the information. Some students may resort to rote memorization because of the overwhelming amount of "stuff" to be learned. Memorization often serves them poorly, however, when they are required to apply pathophysiology concepts in clinical practice. Techniques to stimulate critical thinking in the classroom may facilitate the student's ability to transfer classroom knowledge into clinical situations.

Depending on teaching style, classroom time frame, and class size, individual instructors may wish to stick primarily to the lecture format, with a few techniques to keep students thinking. Others may be ready to abandon didactic teaching altogether in favor of the critical thinking approach. This manual contains supportive materials for both approaches, including example Key Questions that can be used to guide class discussions, suggested lecture outlines, case studies, and exam questions.

## USING THE MANUAL

This instructor's manual is divided into five sections. The content included in each section is detailed below, with suggested applications.

### *Sections One*

Section One includes the present introduction to teaching strategies and a sample course syllabus. This syllabus is for a typical 16-week, three-semester hour course and includes a course description, course objectives, course policies, grading, written assignments, and a topical outline.

### *Section Two*

The organization of this section parallels that of the Copstead textbook. Each unit includes Key Questions to guide critical thinking activities, case examples, and test items with answer keys. These are detailed here.

#### Key Physiology and Pathophysiology Questions

Many students taking an introductory pathophysiology course will need to review normal physiology. Chapters on normal physiology are included in the Copstead textbook for all of the major body systems. Since time constraints will usually not allow devotion of much class time to physiology review, students may be required to accomplish this independently. Key Questions for physiology chapters can be given to students to guide their own review and self-assessment, or they can be administered as a preliminary exam prior to beginning the course content, with specific direction for students to self-remediate areas of weakness.

Key Questions are designed to guide classroom discussions of key pathophysiology concepts. They were written to promote intellectual processing rather than simple recall of information from the text. These questions are linked to the Key Concepts in each chapter of the Copstead textbook. For every unit, students can also be asked the following question, "Are the Key Concepts included in this unit indeed the key points?" To answer this question, students will need to critically read the textbook, formulate their own key ideas, and compare them to the ones identified in the textbook. In addition to stimulating critical reading skills, students will be encouraged to realize that a textbook is only one way of interpreting the "facts."

Key Questions may also serve as a basis for take-home assignments, essay exam questions, and small group work. When engaging in small group work in a larger classroom, it may be useful to tell students that a representative from the group will be randomly selected by the instructor to report back to the larger group. Do not identify the group representative until the time for them to report. This tactic helps keep all students in the group engaged and actively listening.

Although learning objectives have not been included in this manual, the Key Questions can be reworded to formulate objective statements. For example, the Key Question "How does lifestyle contribute to cancer risk?" can be written as a learning objective: "Understands how lifestyle contributes to cancer risk." If behavioral objectives are preferred, "Describes how lifestyle contributes to cancer risk" can be used instead.

#### Case Examples

One or more case examples are included in each unit of Section Two to help students use pathophysiology concepts in practical situations. Case examples can be used for small group work, take-home assignments, or class discussions.

#### Test Items

Each unit includes a number of possible exam questions. Most questions are written in a format amenable to computer grading (multiple choice, true/false, and matching). Questions related to case scenarios are included to help students begin thinking in terms of application.

### *Section Three*

A sample comprehensive exam is included as Section Three which allows assessment of the students' understanding of interrelated systems. These concepts may not be adequately tested in unit exams that cover only one system.

### *Section Four*

A suggested lecture guide or outline is included for instructors using primarily a didactic format. The lecture guide may be copied for students and used as a note-taking outline during lecture. The lecture guide was designed to provide enough structure to keep students on track, yet not enough to encourage skipping class. Students report that lecture outlines help them get back on track when they get behind or distracted. Without lecture outlines, students may furiously take notes, but comprehend little. If the guides are too complete, inattentiveness and poor attendance may result. Lecture guides are not comprehensive but rather focus on important points that may reasonably be covered in a typical class time frame.

### *Section Five*

Section Five includes 74 transparency masters of selected textbook illustrations. Each transparency master is referenced by title and textbook figure number.

## TEACHING STRATEGIES

### *Getting Clear about Purpose*

A stimulating way to begin a pathophysiology class is to have students try to articulate the purpose of learning pathophysiology. This is not easy, but it will help them develop a sense of how the volumes of information in the textbook can be organized in their own thinking so that it can be useful in clinical practice. A beginning articulation might go something like this: "A working knowledge of pathophysiology is requisite for sound clinical practice. Students who have acquired this working knowledge are able to reason about the significance of assessment findings, identify potential links among bits of information, identify potential clinical problems, and predict the consequences of a particular intervention based on logical theories of pathogenesis. When given a known pathology, the student can predict probable clinical manifestations; the student is also adept at posing probable pathologies from a set of clinical findings."

The goal, then, is to enable students to reason through clinical situations using pathophysiology concepts, sorting important from unimportant information, making logical interpretations, and identifying the need for more data to check their assumptions. Of course, critical thinking about pathophysiology requires a large amount of "factual" information that may be gleaned from the textbook. Class time can be used to reinforce textbook information (lecture) or to provide practice with the reasoning aspect: applying knowledge gained from reading to clinical examples. If the lecture format is used, out of class assignments that require reasoning and clinical application may aid retention of information and development of thinking skills.

### *Gearing Up for Critical Thinking*

On the first day of class, it is helpful to let the students know what they are in for. If you intend to rely primarily on lectures, the students will already be comfortable with this approach since most of their college education to this point has probably been delivered in this style. If you plan to use a critical thinking approach, some warning to your students is in order! Here are some ideas that may be useful.

1. A critical thinking approach requires students to complete reading assignments prior to class. This may be a drastic change for most students. Make it clear that unprepared students will be unable to benefit from class discussions.
2. Let students know that you intend to involve the entire class in discussions and will be calling often on students who do not have their hands up. A shuffled deck of index cards containing the students' names may work well for a large group. Students who have already been called on cannot lapse since their names may be called again as cards are shuffled.
3. Let students know that the response, "I don't know" will not get them off the hook. Come back to them later after giving them some time to think.
4. Students may at first be reluctant to speak in class for fear of being wrong. Stress the reality that ignorance coexists with knowledge and that they are expected to make and learn from mistakes. The goal is to move from greater to lesser ignorance. They will never know it all (and neither will the instructor).
5. Requiring students to keep a class notebook that documents their learning and class participation may be useful. For example, students can be encouraged to record questions that occur to

them during class discussions and insights and deeper understandings they acquire as a result of participation in class discussion. Notebooks can be collected without prior notice periodically throughout the semester to motivate students to keep up with written work.

6. Provide students with a clear (written) explanation of evaluation and grading procedures. (See the sample course syllabus at the end of this section.)

Pathophysiology can be a challenging and exciting subject for instructors and students alike. The Copstead textbook has been written to help students focus on and understand the major pathophysiologic concepts. The materials included in this manual are designed to reinforce this conceptual approach. The case studies, exam questions, and key questions for class discussion are all reflective of the key concepts identified in the Copstead textbook.

## *Sample Course Syllabus*

**COURSE TITLE:** Pathophysiology

**COURSE NUMBER:** XXX

**CREDIT HOURS:** 3 Semester/5 Quarter

**PLACE IN CURRICULUM:** First Semester, Junior Year

**FACULTY:** XXXXX

Office Hours: Thursday 11-1

### COURSE DESCRIPTION

Major pathophysiologic concepts are explored using a body systems approach. Theories relating etiology, pathogenesis, and clinical manifestations are used to study common disease processes. Concepts from anatomy and physiology courses provide the foundation for exploring human dysfunction. Concepts learned in this course are basic to nursing practice.

### COURSE OBJECTIVES

1. Understands the etiology, pathogenesis, clinical manifestations, and treatment implications of common disorders of human function.
2. Critically analyzes clinical data to identify logical connections, sort important and unimportant data, and identify potential pathophysiologic processes.
3. Predicts usual clinical manifestations and appropriate treatments for patients with defined medical diagnoses.
4. Predicts the consequences of particular interventions based on logical theories of pathogenesis.

### INSTRUCTIONAL STRATEGIES

Reading assignments, class discussion, case studies, and small group work are used primarily with limited supplemental lecture.

### REQUIRED TEXTS

Copstead, L. E. (1995) *Perspectives on Pathophysiology:* Philadelphia, W. B. Saunders Company.

## EVALUATION

The grade for this course will be determined on the basis of in-class exams, take home assignments, and class participation. An overall average of 73% must be achieved to pass the course.

| | |
|---|---|
| In-Class Exams: | 80% |
| Exam 1 (20%) | |
| Exam 2 (20%) | |
| Exam 3 (20%) | |
| Exam 4 (20%) | |
| Take Home Assignments: | 10% |
| Class Participation: | 10% |
| | 100% |

## COURSE POLICIES

1. Participation in class discussion and small group work is essential to achieving the objectives of this course. It is intended that the entire class will engage in critical listening, critical reading, and critical thinking. Several strategies will be used to facilitate this process:

   a. Readings are to be completed prior to class. Each student will keep a notebook of completed assignments to serve as reference during in class discussions.
   b. Students will be called on randomly to contribute in class.
   c. Students will be expected to critique their own and one another's thinking. This may be done verbally in class or on writing assignments.
   d. The goal is to move from greater ignorance to lesser ignorance. Ignorance co-exists with knowledge in everyone (including the Instructor!). Knowing the "right" answer is of lesser importance than being able to "think through" an answer. A response such as "I don't know" will not get a student off the hook.
   e. Students are expected to help one another achieve the objectives of the course. Each student has areas of strength and weakness that add to the diversity of the class.

2. In-class exams are to be taken at the scheduled time. If a student is unable to take an exam as scheduled, he or she must notify the instructor prior to the exam to make alternate arrangements. All exams are to be the student's own work. Academic dishonesty may result in failure of the course.

## COURSE ASSIGNMENTS

Each student must use an 8-1/2" × 11" college ruled spiral bound notebook for written work in this course. The notebook will be turned in periodically during the course of the semester and will be used to assign a grade for written work which is worth 10% of the total course grade. The notebook will also be a resource for assigning a grade for class participation which is worth 10% of the total course grade. Students should bring notebooks to class each time because they will be collected *without prior notice.*

*Written Work*

### 1. Take Home Questions

For each major body system, take home questions will be distributed. Each student should record the answers to these questions in the class notebook. These should be completed prior to class because they will be discussed in class. Take home questions will guide the students' review of normal physiology.

### 2. Key Concepts

To facilitate the development of critical reading skills, students will identify "Key Concepts" for each chapter of assigned reading. At least ten key concepts must be identified per chapter. Key concepts are to be written in the students' own words and not be copied from the text. Key concepts are to be written in the class notebook prior to class discussion. Additional key concepts may be added to the list as they are discussed during class.

### 3. Case Studies

Three case studies will be completed over the course of the semester. These are to be turned in separately from the class notebook. Detailed instructions will accompany the case study handouts.

## DOCUMENTATION OF CLASS PARTICIPATION (10%)

There are multiple avenues for "actively" participating in class discussions. Not everyone will have an opportunity to contribute verbally in each discussion. It will be helpful in assigning a "Class Participation" grade for the course if students document their weekly participation in the following way:

1. Record questions that occur to you during class discussions and include these in your class notebook.
2. Record insights and deeper understandings that you achieve as a result of critically listening to and thinking about class discussions and include these in your class notebook.

## *COURSE SCHEDULE*

| Date | Class | Readings/Assignments |
|---|---|---|
| **Week 1** | | |
| Aug. 31 | Course Orientation | |
| Sept. 1 | Cell Phys | Chapt 1, 2 |
| **Week 2** | | |
| Sept. 7 | Cell Dysfunction | Chapt 3, 4, 5, 6 |
| Sept. 8 | Neoplasia | |
| **Week 3** | | |
| Sept. 14 | Immune physiology | Chapt 7, 8, 9 |
| Sept. 15 | Immune dysfunction | Chapt 10, 11 |
| **Week 4** | | |
| Sept. 21 | Immune dysfunction | |
| Sept. 22 | Blood and Vascular | Chapt 12, 13, 14, 15 |
| **Week 5** | | |
| Sept. 28 | **EXAM 1** | |
| Sept. 29 | Blood and Vascular | |
| **Week 6** | | |
| Oct. 5 | Cardiac Physiology | Chapt 16 |
| Oct. 6 | Cardiac Physiology | |
| **Week 7** | | |
| Oct. 12 | Cardiac Dysfunction | Chapt 17, 18 |
| Oct. 13 | Cardiac Dysfunction | **Case Study #1 Due** |
| **Week 8** | | |
| Oct. 19 | Respiratory | Chapt 19, 20, 21, 22, 23 |
| Oct. 20 | Respiratory | |
| **Week 9** | | |
| Oct. 26 | Respiratory | |
| Oct. 27 | Acid–Base | Chapt 24, 25 |
| **Week 10** | | |
| Nov. 2 | **EXAM 2** | |
| Nov. 3 | Fluid and Electrolytes | |

*COURSE SCHEDULE (continued)*

| Date | Class | Readings/Assignments |
|---|---|---|
| **Week 11** | | |
| Nov. 9 | Renal | Chapt 26, 27, 28, 29 |
| Nov. 10 | Renal | |
| **Week 12** | | |
| Nov. 16 | GI | **Case Study #2 Due** |
| Nov. 17 | GI | Chapt 35, 36, 37, 38 |
| **Week 13** | Thanksgiving Break | |
| **Week 14** | | |
| Nov. 30 | **EXAM 3** | |
| Dec. 1 | Endocrine | Chapt 39, 40, 41 |
| **Week 15** | | |
| Dec. 7 | Neurophysiology | Chapt 42, 43, 44, 45, 46 |
| Dec. 8 | Neurologic Dysfunction | |
| **Week 16** | | |
| Dec. 14 | Neurologic Dysfunction | **Case Study #3 Due** |
| Dec. 15 | Musculoskeletal | Chapt 49, 50, 51 |
| **Week 17** | | |
| Dec. 21 | **FINAL EXAM**, 8–10 a.m. | |

# SECTION TWO

## *Questions for Class Discussion and Evaluation*

- *Key Questions*
- *Case Examples*
- *Test Items with Answer Keys*

# *Unit I—Central Concepts of Pathophysiology*

## KEY QUESTIONS

### *Chapter 1—Complex Nature of Disease*

1. What is pathophysiology and why is it important for clinical practice?
2. What general factors affect the expression of disease in a particular person?
3. How are normal and abnormal physiologic parameters defined?
4. What factors, other than disease, might result in "abnormal" physiologic values?
5. Why do homeostatic control mechanisms generally function as negative feedback systems?
6. Explain, with examples, two or three homeostatic mechanisms.
7. How might disease disrupt homeostasis?
8. What kinds of information about disease can be gained through epidemiology?
9. Give an example of disease pathogenesis and contrast with etiology.

## TEST ITEMS

### *True/False*

____ 1. Normal ranges for physiologic parameters are arbitrarily defined based on population sampling.

____ 2. Values outside the normal range for a particular variable are always indicative of disease.

____ 3. Illness and disease always coexist.

____ 4. Normalcy is culturally defined.

____ 5. A change in a physiologic variable is more significant than the actual values.

____ 6. Most homeostatic mechanisms function via positive feedback loops.

____ 7. Homeostatic control mechanisms function primarily during disease states.

____ 8. Epidemiology is the study of disease expression in individuals.

____ 9. The etiology and pathogenesis of most disease states have been well defined by research.

____ 10. Individuals experiencing the same disease process will exhibit the same clinical manifestations.

### *Case Scenario*

C. Q. was recently exposed to group A hemolytic streptococcus and subsequently developed a pharyngeal infection. His clinic examination reveals an oral temperature of 102.3°F, skin rash, and reddened throat mucosa with multiple pustules. He complains of sore throat, malaise, and joint stiffness. A throat culture is positive for streptococcus, and antibiotics have been prescribed.

11. The etiology of C. Q.'s disease is
    a. a sore throat.
    b. streptococcal infection.
    c. genetic susceptibility.
    d. pharyngitis.

12. Which of the following is a statement about pathogenesis?
    a. Pharyngitis is caused by group A hemolytic streptococcus infection.
    b. Streptococcal infection activates immune cells leading to inflammation.
    c. Sore throat and mucosal inflammation are common signs and symptoms of pharyngeal infection.
    d. Antibiotics are the treatment of choice for streptococcal infection.

13. Which of the following assessment findings indicates an alteration in C. Q.'s homeostatic control mechanisms?
    a. fever
    b. throat pain
    c. joint stiffness
    d. positive throat culture

## ANSWER KEY

| | | | |
|---|---|---|---|
| 1. | T | 8. | F |
| 2. | F | 9. | F |
| 3. | F | 10. | F |
| 4. | T | 11. | b |
| 5. | T | 12. | b |
| 6. | F | 13. | a |
| 7. | F | | |

# *Unit II—Alterations in Cellular Function*

## KEY QUESTIONS

### *Chapter 2—Cell Structure and Function*

1. How does cell membrane structure lead to selective permeability toward lipid-soluble and lipid-insoluble substances?
2. What are the general functions and structures of the cell cytoskeleton, nucleus, endoplasmic reticulum, Golgi apparatus, lysosomes, peroxisomes, and mitochondria?
3. How is cellular ATP produced and used in a cell?
4. How are large and small molecules transported across cell membranes?
5. How do carrier-mediated transport and channel-mediated transport differ?
6. How do changes in extracellular potassium ion affect the resting membrane potential?
7. What is the role of voltage-gated ion channels in action potential conduction?
8. How do cells in a multicellular organism communicate with one another?
9. How can extracellular signals be transmitted intracellularly?

### *Chapter 3—Cell Injury, Aging, and Death*

1. How can one determine if a person is experiencing cell injury?
2. How would cell death be manifested?
3. To what kinds of injury are cells susceptible?
4. What are some examples of etiologic factors that might injure cells?
5. What are normal aging changes, and how can they be differentiated from disease processes?

### *Chapter 4—Genetic Control—Inheritance*

1. How can the simple four-base structure of DNA serve as a template for synthesis of proteins, which may contain 20 different amino acids?
2. How is DNA replication accomplished?
3. What is a *gene*?
4. How can cells of the same genotype be as different as a skin cell and a liver cell?
5. How do DNA-binding proteins function to regulate gene expression?
6. What are the general structures and functions of the four types of tissues: epithelial, connective, nervous, and muscle?
7. In your own words, define the following terms: *genotype, phenotype, dominant, recessive, autosome, mitosis, meiosis,* and *allele.*

### *Chapter 5—Genetic and Developmental Disorders*

1. Explain, with examples, how pedigree analysis can be used to determine if a trait is inherited as autosomal dominant, autosomal recessive, or X-linked.
2. What is the role of the environment in development of congenital disorders?
3. Under what conditions would it be appropriate to recommend that potential parents receive genetic counseling?

### *Chapter 6—Neoplasia*

1. What are the major differences between benign and malignant tumors?
2. What is the purpose of tumor grading and staging?
3. How do cancer cells differ from normal cells?
4. What are *oncogenes* and how might they be activated within a cell?
5. How might oncogenes lead to inappropriate cell growth?
6. What is meant by the statement, "Cancer is a multistep process"?
7. How might advancing cancer be manifested in the host?
8. How is the appropriate type of cancer therapy determined for a particular patient?
9. How might lifestyle contribute to cancer risk?

## CASE EXAMPLE

K. S. is in for a clinic visit to determine if she is pregnant. She is very concerned because she suspects there may be a genetic disease in her family. Upon further questioning, you find out that her brother's son has the disorder. Her brother's other children (boy and girl) are unaffected. K. S.'s parents, grandparents, and other siblings (a brother and two sisters) do not have signs of the disorder. Her brother's wife has said that she thinks one of her distant relatives may have had the disease.

### *Discussion Questions*

1. If the disorder is indeed inherited as a single gene defect, do you think it is autosomal dominant, autosomal recessive, or X-linked? Justify your answer.
2. Construct a pedigree chart and predict the likelihood that K. S. has the defective gene.

3. If K. S. does carry the defective gene, what are the chances that her offspring would be affected? In making this prediction, what assumptions are you making about K. S.'s mate?
4. What other information would be important to gather from K. S. to further assess her risk of bearing a child with genetic or congenital anomalies?

## TEST ITEMS

### *Multiple Choice*

1. Glycolysis is the metabolic process of breaking down a glucose molecule to form
   a. $CO_2$ and $H_2O$.
   b. 2 ATP and 2 pyruvate.
   c. 34 ATP.
   d. oxygen and ATP.

2. The *primary* purpose of glycolysis is to
   a. produce ATP.
   b. supply substrate to the Kreb's cycle.
   c. produce energy.
   d. supply lactate during anaerobic conditions.

3. The energy derived from the transport of electrons along the electron-transport chain on the inner mitochondrial membrane is used to
   a. synthesize ATP.
   b. generate a proton gradient.
   c. reduce oxygen to water.
   d. produce NADH.

4. Which of the following reactions would occur in the body spontaneously *without* energy input from direct (ATP) or secondary (gradient) energy sources? (Choose *all* the correct answers.)
   a. sodium entry into the cell
   b. calcium extrusion from the cell
   c. translation
   d. endocytosis/exocytosis
   e. osmosis
   f. transcription

5. Repolarization of a neuron after a depolarizing action potential is due to (choose *all* that apply)
   a. activation of the $Na^+/K^+$ pump.
   b. opening of voltage-gated calcium channels.
   c. efflux of potassium.
   d. closure of fast $Na^+$ channels.
   e. extrusion of calcium.

6. Excitable cells are able to conduct action potentials because they
   a. have receptors for neurotransmitters.
   b. have gap junctions.
   c. have ligand-gated channels.
   d. have voltage-gated channels.

7. Hydropic swelling results from
   a. membrane rupture.
   b. ATP accumulation.
   c. oncogene activation.
   d. $Na^+/K^+$ pump dysfunction.

8. Cell division resulting in 23 chromosomes occurs with
   a. transformation.
   b. mitosis.
   c. chromosome lag.
   d. meiosis.

9. Characteristics of X-linked recessive disorders include
   a. all daughters of affected fathers are carriers.
   b. boys and girls are equally affected.
   c. the son of a carrier mother has a 25% chance of being affected.
   d. affected fathers transmit the gene to all of their sons.

10. An increase in cardiac size and function due to increased workload is termed
    a. atrophy.
    b. hypertrophy.
    c. functional.
    d. inflammation.

11. Coagulative necrosis
    a. resembles crumbly cheese.
    b. can result from interrupted blood supply.
    c. is reversible if promptly and agressively treated.
    d. remains functional for 5–7 days.

12. A fetus is most vulnerable to environmental teratogens during
    a. birth.
    b. conception.
    c. the first trimester.
    d. the last trimester.

13. Proto-oncogenes
    a. are synonymous with anti-oncogenes.
    b. are normal cellular genes that promote growth.
    c. always code for viral proteins.
    d. result from severe mutational events.

14. Familial retinoblastoma involves the transmission of which of the following from parent to offspring?
    a. mutant anti-oncogene
    b. cancer-causing virus
    c. oncogene
    d. extra chromosome

15. Cancer can be caused by addition of an (oncogene/anti-oncogene) or by deletion of an (oncogene/anti-oncogene). (Circle the correct answer in each pair.)

16. The TNM tumor classification system describes
    a. types of cancer.
    b. locations of tumors in the body.
    c. cancer histology.
    d. etiology of tumor formation.

### *Case Scenarios*

J. X. and S. X., a married couple, have just delivered their first child, who appears normally developed. Results of biochemical tests indicate that the infant has phenylketonuria (PKU). Questions 17–20 refer to this situation.

17. The parents ask what PKU means. Correct responses would include all the following *except*
    a. PKU is an enzyme deficiency resulting in the inability to metabolize phenylalanine.
    b. PKU is an inborn error of metabolism.
    c. PKU results from a chromosome abnormality called nondisjunction
    d. PKU is transmitted as an autosomal recessive disorder.

18. The parents are concerned about the risk of transmitting the disorder in future pregnancies. What is a correct assessment of the risk?
    a. Each child has a 25% chance of being a carrier.
    b. Each child has a 25% chance of being affected.
    c. Since one child is already affected, her next three children will be unaffected.
    d. One cannot predict the risk for future pregnancies.

19. What information should J. X. and S. X. be given about the consequences of PKU?
    a. High dietary phenylalanine may help induce enzyme production.
    b. PKU is commonly associated with other congenital anomalies.
    c. Failure to avoid phenylalanine results in progressive mental retardation.
    d. Mental retardation is inevitable.

20. Phenylalanine is most likely to be a component of
    a. fat.
    b. sugar.
    c. protein.
    d. carbohydrate.

G. P. is a 63-year-old real estate agent living in an urban area. She reports her diet to be poor, containing "lots of fat." She entertains often and leads a "stressful" life. She has smoked "about two packs a day for the last 40 years." Her chronic morning cough has recently worsened and she is coughing up blood. She also complains of fatigue, frequent respiratory infections, sore throats, and hoarseness. A lung mass is suspected. Questions 21–27 refer to G. P.

21. The most likely contributing factor for development of lung cancer in G. P. is
    a. high fat diet.
    b. urban pollutants.
    c. stressful lifestyle.
    d. cigarette smoking.

22. G. P. underwent bronchoscopy and histologic examination of a suspected tumor. She was diagnosed with primary bronchial carcinoma, which means that the tumor
    a. is benign.
    b. is malignant.
    c. is secondary to cancer elsewhere in the body.
    d. has spread.

23. G. P. is scheduled for a staging procedure. She wants to know what that means. Which response is correct? It is a
    a. procedure for determining the spread of tumor in the body.
    b. histologic examination of tissues to determine the degree of tumor differentiation.
    c. surgical removal of all tumor cells.
    d. biochemical testing of tumor cells to determine the genetic basis of the tumor.

24. G. P.'s tumor is determined to have metastasized, which means that the
    a. tumor cells have invaded locally.
    b. tumor cells have spread contiguously to adjacent tissue.
    c. tumor has become encapsulated.
    d. tumor has spread to distant sites.

25. G. P. wants to know her chances for survival. What information should serve as the basis for a response?
    a. Lung cancer is always fatal.
    b. Lung cancer has about a 10% cure rate.
    c. Lung cancer is highly curable when diagnosed early.
    d. Lung cancer tends to remain localized and responds well to surgical removal.

26. After surgery to remove the lung tumor, G. P. is scheduled for chemotherapy, which will
    a. selectively kill tumor cells.
    b. stimulate immune cells to fight the cancer.
    c. have minimal side effects.
    d. kill rapidly dividing cells.

27. Side effects of chemotherapy include all the following *except*
    a. anemia.
    b. nausea.
    c. leukocytosis.
    d. bleeding.

## *Matching*

Match the descriptions on the left with the terms on the right. (Not all letters will be used.)

| | |
|---|---|
| ____ 28. transmits information about cell configuration to the nucleus | a. actin |
| ____ 29. mediate the movement of chromatids during mitosis | b. microtubules |
| ____ 30. processes and "addresses" proteins for export | c. cytoskeleton |
| ____ 31. contains digestive enzymes of the hydrolytic sort | d. rough ER |
| ____ 32. contains Kreb's cycle enzymes in its matrix | e. mitochondria |
| | f. peroxisomes |
| | g. lysosomes |
| | h. Golgi apparatus |
| | i. smooth ER |

Match the descriptions on the left with the terms on the right. (Not all letters will be used.)

| | |
|---|---|
| ____ 33. carry amino acids in the cytoplasm | a. transcription |
| ____ 34. is a complimentary copy of DNA that contains uracil not thymine | b. translation |
| ____ 35. process of formation of messenger RNA | c. replication |
| ____ 36. process that synthesizes a protein from mRNA | d. messenger RNA |
| | e. transfer RNA |

Match the descriptions on the left with the terms on the right. (Not all letters will be used.)

| | |
|---|---|
| ____ 37. "new growth" of proliferating cells | a. leukemia |
| ____ 38. malignant cancer of glandular origin | b. sarcoma |
| ____ 39. benign tumor | c. adenosarcoma |
| ____ 40. cancer of blood-forming tissue | d. neoplasm |
| | e. fibroma |

### *Short Answer and Essay*

41. List the four types of membrane ion channels classified by their mechanism of regulation (gating).

42. What would the complimentary mRNA sequence be for the gene below.
    Gene: A C T G C A A C T
    mRNA:

43. Draw a Punnett diagram showing the mating of two heterozygous parents (Bb). If b carries a mutation, what are the chances that an offspring would be a carrier of the disorder? What are the chances that an offspring would exhibit the disorder?

## ANSWER KEY

1. b
2. b
3. b
4. a, e
5. c, d
6. d
7. d
8. d
9. a
10. b
11. b
12. c
13. b
14. a
15. oncogene, anti-oncogene
16. b
17. c
18. b
19. c
20. c
21. d
22. b
23. a
24. d
25. b
26. d
27. c
28. c
29. b
30. h
31. g
32. e
33. e
34. d
35. a
36. b
37. d
38. c
39. e
40. a
41. voltage-gated, ligand-gated, mechanically gated, and leak
42. U G A C G U U G A
43.

| | B | b |
|---|---|---|
| B | BB | Bb |
| b | Bb | bb |

carrier = 50% chance
exhibit = 25% chance

# *Unit III—Alterations in Defense*

## KEY QUESTIONS

### *Chapter 7—Stress, Adaptation, and Coping*

1. What role does stress play in development of disease?
2. What is the purpose of the "fight or flight" reaction?
3. What are the neuronal, hormonal, and immune mediators of the stress response?
4. How might the stress response be exhibited in an individual?
5. What interventions might be useful in minimizing the deleterious effects of the stress response?
6. Why might individuals respond to "stressors" differently?
7. What is the difference between *coping* and *adaptation*?
8. What determines if a coping strategy is functional or nonfunctional?

### *Chapter 8—Infectious Processes*

1. What is an *opportunistic infection*?
2. What characteristics differentiate bacteria from viruses?
3. What factors (host, environment, microorganism) influence the likelihood of establishing infection in the host?
4. What are the clinical manifestations of viral and bacterial infections?
5. How does inflammation serve to limit the spread of infection?
6. How do microorganisms cause injury to the host?
7. Under what clinical circumstances might the host's normal defenses against microorganisms be compromised?

### *Chapter 9—Inflammation and Immunity*

1. Draw a diagram of blood cell differentiation beginning with a common stem cell. Label the major differentiated cell types, including B cells, T cells, RBCs, megakaryocytes, monocytes, and granulocytes.
2. Briefly describe the function of each of the major immune cells.
3. What are the functions of complement, and how is the complement cascade activated?
4. How do immune cell cytokines function to coordinate the activities of the immune system?
5. How do specific and nonspecific immune mechanisms differ?
6. Describe inflammation and explain why it is said to be nonspecific.
7. What are inflammatory exudates, and how do the compositions of the various types differ?
8. What is the role of MHC proteins in helping T lymphocytes differentiate self from foreign cells?
9. Why is an immune response usually more effective on second exposure to an antigen than it was on first exposure?
10. How are T-helper cells activated, and what is their role in mounting an immune response?
11. How are B cells stimulated to produce antibody?
12. How does antibody production aid in the immune response?
13. What is the difference between active and passive immunity?
14. Give some examples of interdependent functions of specific and nonspecific immune cells.

### *Chapter 10—Alterations in Immune Function*

1. What are potential mechanisms whereby the immune system erroneously reacts with self tissue leading to autoimmune diseases?
2. What is the role of IgE in anaphylactic reactions (type I hypersensitivity)?
3. How would a type I reaction be manifested clinically?
4. Give an example of a type II hypersensitivity reaction and differentiate from an anaphylactic reaction.
5. What factors predispose an individual to development of type III hypersensitivity reactions?
6. What is the role of T cells in type IV hypersensitivity reactions?
7. What is the difference between transplant rejection and graft-versus-host disease?
8. Use the example of severe combined immunodeficiency (SCID) to describe the clinical consequences of stem cell failure in the bone marrow.
9. What is the etiology of AIDS, and what are the risk factors for acquiring the disease?
10. What are the risks and benefits of HIV testing?
11. What does a "negative" HIV test indicate?
12. How can the spread of HIV infection be prevented?
13. What is the difference between HIV+ and AIDS?
14. How does the HIV retrovirus lead to widespread immunodeficiency?
15. What is the rationale for treating HIV+ patients with AZT?
16. Why is there still no effective HIV vaccine?

### *Chapter 11—Lymphoproliferative Disorders*

1. Given the diagnosis of leukemia, how could one determine its classification as ALL, CLL, ANLL, or CNLL?
2. What is the effect of leukemia on blood cell production by the bone marrow?
3. What clinical data would lead to a suspicion of leukemia?
4. What is *remission*?
5. What are the benefits and risks of using chemotherapy to treat leukemia?
6. What clinical data would lead to a suspicion of Hodgkin's disease, and how would the diagnosis be confirmed?
7. How is staging for Hodgkin's disease used to make a prognosis and guide the choice of treatment?
8. Why is radiation used effectively for Hodgkin's disease and not for leukemia?
9. What are the major differences between Hodgkin's disease and non-Hodgkin's lymphoma?
10. What clinical data would lead to a suspicion of multiple myeloma, and how would the diagnosis be confirmed?
11. What is the rationale for treating multiple myeloma with diuretics and fluid therapy?

## CASE EXAMPLES

M. L. is a 26-year-old homosexual male admitted to the hospital for progressive respiratory distress, fever, weakness, and chronic diarrhea. He tested HIV+ about 3 years ago, but has remained asymptomatic until 2 months prior to admission. Pneumocystis carinii pneumonia was suspected and confirmed by culture. Laboratory analysis demonstrates a low CD4+ count. Treatment with AZT was started 2 months ago.

### *Discussion Questions*

1. M. L.'s mother is concerned about the potential for catching AIDS from her son. What can you tell her about the risk factors and transmission of AIDS?
2. What is the significance of the CD4+ count?
3. PCP is an opportunistic infection to which immunocompetent people are immune. What other opportunistic infections are commonly seen in AIDS patients? Are there any data to suggest that M. L. may have one of these?
4. M. L.'s sexual partner recently tested negative for HIV. What conclusions can be made about his HIV status?
5. Why is M. L. being treated with AZT?
6. A medical student asks you to draw a picture of the HIV virion and a CD4+ cell and explain to her the mechanism of intracellular infection and the role of reverse transcriptase. Show your work.

A. S. was recently diagnosed with Hodgkin's disease and scheduled for a staging procedure. His previous axillary lymph node biopsy was positive for Reed-Sternberg cells. The surgeon charted the results of the staging procedure as "stage I."

### *Discussion Questions*

1. What is the purpose of the staging procedure for A. S.?
2. How does Hodgkin's lymphoma spread in the body, and what does "stage I" signify for A. S.?
3. What is the difference between Hodgkin's disease and non-Hodgkin's lymphoma?
4. What is the prognosis and predicted therapy for A. S. now that she has been diagnosed with stage I Hodgkin's disease?
5. What side effects might A. S. expect from this therapy?

E. O. is an 8-year-old girl with a history of asthma and allergy to bee stings. She has been brought to the clinic complaining of a throat infection. She was treated one time previously with a penicillin antibiotic and developed a slight rash, but no other side effects. Her health-care physician prescribes a course of penicillin to treat her current infection and cautions her parents to watch her closely for a reaction.

### *Discussion Questions*

1. What type of reaction is the physician concerned about and why?
2. Explain the role of IgE and mast cells in type I hypersensitivity reactions. Why might E. O. react adversely to the antibiotic this time when she did not previously?
3. What would you teach E. O.'s parents to look for when they are assessing for a reaction?
4. What would you suggest the parents do if a reaction does occur?

# TEST ITEMS

## *Multiple Choice*

1. Which of the following cell types does not evolve from the myelocytic pathway?
   a. red cells
   b. monocytes
   c. granulocytes
   d. natural killer cells

2. Which of the following cell types is thought to dampen the immune response?
   a. T-helper cells
   b. neutrophils
   c. eosinophils
   d. macrophages

3. Which of the following immune reactions does not require participation by specific immune cells (lymphocytes)?
   a. activation of complement cascade via the classic pathway
   b. mast cell degranulation in response to antigen
   c. phagocytosis of antigen by macrophage
   d. type IV hypersensitivity reaction

4. Inflammation is said to be nonspecific because
   a. specific immune cells do not participate.
   b. the inflammatory reaction is similar regardless of etiology.
   c. inflammation contributes minimally to immune functions.
   d. it is a poorly understood phenomenon.

5. Antigen presenting cells function to
   a. display foreign antigen on their surface in association with MHCII.
   b. stimulate cytokine production by macrophages.
   c. phagocytose and degrade foreign antigens.
   d. initiate the complement cascade by way of the alternate pathway.

6. Which of the following is *not* a function of T-lymphocytes?
   a. antibody synthesis
   b. interleukin-2 production
   c. cell lysis
   d. stimulation of B cells

7. An example of passive immunity would be
   a. vaccination with polio vaccine.
   b. antibody production in response to infection.
   c. immune protection passed through the placenta.
   d. antibiotic administration for strep throat.

8. All of these are actions of antibodies *except*
   a. antigen agglutination.
   b. antigen precipitation.
   c. opsonization.
   d. phagocytosis.

9. Antigen-specific receptors on the surfaces of B- and T cells are produced
   a. in response to interferons.
   b. by MHC genes.
   c. in response to specific antigens.
   d. randomly by genetic recombination.

10. The "classic pathway" for activation of the complement cascade requires
    a. activated T cells.
    b. macrophages.
    c. exposed foreign surfaces.
    d. B cell production of antibodies.

11. Clonal deletion refers to
    a. proliferation of plasma cells in response to antigen.
    b. destruction of self-reacting B- and T-lymphocytes.
    c. desensitization therapy for allergic reactivity.
    d. T-suppressor activity.

12. The reticuloendothelial system consists of
    a. monocytes and fixed tissue macrophages.
    b. specifically activated lymphocytes.
    c. bone marrow stem cells.
    d. antibody-secreting plasma cells.

13. Proteins that are increased in the blood stream during acute inflammation are called
    a. antibody proteins.
    b. lymphokine proteins.
    c. acute phase proteins.
    d. anti-idiotype proteins.

14. Activation of the complement cascade results in
    a. antibody production.
    b. inflammation.
    c. immunosuppression.
    d. autoimmunity.

15. Dramatic hypotension sometimes accompanies type I hypersensitivity reactions because
    a. massive histamine release from mast cells leads to vasodilation.
    b. toxins released into the blood interfere with cardiac function.
    c. anaphylaxis results in large volume losses secondary to sweating.
    d. hypoxia due to bronchoconstriction impairs cardiac function.

16. Autoimmune diseases
    a. are due to increased T-suppressor cell activity associated with aging.
    b. occur only when lymphocytes are in close contact with body cells during embryogenesis.
    c. result from failure of the immune system to differentiate self and nonself molecules.
    d. are often communicable to others by direct contact.

17. The major cause of death from leukemic disease is
    a. infection.
    b. malnutrition.
    c. hemorrhage.
    d. heart failure.

18. The primary reason that an HIV vaccine is difficult to produce is that
    a. HIV is not immunogenic.
    b. B cells are unable to produce antibodies against HIV.
    c. HIV mutates frequently.
    d. reverse transcriptase cleaves the vaccine.

19. Indicators that an individual is experiencing a stress response include all of the following *except*
    a. tachycardia.
    b. diaphoresis.
    c. peripheral vasoconstriction.
    d. pupil constriction.

20. Which of the following is normally *not* secreted in response to stress?
    a. norepinephrine
    b. cortisol
    c. epinephrine
    d. insulin

21. Which of the following may be a characteristic of bacteria?
    a. intracellular parasite
    b. composed of RNA or DNA
    c. contains cell wall endotoxin
    d. cannot replicate extracellularly

22. Clinical data indicating that a patient has an increased risk of infection include
    a. acidic urine.
    b. history of allergy to antibiotics.
    c. closed surgical wound.
    d. WBC count of $10,000/mm^3$.

23. A 58-year-old woman is seen in the clinic for complaints of severe back pain. Her chest x-ray demonstrates generalized bone demineralization and compression fracture. Blood studies demonstrate elevated calcium levels. The most likely diagnosis is
    a. leukemia.
    b. multiple myeloma.
    c. Hodgkin's disease.
    d. back trauma.

24. Fluid and diuretic therapy are used in the treatment of multiple myeloma to
    a. reduce the rate of bone destruction.
    b. dilute plasma cells in the bloodstream.
    c. prevent damage to renal tubules.
    d. improve cardiac function.

## *Case Scenarios*

R. V. is a 28-year-old HIV+ male recently hospitalized for evaluation of symptoms of progressive weakness, dyspnea, weight loss, and low grade fever. Questions 25–28 refer to R. V.

25. A biopsy of R. V's lung tissue reveals Pneumocystis carinii pneumonia. This diagnosis means that R. V.
    a. has AIDS.
    b. has less than 2 years to live.
    c. cannot be treated.
    d. was an intravenous drug abuser.

26. The immune system disorder associated with HIV is
    a. an overactive B cell system.
    b. proliferation of immature WBCs (blasts).
    c. deficiency of helper T-lymphocytes.
    d. a cancerous growth of lymph tissue.

27. Which of the following statements best describes the etiology and transmission of AIDS?
    a. AIDS is caused by a retrovirus and transmitted through body fluids.
    b. The mechanism of AIDS transmission is unknown, therefore AIDS is considered to be highly contagious.
    c. AIDS is an autoimmune disease triggered by a homosexual lifestyle.
    d. AIDS is caused by a virus that can be transmitted only by sexual contact.

28. HIV infection of helper T cells is facilitated by attachment of the viral envelope protein gp120 to
    a. CD8+ proteins on suppressor cells.
    b. reverse transcriptase.
    c. CD4+ proteins on helper cells.
    d. the macrophage lipid bilayer.

J. B. is a 12-year-old boy with acute lymphocytic leukemia (ALL). Questions 29–32 refer to J. B.

29. Manifestations of J. B.'s leukemia prior to treatment would include all of the following *except*
    a. anemia.
    b. leukocytosis.
    c. leukopenia.
    d. thrombocytopenia.

30. As part of J. B.'s treatment, he must undergo several weeks of chemotherapy. The most serious complication of chemotherapy is
    a. nausea and vomiting.
    b. anemia.
    c. alopecia.
    d. immunodepression.

31. While in the hospital, J. B. developed a severe thrombocytopenia. The most appropriate action for this condition would be
    a. anticoagulant therapy.
    b. chemotherapy.
    c. activity restriction.
    d. isolation.

32. J. B. developed an opportunistic infection that is to be treated with an antibiotic. J. B. has received this antibiotic one time previously with no adverse reactions. Which of the following statements should guide the administration of the drug this time?
    a. Minimal chances of anaphylaxis since no reaction the first time the antibiotic was given.
    b. Anaphylaxis is antibody mediated and may occur on second exposure.
    c. Anaphylaxis is T cell mediated and slow to develop.
    d. Antibiotics are rarely associated with anaphylactic reactions.

## *True or False*

____ 33. Immunoglobulins produced by malignant plasma cells are monoclonal.

____ 34. Each B-Lymphocyte is able to bind to and produce antibody against only one specific antigen.

____ 35. Non-Hodgkin's lymphoma tends to spread in a predictable pattern.

____ 36. Clonal expansion of B-lymphocytes upon first exposure to antigen requires T-helper stimulation.

____ 37. The macrophage has little importance in immune function other than phagocytosis.

____ 38. Tolerance to self-tissues only occurs during embryogenesis.

____ 39. HIV causes immunodeficiency by destroying primarily CD8 T-lymphocytes.

____ 40. T-lymphocytes are activated primarily by free viruses.

## *Matching*

Match the terms on the left with their definitions on the right. Use each answer only once.

| | |
|---|---|
| ____ 41. T-lymphocytes | a. membrane attack complex (MAC) |
| ____ 42. histiocytes | b. basophil-like cells in tissues |
| ____ 43. monocytes | c. lymphocyte that lacks B/T markers |
| ____ 44. neutrophils | d. able to bind IgE (Fc end) |
| ____ 45. eosinophils | e. circulating macrophages |
| ____ 46. basophils | f. fixed tissue macrophages |
| ____ 47. plasma cells | g. cause nonspecific dampening of inflammation |
| ____ 48. mast cells | h. express CD4 or CD8 markers |
| ____ 49. natural killers | i. make up 90% of circulating granulocytes |
| ____ 50. complement | j. MHC class I restricted |
| ____ 51. cytotoxic T | k. antibody producing B cells |

## *Short Answer*

52. ________________________ lymphocytes are activated by recognition and binding of antigen in association with MHC II proteins.

53. For T-helper cells to bind a foreign antigen, the antigen must first be processed by a(n) ________________________.

54. MHC I are present on the surface of ______________ cells, whereas MHC II are present on the surface of __________________cells.

55. The "constant" region of an antibody molecule determines (antigen specificity/antibody class).

56. The most prevalent antibody class in the body is ____________________.

57. Give an example of each of the four types of hypersensitivity reactions.

## ANSWER KEY

1. d
2. c
3. c
4. b
5. a
6. a
7. c
8. d
9. d
10. d
11. b
12. a
13. c
14. b
15. a
16. c
17. a
18. c
19. d
20. d
21. c
22. c
23. b
24. c
25. a
26. c
27. a
28. c
29. c
30. d
31. c
32. b
33. T
34. T
35. F
36. T
37. F
38. F
39. F
40. F
41. h
42. f
43. e
44. i
45. g
46. d
47. k
48. b
49. c
50. a
51. j
52. T-helper
53. antigen presenting cell
54. all nucleated cells, certain immune cells
55. antibody class
56. IgG
57. a. type I: drug anaphylaxis
    b. type II: transfusion reaction
    c. type III: post-streptococcal glomerulonephritis
    d. type IV: graft-versus-host disease

# *Unit IV—Alterations in Oxygen Transport, Blood Coagulation, Blood Flow, and Blood Pressure*

## KEY QUESTIONS

### *Chapter 12—Alterations in Oxygen Transport*

1. How does the structure of red cells relate to their functions?
2. What laboratory tests are used to describe blood composition and detect abnormalities?
3. What is the role of erythropoietins in red cell production?
4. Under what conditions might the blood reticulocyte count be elevated?
5. How does hemoglobin bind and release oxygen in the red cell?
6. What factors are necessary for red cell production?
7. How does the fact that mature red cells have no mitochondria or nucleus affect red cell energy metabolism and lifespan?
8. What are the risk factors and manifestations of high serum bilirubin?
9. What is the relative importance of dissolved oxygen versus oxygen bound to hemoglobin in oxygen delivery to cells?
10. Use the oxyhemoglobin saturation curve to explain the relationship between partial pressure of oxygen ($PO_2$) and hemoglobin saturation.
11. How do factors such as blood acidity, carbon dioxide level, and 2,3-DPG affect the affinity of hemoglobin for oxygen?
12. In what way do changes in $PaO_2$, hemoglobin level, and hemoglobin saturation affect blood oxygen content?
13. How does carbon dioxide get excreted from the body?
14. What are the general effects of anemia on the body systems, and how are they manifested?
15. What are the general causes of anemia?
16. How can the different types of anemia be differentiated using history, differential signs and symptoms, and laboratory studies?
17. What treatment measures are appropriate for each of the common types of anemia?
18. How can the different types of polycythemia be differentiated using history, differential signs and symptoms, and laboratory studies?
19. What treatment measures are appropriate for each of the three types of polycythemias?

### *Chapter 13—Alterations in Hemostasis and Blood Coagulation*

1. What are the important steps in hemostasis?
2. How do platelets and clotting factors contribute to hemostasis?
3. Why is fibrinolysis initiated at the same time as clotting?
4. What findings from the patient history, clinical manifestations, and laboratory studies would lead to a suspicion of bleeding disorder?
5. How can laboratory tests be used to help pinpoint the specific coagulation dysfunction?
6. Why might an individual with a normal platelet count have abnormal platelet function and prolonged bleeding time?
7. What are some risk factors for platelet deficiency?
8. What is the etiology of clotting defects in hemophilia A and B and in Von Willebrand's disease?
9. What is the role of vitamin K in preventing clotting dysfunction?
10. What are the risk factors for development of disseminated intravascular clotting (DIC)?
11. How does DIC lead simultaneously to bleeding and thrombosis?
12. How are coagulation screening labs used to diagnose DIC?

### *Chapter 14—Alterations in Blood Flow*

1. How do the structures of arteries, veins, and capillaries differ, reflecting the function of each?
2. What is the relationship among vessel resistance, blood pressure, and blood flow?
3. What are the primary determinants of resistance to flow?
4. How is blood flow through a particular capillary bed controlled by the autonomic nervous system and by autoregulation?
5. Why is blood flow slowest in the capillary beds?
6. What determines the rate of transcapillary exchange of fluids, electrolytes, and nutrients?
7. What are the upstream and downstream consequences of acute and chronic arterial obstruction?
8. What are the upstream and downstream consequences of venous obstruction?
9. How do arterial and venous obstructions develop?
10. What is the usual sequence of events in the development of atherosclerosis?
11. What are the six "P's" that characterize acute arterial obstruction?
12. What are the risk factors and clinical manifestations of deep vein thrombosis?

## *Chapter 15—Alterations in Blood Pressure*

1. What is the relationship between the cardiac cycle and arterial blood pressure?
2. What are the relationships among systolic pressure, diastolic pressure, pulse pressure, and mean pressure?
3. How do changes in cardiac output and systemic vascular resistance affect blood pressure?
4. How do changes in arteriolar diameter affect systemic vascular resistance and blood pressure?
5. How is blood pressure detected and controlled by the autonomic nervous system?
6. How do vasoactive hormones and drugs influence arteriolar diameter?
7. What steps can be taken to minimize the chances of erroneous blood pressure measurement?
8. What are the risk factors for development of primary hypertension?
9. What disorders are associated with the development of secondary hypertension?
10. How is high blood pressure defined?
11. How does failure of normal regulatory control mechanisms contribute to development of hypertension?
12. What is the rationale for using ACE inhibitors, diuretics, calcium channel blockers, and beta-blockers in the treatment of high blood pressure?
13. How is *orthostatic hypotension* defined?
14. What are predisposing factors for development of orthostatic hypotension?

## CASE EXAMPLES

M. B is a generally healthy 36-year-old woman with complaints of persistent generalized fatigue. At her annual checkup, she is noted to have the following vital signs: heart rate 118 beats/min, blood pressure 128/60, oral temperature 37°C, respiratory rate 26 breaths/min. Her skin tones and nail beds are pale. Laboratory results demonstrate hematocrit 31%; hemoglobin 10 g/dL; MCHC 27; MCV 70; total iron-binding capacity 600 mg/dL.

### *Discussion Questions*

1. What type of hematologic disorder would you suspect based on M. B.'s history, physical examination, and laboratory values?
2. What other history data would be helpful in determining the etiology of this disorder?
3. Which of M. B.'s clinical signs are reflective of the body's effort to compensate for decreased oxygen-carrying capacity?
4. How would tissue hypoxia related to decreased oxygen-carrying capacity affect the affinity of hemoglobin for oxygen?
5. M. B. is counseled to increase her dietary intake of iron-containing foods. What kinds of food would be recommended?
6. M. B. is given a prescription for ferrous sulfate 325 mg three times per day. What advise can you give to her about the timing of doses and expected side effects?

N. R. is a 49-year-old lumber worker admitted to the emergency department after a severe laceration of his left thigh. He lost about 4 units of blood prior to effective closure of the wound. He received several hundred milliliters of normal saline during the procedure. Postsurgical clinical data are as follows: vital signs lying down, HR 115, BP 98/60, RR 28; sitting, HR 140, BP 92/62, RR 28; hematocrit 22, hemoglobin 8, $PaO_2$ 90, $SaO_2$ 98% breathing room air. N. R. continues to ooze significantly from his sutured wound postoperatively, prompting his physician to order a coagulation screen: platelet count 250,000, bleeding time >10 min, PT and aPTT within normal ranges.

### *Discussion Questions*

1. In view of N. R.'s history and vital signs, do you think he is hypovolemic? Support your conclusion.
2. Calculate N. R.'s arterial oxygen content ($CaO_2$) using the following formula: $CaO_2 = (PaO_2 \times 0.003) + (Hb \times SaO_2 \times 1.34)$. What does his $CaO_2$ indicate?
3. What would be the effect on N. R.'s $CaO_2$ if he were given a blood transfusion to increase his hemoglobin to 12 g/dL?
4. What would be the effect of administering 100% oxygen to N. R. to increase his $SaO_2$ to 99% and his $PaO_2$ to 500 mm Hg?
5. Do you think N. R. has a bleeding disorder? Support your answer.
6. What information about this patient's history might be helpful in determining the etiology of the prolonged bleeding time?

K. H. is a 67-year-old African-American man with primary hypertension. He is currently taking an angiotensin converting enzyme (ACE) inhibitor and following a salt-restricted weight loss diet. He is about 30 pounds over ideal weight. At his clinic visit, his blood pressure is noted to be 135/96. His heart rate is 70 beats/min. He has no complaints. His wife brought a blood pressure cuff and stethoscope with her in hopes of learning to take her husband's blood pressure at home.

### *Discussion Questions*

1. What risk factors for primary hypertension are evident from K. H.'s history and physical data?
2. What is the rationale for treating K. H. with an ACE inhibitor? What is its mechanism of action?
3. Is K. H.'s hypertension adequately controlled?
4. What tips can you give K. H.'s wife to improve the accuracy of her blood pressure measurement technique?

## TEST ITEMS

### *Multiple Choice*

1. The primary source of erythropoietin is the
   a. bone marrow.
   b. kidney.
   c. lung.
   d. liver.

2. Which of the following conditions is associated with an elevated reticulocyte count?
   a. renal disease
   b. aplastic anemia
   c. hypertension
   d. hemolytic anemia

3. Which of the following conditions is associated with a "shift to the right" of the oxyhemoglobin dissociation curve?
   a. acidemia
   b. alkalemia
   c. hypothermia
   d. low blood $PCO_2$

4. An increase in hemoglobin affinity for oxygen occurs with
   a. hyperthermia
   b. acidosis
   c. elevated $PCO_2$
   d. alkalosis

5. Which of the following is *not* necessary for red blood cell production?
   a. vitamin K
   b. folate
   c. iron
   d. vitamin $B_{12}$

6. Red cells differ from other cell types in the body because they
   a. contain cytoplasmic proteins.
   b. have no cytoplasmic organelles.
   c. have a longer lifespan.
   d. contain glycolytic enzymes.

7. Which of the following is indicative of hemolytic anemia?
   a. increased total iron binding capacity
   b. increased heart rate
   c. hypovolemia
   d. jaundice

8. A low MCHC and MCV are characteristic of which type of anemia?
   a. vitamin $B_{12}$ deficiency
   b. folate deficiency
   c. iron deficiency
   d. erythropoietin deficiency

9. The arterial oxygen content ($CaO_2$) for a patient with $PaO_2$ 100 mm Hg, SaO2 95%, and hemoglobin 15g/dL would be
   a. 19.4 mL oxygen/dL.
   b. 1909.8 mL oxygen/dL.
   c. 210 mL oxygen/dL.
   d. 21.05 mL oxygen/dL.

10. Most carbon dioxide is transported in the bloodstream as
    a. carboxyhemoglobin.
    b. bicarbonate ion.
    c. dissolved carbon dioxide.
    d. carbonic acid.

11. The most appropriate treatment for secondary polycythemia is
    a. volume expansion with saline.
    b. measures to improve oxygenation.
    c. phlebotomy.
    d. chemotherapy.

12. A laboratory test that would be helpful in confirming the diagnosis of iron-deficiency anemia is
    a. elevated total iron binding capacity.
    b. elevated MCHC and MCV.
    c. elevated total and indirect bilirubin.
    d. positive direct or indirect Coombs.

13. A prolonged bleeding time (>10 min) in association with normal platelet count and normal PT and aPTT is indicative of
    a. vitamin K deficiency.
    b. hemophilia B.
    c. hemophilia A.
    d. platelet dysfunction.

14. The final step in clot formation is
    a. conversion of prothrombin to thrombin.
    b. platelet degranulation and adhesion.
    c. conversion of fibrinogen to fibrin.
    d. conversion of plasminogen to plasmin.

15. Dysfunction of which of the following organs would lead to clotting factor deficiency?
    a. liver
    b. kidney
    c. spleen
    d. pancreas

16. The conversion of plasminogen to plasmin results in
    a. clot retraction.
    b. fibrinolysis.
    c. platelet aggregation.
    d. activation of thrombin.

17. Activation of the extrinsic pathway of coagulation is initiated by
    a. platelet factors.
    b. collagen exposure.
    c. tissue thromboplastin.
    d. factor VIII.

18. The prothrombin time (PT) measures the integrity of
    a. platelet function.
    b. extrinsic and common pathway.
    c. intrinsic pathway.
    d. common pathway only.

19. The activated partial thromboplastin time (aPTT) measures the integrity of
    a. the extrinsic pathway.
    b. the intrinsic pathway.
    c. factor VIII synthesis.
    d. plasminogen.

20. A commonly ingested substance associated with prolongation of the bleeding time is
    a. acetominophen.
    b. tobacco.
    c. caffeine.
    d. aspirin.

21. The megakaryocyte is a precursor to
    a. factor IX.
    b. WBCs.
    c. RBCs.
    d. platelets.

22. Causes of thrombocytopenia include
    a. hypoxemia.
    b. reduced erythropoietin.
    c. chemotherapy.
    d. secondary polycythemia.

23. Widespread activation of the clotting cascade secondary to sepsis or massive trauma is called
    a. Von Willebrand's disease.
    b. disseminated intravascular coagulation.
    c. Hageman disease.
    d. ideopathic thrombocytopenia purpura.

24. A 3-year-old boy who exhibits prolonged bleeding after minor trauma and a prolonged aPTT, but normal platelet count, likely has
    a. hemophilia.
    b. liver dysfunction.
    c. disseminated intravascular coagulation.
    d. thrombocytopenia.

25. Treatment for hemophilia A includes
    a. heparin administration.
    b. factor IX replacement.
    c. factor VIII replacement.
    d. platelet transfusion.

26. DIC may be treated with heparin therapy to
    a. enhance fibrinolysis.
    b. inhibit clotting factor consumption.
    c. activate platelets.
    d. enhance liver synthesis of clotting factors.

27. A vessel in which you would expect to find the most rapid blood flow is
    a. an arteriole.
    b. a capillary.
    c. a venule.
    d. the vena cava.

28. Blood pressure is lowest in the
    a. arteries.
    b. capillaries.
    c. veins.
    d. right atrium.

29. Which of the following would cause vasoconstriction?
    a. norepinephrine
    b. calcium channel blocker
    c. alpha adrenergic antagonist
    d. acetylcholine

30. Activation of the aortic and carotid baroreceptors by increased blood pressure results in
    a. vasoconstriction.
    b. reduced heart rate.
    c. sympathetic activation.
    d. hypertension.

31. Blood flow is slow through capillaries because they
    a. are so far away from the heart.
    b. have the largest total cross-sectional area.
    c. are so narrow.
    d. have no smooth muscle.

32. What is the effect on resistance if the radius of a vessel is halved?
    a. resistance doubles
    b. resistance decreases by a factor of 16
    c. resistance decreases by one-half
    d. resistance increases by a factor of 16

33. Clinical manifestations of chronic arterial obstruction include
    a. edema.
    b. intermittent claudication.
    c. decreased pressure proximal to the obstruction.
    d. distal hyperemia.

34. Elevation of an extremity suffering from arterial insufficiency will
    a. increase perfusion to the extremity.
    b. promote circulation distal to the obstruction.
    c. decrease perfusion to the extremity.
    d. relieve ischemic pain.

35. Peripheral edema is a result of
    a. arterial insufficiency.
    b. venous thrombosis.
    c. hypertension.
    d. atherosclerosis.

36. The relationship of blood flow (Q), resistance (R), and pressure (P) in a vessel can be expressed by
    a. $P = Q \times R$.
    b. $Q = R/P$.
    c. $R = P \times Q$.
    d. $P = Q/R$.

37. Risk factors for atherosclerosis include
    a. female gender.
    b. hyperlipidemia.
    c. a high carbohydrate diet.
    d. a low fiber diet.

38. Which of the following is *not* a manifestation of acute arterial obstruction?
    a. pain
    b. purpura
    c. pallor
    d. pulselessness

39. Deep vein thrombosis is treated with heparin to
    a. relieve edema.
    b. prevent clot dislodgment.
    c. dissolve the thrombus.
    d. prevent further clot formation.

40. Which of the following would enhance filtration from the capillary into the tissue?
    a. increased tissue hydrostatic pressure
    b. increased tissue oncotic pressure
    c. decreased capillary hydrostatic pressure
    d. increased capillary oncotic pressure

41. Pulse pressure is defined as
    a. 2/3 systolic plus diastolic pressure.
    b. systolic plus diastolic pressure.
    c. systolic minus diastolic pressure.
    d. systolic pressure times systemic resistance.

42. Which of the following would result in an increase in systemic blood pressure?
    a. hypovolemia
    b. decreased cardiac output
    c. vasoconstriction
    d. decreased vascular resistance

43. An erroneously low blood pressure measurement could be caused by
    a. positioning the arm above the heart level.
    b. using a cuff that is too small.
    c. positioning the arm at heart level.
    d. measuring pressure after exercise.

44. Angiotensin converting enzyme (ACE) inhibitors block
    a. the release of renin.
    b. the conversion of angiotensin I to II.
    c. the conversion of angiotensinogen to angiotensin I.
    d. the effect of aldosterone on the kidney.

45. Which of the following findings is indicative of orthostatic hypotension in a person with a supine blood pressure of 110/70 and a heart rate of 100?
    a. sitting bp 110/72, HR 118
    b. sitting bp 108/68, HR 102
    c. sitting bp 110/78, HR 98
    d. sitting bp 120/80, HR 100

## ANSWER KEY

1. b
2. d
3. a
4. d
5. a
6. b
7. d
8. c
9. a
10. b
11. b
12. a
13. d
14. c
15. a
16. b
17. c
18. b
19. b
20. d
21. d
22. c
23. b
24. a
25. c
26. b
27. d
28. d
29. a
30. b
31. b
32. d
33. b
34. c
35. b
36. a
37. b
38. b
39. d
40. b
41. c
42. c
43. a
44. b
45. a

# *Unit V—Alterations in Cardiac Function*

## KEY QUESTIONS

### *Chapter 16—Cardiac Function*

1. What is the normal pathway of blood as it travels from the right atrium, through the pulmonary and systemic circulations, and back to the right atrium?
2. Where are the anatomical locations of the heart valves, epicardium, endocardium, and pericardium?
3. How are the events of the cardiac cycle reflected in pressure changes within the atria, ventricles, and great vessels?
4. What factors affect blood flow through the coronary arteries?
5. How does the microanatomy of the cardiac muscle cell relate to its contractile function?
6. How does cardiac muscle cell depolarization lead to muscle contraction (excitation–contraction coupling)?
7. What roles do ATP and intracellular calcium ion play in cardiac muscle contraction?
8. Why is muscle relaxation an energy-requiring process?
9. What is the role of creatine phosphate in cardiac energy metabolism?
10. How does serum potassium ion concentration affect the cardiac resting membrane potential?
11. What changes in ion conductance through the cardiac cell membrane are responsible for each phase of the cardiac action potential?
12. How are action potentials generated in automatic pacemaker cells?
13. What is the normal impulse conduction pathway through the heart and how does it relate to the normal ECG?
14. How do heart rate, preload, afterload, and contractile state affect cardiac output and cardiac workload?
15. What diagnostic tests are most useful in evaluating cardiac function?

### *Chapter 17—Alterations in Cardiac Function*

1. What are the risk factors for development of coronary artery disease?
2. What is the role of thrombus formation in acute cardiac ischemia?
3. What are the four ischemic syndromes associated with coronary artery disease?
4. How can angina pectoris and acute myocardial infarction be differentiated?
5. How is myocardial infarction treated?
6. How do the various valvular disorders affect pressure gradients in and workload of the chambers of the heart?
7. What are the common etiologic factors that lead to valvular dysfunction?
8. How do the three types of cardiomyopathy differ?
9. How is myocarditis differentiated from cardiomyopathy?
10. What is cardiac tamponade and how is it clinically manifested?
11. What are the manifestations and complications of acute pericarditis?
12. Which congenital heart defects result in right to left shunting of blood?
13. Which congenital heart defects are usually acyanotic?

### *Chapter 18—Heart Failure and Dysrhythmias: Common Sequelae of Cardiac Diseases*

1. What is *heart failure* and why does it occur?
2. Which cardiac diseases are associated with impaired myocardial contractility or increased cardiac workload?
3. How do the three compensatory mechanisms activated in heart failure serve to increase cardiac output?
4. What are the "forward" and "backward" effects of left-sided heart failure?
5. What are the "forward" and"backward" effects of right-sided heart failure?
6. How are preload, afterload, and myocardial contractility therapeutically managed in the patient with heart failure?
7. What are the characteristics of a normal ECG?
8. Under what cardiac conditions are reentrant circuits likely to occur?
9. What is the etiology, characteristic ECG pattern, clinical significance, and treatment of each of the common cardiac dysrhythmias:
   - sinus tachycardia
   - sinus bradycardia
   - sinus arrhythmia
   - asystole
   - junctional and ventricular escape rhythms
   - premature atrial, junctional, and ventricular complexes
   - atrial fibrillation
   - ventricular tachycardia and ventricular fibrillation

- first-, second-, and third-degree conduction blocks
- pre-excitation syndromes
- intraventricular conduction disturbances

## CASE EXAMPLES

A. O. was an 89-year-old woman with a long history of congestive heart failure secondary to a large left ventricular infarct. She had poor activity tolerance and required assistance with activities of daily living. Even minimal activity was associated with moderately severe dyspnea and exertional chest pain which was relieved by rest. A. O. also exhibited marked pedal edema bilaterally. She took digitalis, lasix, KCl, and sublingual nitroglycerin.

### *Discussion Questions*

1. Which type of heart failure (left- or right-sided) is usually associated with dyspnea? What other clinical findings are likely to be present with this type of heart failure?
2. What compensatory mechanisms are likely to be operative in A. O. to enhance cardiac output?
3. What is the most likely cause of A. O.'s pedal edema?
4. What is the etiology of A. O.'s exertional chest pain? What laboratory tests would be useful to confirm this diagnosis?
5. What is the rationale for the use of each of A. O.'s medications in treating her heart disease?

K. R. was a 46-year-old male admitted to the emergency department with unremitting chest discomfort. The pain started while he was shoveling snow from his front walkway. He had experienced chest discomfort with activity previously, but the pain had subsided with rest and he sought no medical help. This time, the pain did not subside and became increasingly severe, radiating to his left arm and lower jaw. In the emergency department, an ECG and cardiac enzymes were obtained. The cardiac monitor showed sinus tachycardia with occasional premature ventricular complexes. K. R. was treated with 2 liters nasal oxygen, tissue plasminogen activator, sublingual nitroglycerin, and IV morphine sulfate. When he was pain free, he was transferred to the cardiac unit for monitoring.

### *Discussion Questions*

1. What ECG changes would indicate that K. R. had experienced a myocardial infarction (MI)?
2. What changes in "cardiac enzymes" would be consistent with a diagnosis of MI?
3. What is the most common precipitating event for MI?
4. What is the rationale for using tissue plasminogen activator in the treatment of acute MI?
5. Why are morphine and nitroglycerin used to treat ischemic chest pain?

## TEST ITEMS

### *Multiple Choice*

1. The mitral valve
   a. opens during ventricular systole.
   b. is located between the right atrium and ventricle.
   c. has three valve leaflets.
   d. allows blood to flow from the left atrium to the left ventricle.

2. Blood is transported from the right ventricle to the lungs by the
   a. pulmonary veins.
   b. aorta.
   c. pulmonary artery.
   d. bronchial arteries.

3. A vessel that normally contains desaturated (venous) blood is
   a. bronchial arteries.
   b. pulmonary artery.
   c. pulmonary vein.
   d. coronary artery.

4. During which phase of the cardiac cycle is the mitral valve normally open?
   a. atrial systole
   b. isovolumic contraction
   c. isovolumic relaxation
   d. ventricular ejection

5. The "a" wave of the atrial pressure tracing corresponds to
   a. atrial filling.
   b. ventricular systole.
   c. atrial systole.
   d. mitral valve closure.

6. Blood flow through the coronary arteries
   a. occurs primarily during systole because perfusion pressure is high.
   b. is controlled primarily by the autonomic nervous system.
   c. is increased with elevated right atrial pressure.
   d. occurs primarily during ventricular diastole.

7. An increase in intracellular calcium ion results in myocardial contraction because calcium
   a. activates membrane calcium pumps.
   b. binds troponin, causing actin-binding sites to be exposed.
   c. increases affinity of myosin for actin cross-bridge sites.
   d. promotes ATP synthesis.

8. Cardiac muscle relaxation
   a. is an energy-requiring process.
   b. occurs passively following muscle contraction.
   c. is inhibited by cAMP.
   d. is enhanced by intracellular free calcium.

9. Creatine phosphate is
   a. a waste product of cellular metabolism.
   b. synthesized when ATP levels are high.
   c. enzymatically degraded to form creatine kinase.
   d. a marker of myocardial cell damage.

10. Phase 0 of the cardiac muscle cell action potential is associated with
    a. opening of slow calcium ion channels.
    b. opening of fast potassium ion channels.
    c. opening of fast sodium ion channels.
    d. closure of sodium leak channels.

11. Automatic pacemaker cells spontaneously depolarize because
    a. leak channels allow calcium and sodium ions into the cell.
    b. they lack efficient sodium/potassium pumps.
    c. voltage-sensitive sodium channels spontaneously open.
    d. chloride leaks into the cell during rest.

12. Parasympathetic stimulation of the heart generally leads to a decrease in heart rate because acetylcholine
    a. increases intracellular cAMP levels and opens calcium channels.
    b. opens potassium channels allowing potassium ion efflux.
    c. binds and blocks beta receptors on the cell membrane.
    d. inhibits sodium and calcium leak channels in the membrane.

13. One role of ATP in cardiac muscle contraction is
    a. providing energy to pump calcium into the cell.
    b. inducing a conformational change in tropomyosin.
    c. altering myosin affinity for actin binding sites.
    d. releasing sequestered calcium from the sarcoplasmic reticulum.

14. In lead II of the normal ECG, the Q wave is a downward deflection resulting from
    a. atrial depolarization.
    b. apical depolarization.
    c. lateral wall depolarization.
    d. septal depolarization.

15. Which of the following physiologic changes would increase cardiac work, but would not enhance cardiac output?
    a. increased preload
    b. increased heart rate
    c. increased contractility
    d. increased afterload

16. The most reliable indicator that a person has experienced an MI rather than angina pectoris is
    a. severe, crushing chest pain.
    b. ECG abnormalities.
    c. dysrhythmias.
    d. elevated serum creatine kinase (MB).

17. The compensatory mechanisms that are triggered following MI
    a. protect the heart from further ischemia.
    b. increase myocardial oxygen demands.
    c. reduce heart rate and blood pressure.
    d. result from parasympathetic activation.

18. Left heart failure is characterized by
    a. pulmonary congestion.
    b. decreased systemic vascular resistance.
    c. jugular vein distention.
    d. peripheral edema.

19. A therapy that is most likely to *decrease* cardiac output in a patient with heart failure is
    a. afterload reduction.
    b. beta agonist agents.
    c. preload reduction.
    d. digitalis.

20. Hypertrophy of the right ventricle is a compensatory response to
    a. aortic stenosis.
    b. aortic regurgitation.
    c. tricuspid stenosis.
    d. pulmonary stenosis.

21. Rheumatic heart disease is most often a consequence of
    a. chronic intravenous drug abuse.
    b. viral infection with herpes virus.
    c. beta hemolytic streptococcal infection.
    d. cardiomyopathy.

22. Beta adrenergic drug therapy may be indicated in the treatment of MI to
    a. decrease myocardial oxygen demands.
    b. increase myocardial contractility and cardiac output.
    c. decrease aortic resistance to flow (afterload).
    d. increase intracardiac volume (preload).

23. An example of an acyanotic heart defect is
    a. tetralogy of Fallot.
    b. transposition of the great vessels.
    c. ventricular septal defect.
    d. all right-to-left shunt defects.

24. Which of the following is an accurate description of patent ductus arteriosus?
    a. an opening between the atria
    b. a stricture of the aorta that impedes blood flow
    c. a communication between the aorta and pulmonary artery
    d. a cyanotic heart defect associated with right-to-left shunt

25. Decreased cardiac output, muffled heart sounds, and equalized intracardiac pressures are manifestations of
    a. myocardial infarction.
    b. cardiac tamponade.
    c. congestive heart failure.
    d. cardiomyopathy.

26. Restrictive pericarditis is associated with
    a. impaired cardiac filling.
    b. cardiac hypertrophy.
    c. increased cardiac preload.
    d. elevated myocardial oxygen consumption.

27. Mitral stenosis is associated with
    a. systolic murmur.
    b. elevated left atrial/left ventricular diastolic pressure gradient.
    c. left ventricular hypertrophy.
    d. muffled second heart sound (S2).

28. Aortic regurgitation is associated with
    a. diastolic murmur.
    b. elevated left ventricular/aortic systolic pressure gradient.
    c. elevated systemic diastolic blood pressure.
    d. shortened ventricular ejection phase.

29. Which of the following relationships is a statement about the Frank-Starling law of the heart?
    a. Increased diastolic stretching of myocardial fibers produces increased stroke volume.
    b. Sympathetic activation leads to increased myocardial contractility and heart rate.
    c. An increase in heart chamber diameter increases myocardial wall tension.
    d. An increase in coronary artery diameter results in less rapid coronary blood flow.

30. Angina due to coronary artery spasm is called
    a. stable angina.
    b. classic angina.
    c. unstable angina.
    d. Prinzmetals variant angina.

31. The common denominator in all forms of heart failure is
    a. poor diastolic filling.
    b. reduced cardiac output.
    c. pulmonary edema.
    d. tissue ischemia.

32. *Cor pulmonale* refers to
    a. biventricular failure.
    b. left ventricular hypertrophy secondary to lung disease.
    c. right ventricular hypertrophy secondary to pulmonary hypertension.
    d. right ventricular failure secondary to right ventricular infarction.

33. Lusitropic impairment refers to
    a. poor contractile force.
    b. impaired diastolic relaxation.
    c. altered action potential conduction rate.
    d. altered automaticity.

34. First-degree heart block is characterized by
    a. prolonged PR interval.
    b. absent P waves.
    c. widened QRS complex.
    d. variable PR interval.

35. Second-degree heart block type I (Wenckebach) is characterized by
    a. absent P waves.
    b. variable PR interval and dropped QRS complexes.
    c. constant PR interval and dropped QRS complexes.
    d. no correlation between P waves and QRS complexes.

36. All of the following dysrhythmias are thought to be associated with reentrant mechanisms *except*
    a. second-degree AV block.
    b. atrial fibrillation.
    c. premature ventricular complexes.
    d. preexcitation syndrome tachycardia (WPW).

37. In which of the following dysrhythmias should treatment be immediately instituted?
    a. asymptomatic sinus bradycardia at a heart rate of 50 beats/min
    b. fever induced tachycardia at 122 beats/min
    c. premature atrial complexes occurring every 20 sec
    d. atrial fibrillation with a ventricular rate of 220 beats/min

38. An abnormally wide (>1.0 msec) QRS complex is characteristic of
    a. paroxysmal atrial tachycardia.
    b. supraventricular tachycardia.
    c. junctional escape rhythm.
    d. premature ventricular complexes.

39. A laboratory test that should be routinely monitored in patients receiving digitalis therapy is
    a. serum sodium.
    b. albumin level.
    c. serum potassium.
    d. serum calcium.

### *Case Scenario*

F. S. is an elderly man with a long history of coronary artery disease. He recently suffered his third myocardial infarction and was admitted to a long-term care facility after stabilization in the hospital. Questions 40–45 refer to F. S.

40. While hospitalized, F. S. was noted to have high levels of low density lipoproteins (LDLs). What is the significance of this finding?
    a. Increased LDL levels are associated with increased risk of coronary artery disease.
    b. Measures to decrease LDL levels in F. S. would be unlikely to affect the progression of his disease.
    c. Increased LDL levels are indicative of moderate alcohol intake, and F. S. should be advised to abstain.
    d. Elevated LDL levels are an expected finding in the elderly and therefore not particularly significant.

41. F. S. has limited cardiac reserve. What compensatory sign would be expected during periods of physical exertion?
    a. hypertension
    b. bradycardia
    c. aortic regurgitation
    d. tachycardia

42. F. S.'s blood pressure is measured at 160/98. How would his left ventricular function be affected by this level of blood pressure?
    a. This is an expected blood pressure in the elderly and has little effect on left ventricular function.
    b. Left ventricular workload is increased with high afterload.
    c. High blood pressure will enhance left ventricular perfusion during systole.
    d. High pressure work will lead to left ventricular atrophy.

43. F. S. continues to complain of intermittent chest pain brought on by exertion and relieved by rest. The likely etiology of this pain is
    a. stable angina.
    b. myocardial infarction.
    c. coronary vasospasm.
    d. unstable angina.

44. After sitting in a chair for an hour, F. S. develops moderate lower extremity edema. His edema is most likely a consequence of
    a. arterial obstruction.
    b. isolated left heart failure.
    c. right heart failure.
    d. peripheral vascular disease.

45. F. S. receives an ACE inhibiting agent to treat his cardiovascular disease. Which of the following is *not* an expected result of ACE inhibitor therapy?
   a. diuresis
   b. afterload reduction
   c. enhanced sodium excretion
   d. increased cardiac preload

### *True/False*

____ 46. Acute angina pectoris may produce significantly elevated serum cardiac enzymes.

____ 47. Although smoking has been linked to heart disease, it is no longer considered a major risk factor.

____ 48. Calcium entry from the extracellular fluid into the myocardial cytoplasm is an energy-requiring process.

____ 49. Pulmonary valvular stenosis is characterized by a high right atrial/right ventricular pressure gradient during diastole.

____ 50. The heart sound S2 is due to closing of the aortic and pulmonic valves.

## ANSWER KEY

1. d
2. c
3. b
4. a
5. c
6. d
7. b
8. a
9. b
10. c
11. a
12. b
13. c
14. d
15. d
16. d
17. b
18. a
19. c
20. d
21. c
22. b
23. c
24. c
25. b
26. a
27. b
28. a
29. a
30. d
31. b
32. c
33. b
34. a
35. b
36. a
37. d
38. d
39. c
40. a
41. d
42. b
43. a
44. c
45. d
46. F
47. F
48. F
49. F
50. T

# *Unit VI—Alterations in Respiratory Function*

## KEY QUESTIONS

### *Chapter 19—Respiratory Function*

1. During which embryologic stage does alveolar development and surfactant production occur?
2. Which structures are considered upper airway and which are considered lower airway?
3. Which respiratory system structures engage in gas exchange?
4. What is the difference between a type I and a type II pneumocyte?
5. What are the effects of sympathetic and parasympathetic stimulation of the respiratory airways?
6. What are the functions of the bronchial and pulmonary circulations?
7. How does the lung increase diffusion under conditions of increased pulmonary blood flow?
8. How do hydrostatic pressure and colloid osmotic pressure influence filtration across pulmonary capillaries?
9. What factors affect anatomic and physiologic deadspace in the lung?
10. How is the oxygen content of the blood calculated, and what factors would lead to decreased arterial oxygen content?
11. What factors and physiologic conditions lead to changes in affinity or "shifts" in the oxyhemoglobin saturation curve?
12. What is the effect of gravity on the distribution of ventilation and perfusion in the lung?
13. What is A-a$DO_2$? What is the significance of a large alveolar–arterial oxygen difference?
14. What physiologic conditions can lead to tissue hypoxia?
15. How is carbon dioxide transported in the blood?
16. What is the function of the brainstem "respiratory center"?
17. How do chemoreceptors, baroreceptors, proprioceptors, and pulmonary stretch receptors influence the brainstem respiratory neurons?
18. How do central and peripheral chemoreceptors differ in their responsiveness to pH, $PCO_2$, and $PO_2$?
19. How does respiratory muscle contraction lead to inspiration?
20. What are the major factors contributing to resistance to airflow through the airways?
21. What roles do surfactant and elastic properties of the lung play in determination of lung compliance?
22. How is ventilatory failure differentiated from oxygenation failure?

### *Chapter 20—Obstructive Pulmonary Disorders*

1. Why do people with obstructive airway diseases typically have air trapping within the lungs?
2. How do *bronchiectasis* and *bronchiolitis* differ?
3. What are the clinical manifestations of acute airway obstruction?
4. What is the etiology of and treatment for cystic fibrosis?
5. How do the precipitating factors for intrinsic and extrinsic asthma differ?
6. What three pathophysiologic airway changes occur during an acute episode of asthma?
7. What is the role of IgE in extrinsic asthma?
8. How can asthma attacks be prevented and treated?
9. What is the definition of *chronic bronchitis*?
10. What are the usual pathologic airway changes of chronic bronchitis?
11. Why does chronic bronchitis often result in cor pulmonale and polycythemia?
12. How are acute and chronic bronchitis treated?
13. How do the clinical presentations of emphysema and chronic bronchitis differ?
14. What is the pathogenesis of alveolar destruction associated with emphysema?
15. What characteristic pulmonary function test abnormalities are associated with obstructive respiratory disorders?

### *Chapter 21—Restrictive Pulmonary Disorders*

1. How do the restrictive disorders (a) diffuse interstitial pulmonary fibrosis, (b) sarcoidosis, and (c) hypersensitivity pneumonitis differ with regard to etiology, clinical findings, and treatment?
2. What pathophysiologic factors can lead to abnormal accumulations of pleural fluid or air?
3. How can simple pneumothorax and tension pneumothorax be differentiated?
4. Why are abnormal pleural accumulations classified as restrictive pulmonary disorders?
5. How do chest wall abnormalities such as kyphoscoliosis, ankylosing spondylitis, and extreme obesity affect respiratory function?

### *Chapter 22—Ventilation and Respiratory Failure*

1. How can arterial blood gases be used to define acute respiratory failure?
2. What conditions predispose to development of acute respiratory failure?
3. What clinical manifestations are commonly associated with respiratory failure?
4. How is respiratory failure generally treated?
5. What conditions predispose to development of ARDS?
6. What three major pathologic changes occur in the lung as a consequence of the inflammatory changes of ARDS?
7. What characteristic changes in pulmonary function are associated with ARDS?
8. What are the usual clinical manifestations of ARDS?
9. How is ARDS treated?
10. What role does surfactant deficiency have in the development of IRDS?
11. In what respect are ARDS and IRDS similar?

### *Chapter 23—Other Respiratory Disorders*

1. How do bacterial and viral pneumonias differ in clinical manifestations, severity, and treatment?
2. What are the etiology, clinical and diagnostic findings, and treatment protocols for tuberculosis?
3. What is the major etiologic factor in development of lung cancer?
4. When should lung cancer be suspected, and how can the diagnosis be confirmed?
5. What is the relationship between reduced cross-sectional area of the pulmonary capillaries and pulmonary hypertension?
6. What factors can lead to pulmonary hypertension?
7. What complications can arise from untreated pulmonary hypertension?
8. What compounds have been linked to development of occupational lung diseases?
9. How does chronic inhalation of inert particles lead to development of pulmonary fibrosis?
10. What are the usual clinical manifestations of the pneumoconioses?
11. What factors predispose to development of pulmonary embolism?
12. When should pulmonary embolism be suspected, and how can the diagnosis be confirmed?
13. How can pulmonary emboli be prevented and treated?

## CASE EXAMPLES

R. S. is a long time smoker who developed bronchitic COPD. He also has a history of coronary artery disease and peripheral vascular disease. His arterial blood gas values are pH = 7.32, $PaCO_2$ = 60 mm Hg, $PaO_2$ = 50 mm Hg, $HCO_3^-$ = 30 mEq/L. His hematocrit is 52% with normal red cell indices. He is taking an inhaled beta agonist and theophylline to treat his respiratory condition. At his clinic visit, it is noted that R. S. has an area of consolidation in his right lower lobe thought to be consistent with pneumonia.

### *Discussion Questions*

1. What clinical findings are likely in R. S. as a consequence of his bronchitic COPD? How would these differ from emphysematous COPD?
2. Interpret R. S.'s laboratory results. How would his acid–base disorder be classified? What is the most likely etiology of his polycythemia?
3. What is the rationale for treating R. S. with theophylline and a beta agonist?
4. What effects would these medications have on R. S.'s cardiovascular function?
5. In what position would R. S. have the worst ventilation–perfusion matching?

T. V. is hospitalized with deep vein thrombosis in her left leg as a complication of abdominal surgery. She is being treated with bed rest and anticoagulant therapy. On the third postoperative day, she suddenly experiences severe dyspnea and is placed on supplemental oxygen. A blood gas is drawn which demonstrates hypoxemia and mild respiratory alkalosis.

### *Discussion Questions*

1. Considering T. V.'s history, what is the most likely etiology of her respiratory distress?
2. What diagnostic findings would help confirm this diagnosis?
3. What is the pathogenesis of the hypoxemia in this disorder?
4. How will T. V.'s respiratory disorder likely be treated?

## TEST ITEMS

### *Multiple Choice*

1. The amount of air remaining in the lungs after a maximal exhalation is called the
   a. residual volume.
   b. functional residual capacity.
   c. expiratory reserve volume.
   d. residual capacity.

2. Surfactant is a phospholipid that reduces
   a. pulmonary vascular capacitance.
   b. elastic recoil force.
   c. alveolar surface tension.
   d. pulmonary capillary fragility.

3. A condition that results in increased pulmonary vascular resistance is
   a. anemia.
   b. pulmonary hypoxemia.
   c. calcium channel-blocking agents.
   d. parasympathetic activity.

4. Restrictive pulmonary disorders are characterized by
   a. increased compliance.
   b. increased residual volume.
   c. decreased respiratory rate.
   d. decreased tidal volume.

5. A structure that participates in diffusion of respiratory gases is the
   a. alveolus.
   b. bronchiole.
   c. trachea.
   d. pharynx.

6. An increase in filtration of fluid from the pulmonary capillaries occurs with
   a. increased capillary oncotic pressure.
   b. increased capillary hydrostatic pressure.
   c. decreased capillary hydrostatic pressure.
   d. decreased interstitial oncotic pressure.

7. Which of the following therapies would be associated with the largest increase in arterial oxygen content in a patient with a $PaO_2$ of 70 mm Hg and a hemoglobin of 10 g/dL?
   a. oxygen administration to increase $PaO_2$ to 200 mm Hg
   b. bicarbonate administration to raise hemoglobin affinity for oxygen
   c. blood transfusion to raise hemoglobin to 14 g/dL.
   d. normal saline administration to raise cardiac output.

8. In zone 1 of the lung,
   a. no air is moving.
   b. circulation is highest.
   c. venous pressure is high.
   d. dead space is high.
   e. shunting is high.

9. In zone 2 of the lung,
   a. alveolar volume does not affect blood flow.
   b. venous pressure is high.
   c. dead space is high.
   d. pulmonary vessels are collapsed.
   e. blood flow is determined by pulmonary artery and alveolar pressure.

10. In zone 3 of the lung,
    a. dead space is high.
    b. alveolar pressure is high.
    c. venous pressure is lowest.
    d. the greatest blood flow occurs.

11. The major reason for air trapping in emphysema is
    a. bronchoconstriction.
    b. bronchial edema.
    c. loss of radial traction.
    d. excessive mucus secretion.

12. Viral pneumonia is characterized by
    a. a productive cough.
    b. a dry cough.
    c. exudative consolidation.
    d. significant ventilation-perfusion imbalance.

13. The characteristic x-ray findings in tuberculosis include
    a. diffuse white out.
    b. Ghon tubercules.
    c. bibasilar infiltrates.
    d. tracheal deviation.

14. Extrinsic asthma is associated with
    a. decreased functional residual capacity.
    b. unknown precipitating factors.
    c. IgE-mediated airway inflammation.
    d. irreversible airway obstruction.

15. Widespread atelectasis, noncardiogenic pulmonary edema, and fibrosis are characteristic of
    a. ARDS.
    b. COPD.
    c. asthma.
    d. cor pulmonale.

16. Copious, foul smelling respiratory secretions are generally associated with
    a. emphysema.
    b. pneumoconioses.
    c. pulmonary edema.
    d. bronchiectasis.

17. Which of the following would be indicative of a left tension pneumothorax?
    a. course crackles throughout the left chest
    b. tracheal deviation to the left
    c. absent breath sounds on the left
    d. increased lung density on the left

18. To maximize V/Q matching in a person with unilateral lung disease, one would
    a. ventilate with PEEP.
    b. position with the "good" lung down.
    c. administer vasodilating agents.
    d. position with the diseased lung dependent.

19. Cardiogenic pulmonary edema results from
    a. "leaky" pulmonary capillary membranes.
    b. increased pulmonary capillary hydrostatic pressure.
    c. exudation of protein-rich fluid into alveoli.
    d. inflammatory injury to the capillary basement membrane.

20. The classic features of ARDS include
    a. increased FRC.
    b. increased compliance.
    c. hyperinflated terminal air sacs.
    d. large pulmonary shunt fraction.

21. Emphysema results from destruction of alveolar walls and capillaries, which is due to
    a. release of proteolytic enzymes from immune cells.
    b. air trapping with resultant excessive alveolar pressure.
    c. excessive alpha-1-antitrypsin.
    d. autoantibodies against pulmonary basement membrane.

22. The central chemoreceptors for respiratory control are
    a. located in the carotid artery.
    b. responsive primarily to changes in pH and $CO_2$.
    c. responsive primarily to hypoxemia.
    d. deactivated by chronic hypercapnia.

23. The peripheral chemoreceptors are
    a. located in the medulla oblongata.
    b. poorly perfused and have a slow response time.
    c. primarily responsible for the hypoxic drive to breathe.
    d. unimportant in the adult human.

24. Distribution of ventilation in the upright lung is such that
    a. the apical portions are better ventilated.
    b. the diaphragmatic areas are better ventilated.
    c. all areas are ventilated equally.
    d. ventilation is not affected by position.

25. All of the following contribute to physiologic shunt except
    a. bronchial veins.
    b. thebesian veins.
    c. arteriovenous shunt.
    d. nonperfused alveoli.

26. Hypoxic pulmonary vasoconstriction
    a. diverts blood to nonhypoxic regions.
    b. increases blood flow to the base of the lung.
    c. is active only at high altitudes.
    d. is always detrimental to the patient.

27. The pulmonary vascular system
    a. has no alpha or beta receptors.
    b. has no parasympathetic innervation.
    c. responds to NE with vasoconstriction.
    d. has very low compliance.

28. In the lateral decubitus position
    a. perfusion is greater in the dependent lung.
    b. perfusion is greater in the upper lung.
    c. ventilation is greatest at the apex.
    d. distribution of ventilation and perfusion are the same as in the upright lung.

29. Intrapulmonary shunting refers to
    a. anatomic dead space.
    b. alveolar dead space.
    c. ventilation without perfusion.
    d. perfusion without ventilation.

30. As one moves from the apex of the lung to the dependent areas,
    a. the alveoli become larger.
    b. pleural pressure becomes more negative.
    c. compliance becomes greater.
    d. alveolar ventilation decreases.

31. Which of the following statements about the oxyhemoglobin dissociation curve is true?
    a. Increasing $PaO_2$ above 90 mm Hg greatly improves saturation.
    b. The curve shifts to the left with acidemia.
    c. The curve shifts to the right with hypercarbia (increased $CO_2$).
    d. An increase in $PaO_2$ causes a linear increase in $SaO_2$.
    e. The oxyhemoglobin curve is affected by hemoglobin level.

32. Most of the carbon dioxide in blood is transported
    a. as bicarbonate.
    b. in physical solution.
    c. as carbonic acid.
    d. as carbaminohemoglobin.

33. Shifts in the oxyhemoglobin dissociation curve represent the
    a. effect of carbonic anhydrase on the uptake of $CO_2$.
    b. ability of blood to pick up more $CO_2$ when $PaO_2$ is low.
    c. amount of hydrogen in solution in the blood.
    d. changes in hemoglobin affinity for oxygen.

34. Chronic bronchitis often leads to cor pulmonale because of
    a. ventricular hypoxia.
    b. increased pulmonary vascular resistance.
    c. left ventricular strain.
    d. hypervolemia.

35. Chronic obstructive pulmonary disorders are characterized by
    a. hyperinflation.
    b. tachypnea.
    c. decrease residual volumes.
    d. decreased lung compliance.

## ANSWER KEY

1. a
2. c
3. b
4. d
5. a
6. b
7. c
8. d
9. e
10. d
11. c
12. b
13. b
14. c
15. a
16. d
17. c
18. b
19. b
20. d
21. a
22. b
23. c
24. b
25. d
26. a
27. c
28. a
29. d
30. c
31. c
32. a
33. d
34. b
35. a

# Unit VII—Alterations in Fluid, Electrolyte, and Acid–Base Homeostasis

## KEY QUESTIONS

### Chapter 24—Fluid and Electrolyte Homeostasis and Imbalances

1. What physiologic and psychologic conditions predispose an individual to disturbances in fluid intake?
2. What factors influence the filtration of fluid across the capillary wall?
3. How do the compositions of capillary and interstitial fluids differ? How are they similar?
4. How is water and electrolyte movement across cell membranes regulated?
5. What are the usual and pathologic routes of fluid loss from the body?
6. How is fluid balance regulated by the kidney?
7. What are the effects of aldosterone, ADH, and ANP on fluid regulation?
8. Under what conditions is saline deficit likely to occur, and what are the characteristic clinical findings?
9. Under what conditions is saline excess likely to occur, and what are the characteristic clinical findings?
10. Under what conditions are water excess (hyponatremia) and water deficit (hypernatremia) likely to occur?
11. What are the effects of hypernatremia and hyponatremia on neuronal cells?
12. What physiologic and pathologic conditions can lead to alterations in electrolyte intake, absorption, distribution, or excretion?
13. How do alterations in serum potassium affect the resting membrane potential, and how are these effects clinically manifested?
14. How do alterations in serum calcium ion affect the threshold potential of nerve and muscle, and how are these effects clinically manifested?
15. What is the effect of magnesium ion on release of acetylcholine at the neuromuscular junction, and how are hyper- and hypomagnesemia clinically manifested?
16. What are the major cellular functions of phosphate ion, and how are phosphate imbalances clinically manifested?

### Chapter 25—Acid–Base Homeostasis and Imbalances

1. What is the chemistry and functional importance of the bicarbonate buffer system?
2. What is the role of the respiratory system in regulating carbonic acid (carbon dioxide)?
3. What is the role of the kidneys in regulating noncarbonic acid and bicarbonate ion?
4. How do the lungs compensate for acid–base disturbances resulting from altered levels of metabolic acids?
5. How do the kidneys compensate for acid–base disturbances resulting from altered levels of carbonic acid?
6. How are arterial blood gas values used to categorize an acid–base disorder as acidosis or alkalosis, respiratory or metabolic, compensated or not?
7. What pathophysiologic conditions predispose an individual to development of an acid–base imbalance?
8. What is the significance of a mixed acid–base disorder?

## CASE EXAMPLES

A. C. is a 79-year-old man living in a long-term care facility. He has had multiple medical diagnoses, including congestive heart failure, chronic obstructive pulmonary disease, and stroke. He is bedridden and receiving enteral tube feedings. He has chronic diarrhea thought to be related to his tube feedings. He receives digoxin and lasix to treat his congestive heart failure.

### Discussion Questions

1. A. C. is prone to several acid-base and fluid–electrolyte disorders. Explain why he is at risk for each of the following disorders, and what the laboratory and clinical findings would likely be.
   - saline excess
   - hypokalemia
   - hypercalcemia
   - hypernatremia
   - respiratory acidosis
2. How would A. C. attempt to compensate for a respiratory acidosis should it occur?
3. What acid–base imbalance might occur as a result of A. C.'s chronic diarrhea?

L. S. is brought to the emergency department for treatment of acute mushroom poisoning. Her respirations are slow and shallow and she is nonresponsive. She is admitted to the critical care unit to be closely monitored for the development of ventilatory failure and renal failure which often accompany mushroom poisoning. Her urine output is decreased, at about 20 mL/hr. Her laboratory values are serum $K^+$ = 5.7 mEq/L; arterial blood gases: pH = 7.13, $PaCO_2$ = 56 mm Hg, $PaO_2$ = 89 mm Hg, $HCO_3^-$ = 18 mEq/L.

### *Discussion Questions*

1. What is the most likely cause of L. S.'s potassium imbalance? Explain the role of the kidney in potassium excretion.
2. What is the relationship between acid–base balance and serum potassium level?
3. What is the reason for her low urine output? How should L. S.'s fluids be managed?
3. Categorize and explain the probable etiology of L. S.'s acid–base disorder.
4. Can L. S. compensate for her acid–base disorder? Why or why not?
5. How should her acid–base imbalance be medically managed?

## TEST ITEMS

### *Multiple Choice*

1. Osmoreceptors located in the hypothalamus control the release of
   a. angiotensin.
   b. atrial natriuretic peptide.
   c. aldosterone.
   d. vasopressin (ADH).

2. The best indicator of extracellular (saline) volume status would be
   a. serum sodium ion.
   b. serum osmolality.
   c. weight change.
   d. serum potassium ion.

3. The most appropriate therapy for an individual with hypernatremia is
   a. volume expansion with normal saline.
   b. administration of colloids.
   c. hypotonic fluids.
   d. diuretics.

4. If an individual with normal fluid balance is given 2 liters of normal saline, how will this fluid distribute in the body (assuming no excretion)?
   a. 50% extracellular, 50% intracellular
   b. 2/3 extracellular, 1/3 intracellular
   c. all intravascular
   d. all extracellular

5. Decreased neuromuscular excitability can be seen in which two electrolyte disorders?
   a. hypercalcemia and hypermagnesemia
   b. hyponatremia and hyperkalemia
   c. hypocalcemia and hypokalemia
   d. hypernatremia and hypomagnesemia

6. Which of the following statements best describes the pathophysiology of hypernatremia?
   a. Saline excess leads to weight gain, edema, and congestive failure.
   b. Increased extracellular osmolality leads to cellular shriveling.
   c. Excess extracellular water leads to swelling of body cells.
   d. Sodium excess leads to excessive water retention.

7. Which of the following is likely to lead to hyponatremia?
   a. insufficient ADH secretion
   b. excess aldosterone secretion
   c. administration of intravenous normal saline
   d. frequent nasogastric tube irrigation with water

8. Which of the following serum electrolyte values is abnormal?
   a. magnesium 2.0 mEq/L
   b. potassium 4.0 mEq/L
   c. calcium 10.0 mEq/L
   d. phosphate 4.0 mg/dL

9. An increase in the resting membrane potential (hyperpolarized) is associated with
   a. hypokalemia.
   b. hyperkalemia.
   c. hypocalcemia.
   d. hypercalcemia.

10. Abnormalities in intracellular regulation of enzyme activity and cellular production of ATP are associated with
    a. hyponatremia.
    b. hypocalcemia.
    c. hypophosphatemia.
    d. hypokalemia.

11. Two important renal buffers are
    a. $NaHCO_3$ and hemoglobin.
    b. $NH_3$ and $HPO_4^-$.
    c. $CO_2$ and $H_2O$.
    d. BUN and creatinine.

12. The body compensates for metabolic alkalosis by
    a. hypoventilation.
    b. decreasing arterial carbon dioxide.
    c. increasing bicarbonate ion excretion.
    d. hyperventilation.

13. Classify the following arterial blood gas: pH = 7.52, $PaCO_2$ = 30 mm Hg, $HCO_3^-$ = 24 mEq/L.
    a. metabolic acidosis
    b. metabolic alkalosis
    c. respiratory acidosis
    d. respiratory alkalosis
    e. mixed alkalosis

14. Classify the following arterial blood gas: pH = 7.19, $PaCO_2$ = 49 mm Hg, $HCO_3^-$ = 18 mEq/L.
    a. metabolic acidosis
    b. metabolic alkalosis
    c. respiratory acidosis
    d. respiratory alkalosis
    e. mixed acidosis

15. Administration of sodium bicarbonate to an individual with acidosis will
    a. exacerbate hyperkalemia.
    b. enhance release of oxygen from hemoglobin to the tissues.
    c. increase formation of carbon dioxide in the blood.
    d. decrease ventilatory requirements.

16. Diarrhea and other lower intestinal fluid losses will contribute to
    a. metabolic akalosis.
    b. metabolic acidosis.
    c. respiratory acidosis.
    d. mixed acid–base disorders.

17. Which of the following arterial blood gases indicates a compensated respiratory acidosis?
    a. pH 7.36, $PaCO_2$ 55, $HCO_3^-$ 30
    b. pH 7.45, $PaCO_2$ 40, $HCO_3^-$ 28
    c. pH 7.26, $PaCO_2$ 60, $HCO_3^-$ 26
    d. pH 7.40, $PaCO_2$ 40, $HCO_3^-$ 24

18. Acidosis is commonly associated with
    a. hyperkalemia.
    b. hypokalemia.
    c. increased neuromuscular excitability.
    d. hypocalcemia.

19. In which of the following acid–base disturbances would compensation occur most quickly?
    a. hypoventilation due to CNS depression
    b. cardiopulmonary arrest
    c. acute bronchoconstriction
    d. ketoacidosis

20. Vomiting of stomach contents or continuous nasogastric suctioning may predispose to development of
    a. carbonic acid deficit.
    b. metabolic acid deficit.
    c. metabolic acidosis.
    d. carbonic acid excess.

## ANSWER KEY

1. d
2. c
3. c
4. d
5. a
6. b
7. d
8. c
9. a
10. c
11. b
12. a
13. d
14. e
15. c
16. b
17. a
18. a
19. d
20. b

# *Unit VIII—Alterations in Intra- and Suprarenal Function*

## KEY QUESTIONS

### *Chapter 26—Renal Function*

1. Which kidney structures are located in the cortex and which in the medulla?
2. What are the functional parts of the kidney nephron?
3. How do the arterial and venous circulations of the kidney relate to the kidneys filtering and absorptive functions?
4. What is the role of renin in kidney function, and what factors stimulate its release from kidney juxtaglomerular cells?
5. What physiologic and pathologic factors can affect glomerular filtration rate?
6. Why is autoregulation of kidney blood flow important?
7. Why does a decrease in glomerular filtration rate lead to accumulation of nitrogenous wastes in the blood?
8. What are the major transport processes in each section of the nephron: proximal tubule, loop of Henle, distal tubule, and collecting duct?
9. How does the kidney regulate metabolic acids and bicarbonate ion concentration?
10. How does the kidney compensate for respiratory acidosis and alkalosis?
11. What is the effect of angiotensin II and aldosterone on kidney function?
12. What are the characteristics of normal urine?
13. What are the potential causes of fixed urine specific gravity, cloudy urine, urine casts, proteins, red cells, glucose, stones, and crystals?
14. How is creatinine clearance used to estimate glomerular filtration rate?
15. What diagnostic studies are useful for evaluating renal structure and function?

### *Chapter 27—Intrarenal Disorders*

1. Where is renal pain generally perceived in men and women?
2. How does renal pain of kidney origin differ from pain involving the ureters?
3. What is the etiology and clinical presentation of polycystic kidney disease?
4. How does the significance of unilateral renal agenesis compare to bilateral renal agenesis?
5. What is the usual etiology and clinical presentation of pyelonephritis?
6. How can pyelonephritis be differentiated from lower urinary tract infection?
7. What is the significance of chronic pyelonephritis?
8. How is acute pyelonephritis generally treated?
9. What physiologic and pathologic conditions predispose to formation of renal calculi?
10. What effect does urinary tract obstruction have on glomerular filtration, urinary stasis, and urinary tract infection?
11. How are renal calculi detected and treated?
12. How are renal tumors detected and treated?
13. How does glomerulonephritis affect the glomerular basement membrane and its filtering function?
14. How can glomerulonephritis and pyelonephritis be differentiated?
15. What are the typical clinical manifestations and treatment of glomerulonephritis?
16. How is nephrosis defined and clinically manifested?

### *Chapter 28—Renal Failure*

1. How are prerenal, intrarenal, and postrenal types of acute renal failure different in etiology, reversibility, clinical and laboratory findings, and treatment?
2. How are the three characteristic phases of acute renal failure differentiated?
3. What are the four progressive phases of chronic renal failure, and how do they relate to the degree of functional nephron loss?
4. What clinical and laboratory findings are characteristic of each stage of chronic renal failure?
5. How do decreased GFR and loss of kidney endocrine function (erythropoietin, vitamin D) contribute to the typical manifestations of end-stage renal failure?
6. What is the rationale for using diuretics in the management of prerenal oliguria?
7. What is the tubular site and mechanism of action of each of the common classes of diuretics?
8. What physiologic and laboratory indices are important to monitor during diuretic therapy?
9. What are the goals of fluid management in the patient with acute or end-stage renal failure?
10. How are hyperkalemia, hyperphosphatemia, hypocalcemia, and metabolic acidosis managed in the patient with renal failure?
11. What is the rationale for prescribing a low protein diet for people with renal failure?
12. What are the indications for instituting hemodialysis or peritoneal dialysis in patients with renal dysfunction?

## *Chapter 29—Disorders of the Bladder*

1. What are the functions of sympathetic and parasympathetic innervation in controlling bladder function?
2. What are the potential etiologies and consequences of neurogenic bladder?
3. How are bladder stones detected and treated?
4. What are the common predisposing factors for development of cystitis?
5. What are the typical clinical and laboratory findings associated with cystitis?
6. How does the typical presentation of cystitis differ in the elderly and in small children?
7. How are bladder tumors detected?
8. How does the treatment of benign and malignant tumors of the bladder differ?
9. Which congenital abnormalities of the bladder predispose to urinary obstruction, stasis, and infection?

# CASE EXAMPLES

J. H. is a 12-year-old boy diagnosed with glomerulonephritis thought to be secondary to a streptococcal throat infection. J. H. had been diagnosed with nephrotic syndrome several months prior to his most recent clinic visit. At his latest clinic visit, a decrease in urine output, increasing lethargy, hyperventilation, and generalized edema are noted. Trace amounts of protein are detected in J. H.'s urine. Blood is drawn for laboratory analysis, which reveal the following:

pH = 7.36
$PaCO_2$ = 33 mm Hg
$PaO_2$ = 100 mm Hg
$HCO_3^-$ = 18 mEq/L
Hct = 30%
$Na^+$ = 130 mEq/L
$K^+$ = 5.4 mEq/L
BUN = 58 mg/dL
creatinine = 3.9 mg/dL
albumin = 2.0 g/dL

### *Discussion Questions*

1. How does streptococcal infection lead to glomerulonephritis?
2. Interpret J. H.'s laboratory values for likely etiology and significance. Is J. H. still experiencing nephrosis or is he progressing to uremia?
3. What additional physical or laboratory findings would be helpful in determining J. H.'s stage of renal impairment?
4. How will J. H.'s therapy change if he has progressed from nephrosis to uremia?

D. K. is being seen in the clinic for complaints of urinary frequency, urgency, and burning. She reports that her urine appears cloudy and smells abnormal. A urine culture is obtained, and D. K is given a prescription for antibiotics.

### *Discussion Questions*

1. What is the most likely etiology of D. K.'s signs and symptoms?
2. Was antibiotic therapy the appropriate treatment? What organism should the antibiotic be effective against since it is the most common cause of this disorder?
3. What factors predispose to development of this urinary tract disorder?
4. What strategies could be suggested to help D. K. avoid reoccurrences of this problem?

# TEST ITEMS

### *Multiple Choice*

1. The primary selectivity barrier for glomerular filtration is the
   a. glomerular basement membrane.
   b. endothelial tight junctions.
   c. epithelial fenestra.
   d. mesangial cells.

2. The glucose transporter in the proximal tubule
   a. has no transport maximum.
   b. does not depend on sodium reabsorption.
   c. is ATP dependent.
   d. may be saturated at high filtered glucose loads.

3. A high urine sodium and a fractional sodium excretion of >1 is associated with
   a. hypovolemia.
   b. acute tubular necrosis.
   c. prerenal oliguria.
   d. activation of the renin-angiotensin-aldosterone cascade.

4. The primary function of the vasa recta is to
   a. secrete renin.
   b. reabsorb NaCl.
   c. reabsorb interstitial water.
   d. secrete urea.

5. A total of 70–80% of the water and electrolytes filtered by the kidney are reabsorbed by the
   a. loop of Henle.
   b. collecting tubule.
   c. distal tubule.
   d. proximal tubule.

6. If normal GFR is maintained but tubular reabsorption is completely blocked, how long does it take to lose 5 liters of fluid?
   a. 10 min
   b. 40 min
   c. 4 hr
   d. 6 hr

7. Which of the following is *not* usually associated with nephrosis?
   a. hyperlipidemia
   b. proteinuria
   c. hematuria
   d. generalized edema

8. The oliguric phase of acute tubular necrosis (ATN) is characterized by
   a. polyuria and nocturia.
   b. rapidly developing uremia.
   c. inability to concentrate urine.
   d. enhanced glomerular filtration.

9. Which of the following conditions would result in increased glomerular filtration rate?
   a. hyperglycemia
   b. increased hydrostatic pressure in Bowman's space
   c. increased glomerular oncotic pressure
   d. increased glomerular hydrostatic pressure

10. A person with acute pyelonephritis would most typically have
    a. fever.
    b. oliguria.
    c. edema.
    d. hypertension.

11. The stage of renal insufficiency is associated with
    a. destruction of more than 90% of the total nephrons.
    b. uremic syndrome.
    c. polyuria and nocturia.
    d. proteinuria and hypoproteinemia.

12. The organism most commonly associated with acute pyelonephritis is
    a. streptococcus.
    b. E. coli.
    c. klebsiella.
    d. enterobacter.

13. Osteodystrophy commonly occurs in patients with chronic renal failure because of
    a. hypoparathyroidism.
    b. hypercalcemia.
    c. insufficient active vitamin D.
    d. phosphate deficiency.

14. Renal artery stenosis, hypertension, and nephrosclerosis may all contribute to renal failure by causing
    a. hydronephrosis.
    b. renal ischemia.
    c. nephrosis.
    d. renal inflammation.

15. Polycystic kidney disease is
    a. always rapidly fatal.
    b. due to a streptococcal infection.
    c. associated with supernumery kidney.
    d. genetically transmitted.

16. Appropriate therapy for prerenal oliguria includes
    a. fluid administration.
    b. potassium supplementation.
    c. fluid restriction.
    d. protein restriction.

### Case Scenario

M. W. is an 8-year-old boy with a history of recurrent streptococcal throat infections. He developed glomerulonephritis 3 months after his last throat infection. Over the next 6 months, M. W.'s renal function progressively deteriorates. His hematocrit falls to 18%, and his arterial blood gases show a compensated acidosis. Questions 17–23 refer to M. W.

17. Renal involvement after streptococcal infection is associated with
    a. renal ischemia.
    b. bacterial invasion of the glomerulus.
    c. an anaphylactic reaction.
    d. an immune-complex reaction.

18. Which of the following signs is consistent with a diagnosis of glomerulonephritis?
    a. pyuria
    b. proteinuria
    c. white cell casts in the urine
    d. foul-smelling urine

19. M. W. is at risk for development of uremia as his nephrons progressively deteriorate because
    a. the basement membrane becomes increasingly permeable.
    b. filtration exceeds secretory and reabsorptive capacity.
    c. excessive solute and water are lost in the urine.
    d. glomerular filtration rate declines.

20. Considering M. W.'s history, the most likely etiology of his anemia is
    a. insufficient erythropoietin.
    b. blood loss secondary to hematuria.
    c. vitamin $B_{12}$ deficiency secondary to deficient intrinsic factor.
    d. iron deficiency.

21. The most likely etiology of M. W.'s compensated acidosis is
    a. insufficient filtration of bicarbonate ion at the glomerulus.
    b. excessive production of respiratory and metabolic acids.
    c. insufficient metabolic acid excretion due to nephron loss.
    d. hypoventilation secondary to uremic CNS depression.

22. The most helpful laboratory value in monitoring the progression of M. W.'s renal failure is
    a. serum creatinine.
    b. serum potassium.
    c. blood urea nitrogen (BUN).
    d. mental status changes.

23. Appropriate management of M. W.'s progressive renal failure includes
    a. potassium supplementation.
    b. high protein diet.
    c. erythropoietin administration.
    d. high phosphate diet.

## *Matching*

Match the predisposing factors on the right with the types of acute renal failure on the left.

| | |
|---|---|
| ____ 24. prerenal | a. nephrotoxic antibiotic |
| ____ 25. intrarenal | b. shock |
| ____ 26. postrenal | c. prostatic hyperplasia |

Match the disease processes on the right with their clinical manifestations on the left. Answers are used more than once.

| | |
|---|---|
| ____ 27. proteinuria | a. nephrotic syndrome |
| ____ 28. azotemia | b. uremic syndrome |
| ____ 29. oliguria | |
| ____ 30. hyperlipidemia | |

## ANSWER KEY

| | |
|---|---|
| 1. a | 16. a |
| 2. d | 17. d |
| 3. b | 18. b |
| 4. c | 19. d |
| 5. d | 20. a |
| 6. b | 21. c |
| 7. c | 22. a |
| 8. b | 23. c |
| 9. d | 24. b |
| 10. a | 25. a |
| 11. c | 26. c |
| 12. b | 27. a |
| 13. c | 28. b |
| 14. b | 29. b |
| 15. d | 30. a |

# *Unit IX—Alterations in Genitourinary Function*

## KEY QUESTIONS

### *Chapter 30—Structure and Function of the Male Genitourinary System*

1. What is the effect of parasympathetic stimulation on the bladder musculature?
2. Which ducts empty fluids into the male urethra?
3. What is the role of the Sertoli cells in spermatogenesis?
4. What is the function of Leydig cells?
5. How are sperm transported from the testis to the urethral duct?
6. Which branch of the autonomic nervous system is responsible for penile erection? Ejaculation?
7. Which genitourinary structures develop embryologically from the Wolffian ductal system in males?
8. How is male and female embryologic reproductive development similar?
9. How do the hypothalamic–pituitary gonadotropic hormones influence male reproductive function?
10. How do the processes of capacitation and acrosome reaction affect the fertilization process?

### *Chapter 31—Alterations in Structure and Function of the Male Genitourinary System*

1. What are the common etiologies of priapism?
2. How do phimosis and paraphimosis differ?
3. Is impotence usually primary or secondary? What are the common causes of secondary impotence?
4. Which sexually transmitted diseases have typical penile lesions?
5. What is the rationale for treating cryptorchidism?
6. What is the clinical significance of hydrocele or spermatocele?
7. What is the usual clinical presentation and significance of testicular torsion?
8. What clinical manifestations would lead to a suspicion of infectious epididymitis, and how would confirmed epididymitis be treated?
9. Which testicular cell is most prone to malignant transformation?
10. What clinical manifestations would lead to a suspicion of prostatitis, and how would confirmed prostatitis be treated?
11. How can benign prostatic hyperplasia be differentiated from prostate cancer?
12. What clinical manifestations are indicative of prostatic enlargement?

### *Chapter 32—Structure and Function of the Female Reproductive System*

1. What are the major structures of the internal and external female reproductive tract?
2. What are the major hormonal events of the female reproductive cycle?
3. What is the role of human chorionic gonadotropin in preventing endometrial sloughing?
4. Which hormones are involved in breast development during pregnancy and lactation, and what are their specific functions?
5. What are the physiologic changes associated with pregnancy?
6. What gestational events occur in the fetus during each of the three trimesters of pregnancy?
7. What hormonal changes lead to menopause?
8. What physiologic changes and complications may result from menopausal hormone deficiencies?

### *Chapter 33—Alterations in Structure and Function of the Female Reproductive System*

1. What are the differentiating factors of the common menstrual disorders, including amenorrhea, metrorrhagia, hypomenorrhea, oligomenorrhea, polymenorrhea, menorrhagia, dysfunctional uterine bleeding, and dysmenorrhea?
2. What are the common etiologic factors leading to uterine prolapse, uterine retrodisplacement, cystocele, and rectocele?
3. What are the predisposing factors, usual causative organisms, clinical manifestations, and complications of pelvic inflammatory disease?
4. What factors predispose to development of vulvovaginitis?
5. How can the pain of endometriosis be differentiated from that of dysmenorrhea?
6. What are the usual sites of endometrial tissue growth in women with endometriosis?
7. What is the rationale for hormone therapy to treat endometriosis?
8. What is the rationale for routine PAP testing for cervical cancer?
9. What factors contribute to the high mortality rate of ovarian cancer?
10. How do placenta previa and abruptio placentae differ?

11. What clinical findings would indicate the development of PIH in a pregnant woman?
12. How can benign and malignant breast lumps be clinically differentiated?
13. How does the treatment for breast cancer differ depending on the extent of tumor spread?

### *Chapter 34—Sexually Transmitted Diseases*

1. What are the characteristic clinical manifestations and lesions of gonorrhea and chlamydia?
2. How do the pathologic changes and clinical manifestations of syphilis differ during the incubation, primary, secondary, and tertiary phases?
3. How do the lesions of herpes simplex, syphilis, and lymphogranuloma venereum differ?
4. Which sexually transmitted diseases remain localized and which have systemic consequences?
5. What are the causative organisms and characteristic lesions of the following localized STDs: chanchroid, granuloma inguinale, molluscum contagiosum, and chondylomata acuminata (genital warts)?

## CASE EXAMPLES

J. Y. is a 43-year-old woman who has detected a lump in the upper outer quadrant of her left breast while performing her monthly self-breast examination. She is examined by her primary physician who finds a single mobile, painless lump. A biopsy is done that shows probable malignancy. J. Y. is scheduled for surgery. There is no evidence of regional lymph node involvement. J. Y.'s tumor is thought to be responsive to estrogen.

### *Discussion Questions*

1. Based on the above information, what type of breast surgery is indicated for J. Y.?
2. What treatment besides surgery is J. Y. likely to receive?
3. What implications does J. Y.'s breast cancer have for the use of estrogen therapy when she becomes menopausal?
4. How often should J. Y. have a mammogram?

C. M. is a 28-year-old woman with a long history of dysmenorrhea treated for many years with oral contraceptives. She stopped the pill 8 months ago in anticipation of becoming pregnant with her first child. After stopping the contraceptives, C. M. experiences diffuse abdominal and back pain beginning about a week before menses. Her periods became very heavy. An initial diagnosis of endometriosis is made.

### *Discussion Questions*

1. What is endometriosis and how is it different from primary dysmenorrhea?
2. What implication does a diagnosis of endometriosis have for C. M.'s plans to become pregnant?
3. What informations should C. M. be given regarding the prognosis, potential complications, and treatment options for endometriosis?

## TEST ITEMS

### *Multiple Choice*

1. In males, pituitary leutinizing hormone (LH)
   a. induces Leydig cells in the testes to produce testosterone.
   b. induces Sertoli cells to produce sperm.
   c. stimulates ejaculation of semen.
   d. has no known reproductive function.

2. Disruption of sympathetic genital innervation in males results in
   a. premature ejaculation.
   b. inability to achieve penile erection.
   c. disrupted ejaculation.
   d. reduced testosterone production.

3. Impotence is rarely due to
   a. drug side effects.
   b. psychologic factors.
   c. primary causes.
   d. vascular diseases.

4. Phimosis is a disorder of the penis characterized by
   a. sustained, painful erection.
   b. inability to retract the foreskin.
   c. inability to achieve erection.
   d. malpositioning of the urinary meatus.

5. Cryptorchidism is
   a. associated with an increased incidence of testicular cancer.
   b. an extremely uncommon disorder.
   c. rarely treated.
   d. a consequence of gonorrhea.

6. Sudden, severe testicular pain is indicative of
   a. prostatitis.
   b. testicular cancer.
   c. testicular torsion.
   d. epididymitis.

7. A progressive decrease in force of the urinary stream, dribbling of urine, and difficulty initiating the urinary stream are characteristic of
   a. prostatitis.
   b. urinary calculi.
   c. bladder carcinoma.
   d. prostatic enlargement.

8. At the midpoint of the menstrual cycle, ovulation occurs in response to
   a. an increase in progesterone.
   b. an increase in LH and FSH secretion.
   c. a drop in estrogen.
   d. a drop in gonadotropin.

9. Estrogen therapy is indicated during menopause to prevent each of the following disorders *except*
   a. breast cancer.
   b. osteoporosis.
   c. heart disease.
   d. hot flushes.

10. Endometriosis is a condition in which
    a. the endometrium sloughs continuously.
    b. ectopic endometrial tissue is present.
    c. an abnormal PAP smear is diagnostic.
    d. the endometrium proliferates and does not shed.

11. A change occurring in a pregnant woman that is indicative of a potential disorder is
    a. increased metabolic rate.
    b. 30–40% increase in cardiac output.
    c. increased oxygen consumption.
    d. increased urinary protein.

12. Absence of menstruation is called
    a. amenorrhea.
    b. metrorrhagia.
    c. menorrhagia.
    d. dysmenorrhea.

13. Dysfunctional uterine bleeding (DUB) is due to
    a. endometrial inflammation.
    b. reproductive tract malignancies.
    c. endometrial fibroid tumors.
    d. irregular secretion of reproductive hormones.

14. Which of the following reproductive tract disorders is most likely to be associated with urinary stress incontinence?
    a. rectocele
    b. menopause
    c. cystocele
    d. cervicitis

15. The organism most commonly associated with pelvic inflammatory disease is
    a. *N. gonorrhoeae.*
    b. *Treponema pallidum.*
    c. *E. coli.*
    d. chlamydia.

16. Fibrocystic breast disease
    a. commonly progresses to breast cancer.
    b. may be exacerbated by methylxanthines.
    c. is characterized by painless breast lumps.
    d. is a contraindication for progesterone birth control pills.

17. Risk factors for breast cancer include
    a. a history of fibrocystic breast disease.
    b. more than three pregnancies prior to age 35.
    c. malnourishment.
    d. high fat diet.

18. A long asymptomatic latent phase is characteristic of which of the following sexually transmitted diseases?
    a. gonorrhea
    b. syphilis
    c. chlamydia
    d. hepatitis B

## ANSWER KEY

1. a
2. c
3. c
4. b
5. a
6. c
7. d
8. b
9. a
10. b
11. d
12. a
13. d
14. c
15. a
16. b
17. d
18. b

# *Unit X—Alterations in Gastrointestinal Function*

## KEY QUESTIONS

### *Chapter 35—Gastrointestinal Function*

1. What congenital disorders of the GI tract commonly present with manifestations of obstruction?
2. What are the major structures of the GI tract and their corresponding functions?
3. What is the role of calcium ions in contraction of intestinal smooth muscle:
4. What types of movements correspond to contraction of the circular and longitudinal smooth muscle layers?
5. How does the autonomic nervous system influence GI motility?
6. How does the enteric nervous system coordinate and regulate GI motility?
7. What are the effects of the hormones, gastrin, gastric inhibitory peptide, cholecystokinin, and secretin on GI motility?
8. Which cranial nerves mediate the swallowing reflex?
9. How is gastric emptying regulated?
10. How do segmental and propulsive movements influence the digestive and absorptive functions of the small intestine?
11. How do the ileocecal and gastrocolic reflexes influence movement in the GI tract?
12. What are the major secretions of each of the following secretory cells and glands: salivary, gastric, intestinal epithelium, pancreas, and gallbladder?
13. How and where are complex carbohydrates digested and absorbed?
14. How and where are proteins digested and absorbed?
15. How and where are lipids digested and absorbed?
16. How and where are water and electrolytes absorbed?
17. What alterations in GI function occur in association with very young or very old age?

### *Chapter 36—Gastrointestinal Disorders*

1. How are the various causes of dysphagia differentiated?
2. What are the common etiologies of these general manifestations of GI disorders: pain, nausea, vomiting, diarrhea, and constipation?
3. What clinical and history data would lead to a suspicion of hiatal hernia and/or esophageal reflux?
4. What factors predispose to life-threatening esophageal bleeding?
5. What are the predisposing factors and characteristic manifestations of peptic ulcer disease?
6. How is peptic ulcer disease diagnosed and treated?
7. In what ways are Crohn's disease and ulcerative colitis similar and dissimilar?
8. What are the classic manifestations of appendicitis?
9. What is the difference between diverticulosis and diverticulitis?
10. What are the predisposing factors for development of acute and chronic gastritis?
11. What is the recommended therapy for irritable bowel syndrome?
12. How are mechanical and functional bowel obstructions differentiated?
13. What are the common causes of mechanical bowel obstruction, and how are they treated?
14. What is the mechanism of megacolon in patients with Hirschsprung's disease?
15. What are the common causes and clinical findings of malabsorption?
16. What warning signs may indicate cancer of the GI tract?

### *Chapter 37—Alterations in Function of the Gallbladder and Exocrine Pancreas*

1. How is bile produced, stored, and secreted?
2. How is pancreatic enzyme secretion regulated?
3. Which pancreatic enzymes are synthesized in an active form and which in an inactive form?
4. What factors predispose to formation of cholesterol gallstones?
5. What clinical manifestations are indicative of gallstones?
6. What is the relationship between cholecystitis and cholelithiasis?
7. What is the treatment of choice for cholecystitis?
8. What clinical and laboratory findings are indicative of acute pancreatitis?
9. What is the rationale for withholding food, instituting continuous nasogastric suction, and administering pancreatic enzymes in treating acute pancreatitis?
10. What serious complications may result from acute pancreatitis?
11. How do the etiology, clinical presentation, and treatment of chronic pancreatitis differ from that of acute pancreatitis?

## *Chapter 38—Liver Disease*

1. What are the two sources of blood supply to the liver and how do they differ?
2. What roles does the liver play in nutrient metabolism, bile synthesis, storage of vitamins and minerals, urea synthesis, clotting factor synthesis, and detoxification?
3. Which manifestations of liver disease are due to hepatocellular failure?
4. Which manifestations of liver disease are due to portal hypertension?
5. What is the pathophysiology of hepatic encephalopathy?
6. What is the pathophysiology of ascites formation?
7. How do the different types of viral hepatitis vary with regard to mode of transmission and severity of symptoms?
8. How can hepatitis be prevented?
9. What clinical and laboratory findings would lead to a diagnosis of liver cirrhosis?
10. Why does acetaminophen overdose cause liver damage?
11. Which genetic disorders are associated with excessive accumulations of iron and copper in the liver?
12. What clinical and history information would lead to a suspicion of liver trauma?
13. What are the usual sources of secondary liver cancer?
14. What treatment modalities are available to the patient with end-stage liver failure?

# CASE EXAMPLES

L. B. is a 45-year-old woman with three children ages 4, 6, and 10 years. She works long hours as an instructor at a local college to support her children and husband, who is chronically unemployed. She has had a 6-month history of severe bouts of abdominal pain associated with indigestion, gas, and steatorrhea. Fatty foods seem to exacerbate the symptoms. L. B. is about 40 pounds overweight. An ultrasound of L. B.'s abdomen reveals multiple stones in her gallbladder. She was scheduled for a cholecystectomy.

### *Discussion Questions*

1. What risk factors does L. B. have that predispose her to development of gallstones?
2. Why are fatty foods often associated with an exacerbation of symptoms?
3. What is the relationship between gallstones and cholecystitis?
4. Will L. B. continue to secrete bile after her surgery? How?
5. How should L. B.'s diet be changed in response to her cholecystectomy?

F. C. is a 54-year-old man with a history of chronic heavy alcohol use. He has frequent bouts of gastrointestinal bleeding for which he has been hospitalized on six separate occasions. He continues to drink and exhibits most of the common manifestations of alcoholic cirrhosis. He was recently hit by a car and was hospitalized for a broken leg. He appeared to be under the influence of alcohol at the time of the accident and had a blood alcohol level of 1.8. F. C.'s family reports that his mental functions have deteriorated significantly over the past few months.

### *Discussion Questions*

1. What are the common manifestations of alcoholic cirrhosis? Which are secondary to hepatocellular failure? Which are secondary to portal hypertension?
2. Why is F. C. at particular risk for GI bleeding?
3. What is the probable etiology of F. C.'s progressive mental deterioration? How might his mental deterioration be medically treated?
4. What problems might be precipitated by F. C.'s abrupt cessation of alcohol intake while hospitalized?

# TEST ITEMS

### *Multiple Choice*

1. The structure and secretions of the salivary gland most closely resemble those of the
   a. gastric gland.
   b. exocrine pancreas.
   c. liver.
   d. gallbladder.

2. The primary stimulus for pancreatic secretion is
   a. gastrin.
   b. histamine.
   c. acetylcholine.
   d. secretin.

3. Bile is manufactured by
   a. hepatocytes.
   b. biliary acini.
   c. pancreatic delta cells.
   d. gallbladder epithelia.

4. All of the following would stimulate secretion from gastric parietal cells *except*
   a. acetylcholine.
   b. histamine.
   c. gastrin.
   d. norepinephrine.

5. Chief cells secrete
   a. pepsinogen.
   b. HCl.
   c. intrinsic factor.
   d. gastrin.

6. Parasympathetic stimulation of the stomach would
   a. decrease motility.
   b. decrease HCl secretion.
   c. inhibit acidity.
   d. stimulate motility.

7. Most of the parasympathetic innervation of the GI tract is supplied by the
   a. hypoglossal nerves.
   b. enteric nervous system.
   c. vagus nerves.
   d. celiac ganglia.

8. Most nutrient digestion and absorption occurs in the
   a. stomach.
   b. small intestine.
   c. large intestine.
   d. cecum.

9. Brush border enzymes are produced by
   a. pancreatic acinar cells.
   b. gastric mucosa cells.
   c. intestinal epithelial cells.
   d. goblet cells.

10. Which of the following statements about pepsin is true?
    a. It is secreted by parietal cells in gastric pits.
    b. It is secreted as an inactive proenzyme.
    c. It accomplishes most of the digestion of dietary protein.
    d. It is permanently denatured by a pH less than 4.0.

11. Which of the following is associated with relaxation of the sphincter of Oddi?
    a. cholecystokinin
    b. morphine
    c. norepinephrine
    d. gastrin

12. Which of the following can be absorbed through the intestinal epithelia without further digestion?
    a. sucrose
    b. lactose
    c. glucose
    d. glycogen

13. Which of the following enzymes is proteolytic?
    a. amylase
    b. chymotrypsin
    c. lactase
    d. lipase

14. A deficiency of lipid digestion or absorption commonly results in
    a. steatorrhea.
    b. constipation.
    c. hyperlipidemia.
    d. cholelithiasis.

15. Which of the following symptoms suggests the presence of a hiatal hernia?
    a. nausea
    b. heartburn
    c. diarrhea
    d. abdominal cramps

16. Histamine antagonists may be used in the treatment of peptic ulcer disease to
    a. increase gastric motility.
    b. inhibit secretion of pepsinogen.
    c. neutralize gastric acid.
    d. decrease HCl secretion.

17. Epigastric pain that is relieved by food is suggestive of
    a. pancreatitis.
    b. cardiac angina.
    c. gastric ulcer.
    d. dysphagia.

18. Acute right lower quadrant pain associated with rebound tenderness and systemic signs of inflammation is indicative of
    a. appendicitis.
    b. peritonitis.
    c. cholecystitis.
    d. gastritis.

19. A silent abdomen 3 hours after bowel surgery most likely indicates
    a. peritonitis.
    b. mechanical bowel obstruction.
    c. perforated bowel.
    d. functional bowel obstruction.

20. Jaundice is a common manifestation of
    a. malabsorption syndromes.
    b. anemia.
    c. liver disease.
    d. cholecystitis.

21. A complication of liver disease that is attributed to portal hypertension is
    a. jaundice.
    b. gonadal hypofunction.
    c. encephalopathy.
    d. esophageal varicies.

22. Hepatitis B is usually transmitted by exposure to
    a. hepatitis vaccine.
    b. feces.
    c. blood or semen.
    d. contaminated food.

23. Patients with acute pancreatitis are generally not allowed to eat and may require continuous gastric suctioning to
    a. prevent abdominal distention.
    b. remove the usual stimuli for pancreatic secretion.
    c. prevent hyperglycemia associated with loss of insulin secretion.
    d. prevent mechanical obstruction of the intestine.

24. Most gallstones are composed of
    a. bile.
    b. cholesterol.
    c. calcium.
    d. uric acid salts.

25. Ulcerative colitis is commonly associated with
    a. bloody diarrhea.
    b. malabsorption of nutrients.
    c. fistula formation between loops of bowel.
    d. inflammation and scarring of the submucosal layer of the bowel.

26. An early indicator of colon cancer is
    a. rectal pain.
    b. bloody diarrhea.
    c. a change in bowel habits.
    d. jaundice.

27. Hepatic encephalopathy is a consequence of
    a. hyperbilirubinemia.
    b. hyperuricemia.
    c. toxic effects of alcohol on brain cells.
    d. increased blood ammonia levels.

28. Elevated serum lipase and amylase levels are indicative of
    a. gallbladder disease.
    b. appendicitis.
    c. pancreatitis.
    d. peritonitis.

29. A patient who should be routinely treated prophylactically for peptic ulcer disease is one one who is
    a. taking six to eight tablets of acetaminophen per day.
    b. being treated with high dose oral glucocorticoids.
    c. experiencing work-related stress.
    d. routinely drinking alcohol.

30. Celiac sprue is a malabsorptive disorder associated with
    a. inflammatory reaction to gluten-containing foods.
    b. megacolon at regions of autonomic denervation.
    c. ulceration of the distal colon and rectum.
    d. deficient production of pancreatic enzymes.

## ANSWER KEY

1. b
2. d
3. a
4. d
5. a
6. d
7. c
8. b
9. c
10. b
11. a
12. c
13. b
14. a
15. b
16. d
17. c
18. a
19. d
20. c
21. d
22. c
23. b
24. b
25. a
26. c
27. d
28. c
29. b
30. a

# *Unit XI—Alterations in Endocrine Function and Metabolism*

## KEY QUESTIONS

### *Chapter 39—Mechanisms of Endocrine Control and Metabolism*

1. How does the solubility of a hormone (lipid or water soluble) affect its transport in the bloodstream and mechanism of action at the target cell?
2. Which hormones are lipid soluble and which are water soluble?
3. How do target cells regulate their responsiveness to endocrine hormones?
4. How do negative feedback mechanisms function to control the secretion of hormones?
5. What are the anterior and posterior pituitary hormones, their target tissues, and their negative feedback mechanisms?
6. How do the hormones insulin, glucagon, catecholamines, thyroid, cortisol, and growth hormone affect metabolism of fats, sugars, and proteins?

### *Chapter 40—Alterations in Endocrine Control of Growth and Metabolism*

1. How can primary and secondary endocrine disorders be differentiated?
2. What etiologic factors would lead to clinical manifestations of hormone excess or deficit?
3. What are the normal functions of growth hormone?
4. What are the etiology, clinical findings, and treatment of growth hormone excess in adults and children?
5. What are the etiology, clinical findings, and treatment of growth hormone deficit in children?
6. What are the normal functions of antidiuretic hormone (ADH)?
7. What are the etiology, clinical findings, and treatment of diabetes insipidus (DI)?
8. What are the etiology, clinical findings, and treatment of the syndrome of inappropriate ADH (SIADH)?
9. How is thyroid hormone synthesized and secreted?
10. What are the normal functions of thyroid hormone?
11. What are the etiology, clinical findings, and treatment of thyroid hormone excess?
12. What are the etiology, clinical findings, and treatment of thyroid hormone deficit in children and adults?
13. What are the normal functions of parathyroid hormone?
14. What are the etiology, clinical findings, and treatment of hyperparathyroidism?
15. What are the etiology, clinical findings, and treatment of hypoparathyroidism?
16. What three classes of steroid hormones are synthesized in the adrenal cortex, and what are their general functions in the body?
17. What are the etiology, clinical findings, and treatment for adrenocortical hormone excess?
18. What are the etiology, clinical findings, and treatment for adrenocortical hormone deficit?
19. Why does congenital adrenal hyperplasia result in development of male secondary sex characteristics?
20. What are the clinical manifestations and therapy for pheochromocytoma?

### *Chapter 41—Diabetes Mellitus*

1. Which hormones are involved in regulation of serum glucose, and under what physiologic conditions would each be secreted?
2. What is the mechanism of action of insulin on target cells?
3. How is insulin secretion regulated?
4. What are the differentiating characteristics of NIDDM and IDDM?
5. What clinical findings are associated with hyperglycemia, and how do they differ from those of hypoglycemia?
6. How is impaired glucose tolerance diagnosed?
7. Why does ketoacidosis tend to occur with IDDM and not with NIDDM?
8. Why does hyperosmolar coma tend to occur with NIDDM and not with IDDM?
9. How is diabetes mellitus treated?
10. How can the efficacy of treatment be monitored?
11. What are the acute and chronic complications of diabetes mellitus?
12. What is the mechanism of diabetic vascular complications?
13. What is the mechanism of diabetic neuropathy?
14. Why can oral hypoglycemic agents be effective for NIDDM but not for IDDM?
15. How are insulins classified, dosed, and administered?

## CASE EXAMPLES

B. J. is a 54-year-old attorney who has been experiencing generalized headaches over several months that have responded poorly to nonnarcotic analgesics. He is also experiencing visual disturbances including blurred vision and double vision. Upon questioning, B. J. reports that he has gained 20 pounds over the previous 2 years despite no change in activity or eating patterns. About his weight gain, B. J. jokes, "I guess its all in my feet. I had to buy new shoes, and my shoe size went from a size 10 to a size 12." It was determined that B. J. should have a CT scan of his head to assess for pituitary adenoma.

### *Discussion Questions*

1. What information from the above scenario would indicate a possible pituitary adenoma?
2. What other signs or symptoms might be apparent if B. J. does indeed have a pituitary adenoma?
3. B. J. is diagnosed with pituitary adenoma and undergoes a transsphenoidal hypophysectomy to remove the tumor. After surgery, he has huge urinary outputs of 500-600 mL/hr. What is the most likely etiology of this high urine output? What other clinical data support this diagnosis?
4. B. J. receives subcutaneous ddAVP to treat his high urine output. What is the rationale for this therapy? How can effectiveness be assessed?
5. It is expected that after his transsphenoidal hypophysectomy, all of B. J.'s anterior pituitary hormones will be deficient (panhypopituitarism). What type of hormone replacement will be necessary for him?
6. What information should be given to B. J. about the expected duration of hormone therapy and monitoring of treatment efficacy?
7. During periods of stress, B. J. is likely to require an adjustment in hormone therapy. Which hormone is most critical and why?

D. K. is a 35-year-old high school secretary who began to experience weight loss despite ravenous appetite and increased dietary intake. She has to make frequent trips to the bathroom to urinate and has difficulty concentrating on her work because of fatigue. She drinks large volumes of coffee to help with a constant dry mouth and to combat her fatigue. At a clinic appointment, it was noted that D. K.'s weight has dropped from 140 to 128 pounds. She is 5′ 7″ tall. Her urine is positive for sugar (2%) and ketones. A chemstick blood glucose level is 412 mg/dL. D. K. had eaten breakfast 3 hours prior to the chemstick blood test.

### *Discussion Questions*

1. Considering D. K.'s presenting history and physical data, what form of diabetes mellitus is indicated?
2. What are the physiologic mechanisms of polydipsia, polyuria, and polyphagia in diabetes mellitus?
3. What immediate and long-term therapy will D. K. need to treat her disorder?
4. D. K. must frequently monitor her own glucose levels to evaluate her diabetic control. What range of blood glucose should she be advised to aim for?
5. D. K. needs to understand the signs and symptoms of hypoglycemia so that she can quickly intervene to prevent life-threatening complications. How can she recognize hypoglycemia and what should she do?
6. D. K.'s health-care provider plans to routinely monitor glycosylated hemoglobin levels ($HB_{A1c}$). What information can be gained from this laboratory test?
7. D. K. should be aware of the potential acute and long-term complications of diabetes mellitus. What are they?

## TEST ITEMS

### *Multiple Choice*

1. Which of the following is a characteristic of lipid-soluble hormones?
   a. transported in a free state in the bloodstream
   b. bind to receptors on the plasma membrane of target cells
   c. diffuse through cell membranes and bind intracellular receptors
   d. activate second messenger cascades within the target cell

2. An example of a lipid-soluble hormone is
   a. catecholamine.
   b. thyroid hormone.
   c. peptide hormone.
   d. pituitary hormone.

3. An example of a secondary endocrine disorder is
   a. pituitary hypersecretion of TSH.
   b. adrenal insufficiency following adrenalectomy.
   c. congenital adrenal hyperplasia.
   d. pheochromocytoma.

4. Upregulation of target cell receptors results in
   a. decreased target cell sensitivity to hormone.
   b. reduced production of hormone.
   c. increased target cell responsiveness to hormone.
   d. an increased hormone half-life ($T_{1/2}$).

5. Growth hormone has several effects on the body, including
   a. decreasing plasma glucose level.
   b. increasing lean body mass.
   c. enhancing deposition of fat.
   d. depressing immune function.

6. Growth hormone stimulates the liver to release
   a. ketones.
   b. insulin.
   c. bile.
   d. somatomedins.

7. Growth hormone excess in adults
   a. results in the condition of acromegaly.
   b. leads to abnormally tall stature.
   c. is associated with hypoglycemia.
   d. is usually asymptomatic.

8. An increase in antidiuretic hormone secretion occurs in response to
   a. a decrease in serum osmolality.
   b. dehydration.
   c. hypervolemia.
   d. hyponatremia.

9. Antidiuretic hormone
   a. increases sodium reabsorption in the distal tubule of the kidney.
   b. increases potassium secretion in the distal tubule of the kidney.
   c. increases water reabsorption in the collecting tubule of the kidney.
   d. increases urinary output.

10. A clinical finding consistent with a diagnosis of syndrome of inappropriate ADH secretion (SIADH) is
    a. hypovolemia.
    b. hyponatremia.
    c. increased osmolality.
    d. dehydration.

11. Diabetes insipidus is a condition
    a. resulting from inadequate ADH secretion.
    b. characterized by oliguria.
    c. associated with anterior pituitary dysfunction.
    d. characterized by glycosuria.

12. Synthesis of thyroid hormones
    a. is increased by thyrotropin-inhibiting factor.
    b. occurs in perifollicular C cells.
    c. is stimulated by ACTH.
    d. is inhibited by iodine deficiency.

13. In comparison to T3, thyroxine (T4)
    a. has greater biological activity.
    b. is more abundant in the circulation.
    c. has a shorter half-life.
    d. binds nuclear receptors with greater affinity.

14. Clinical manifestations of Grave's disease may include
    a. tremor.
    b. cold intolerance.
    c. lethargy.
    d. weight gain.

15. Grave's disease is
    a. a secondary endocrine disorder.
    b. associated with autoantibodies to TSH receptors.
    c. characterized by high serum TSH levels.
    d. untreatable.

16. Propylthiouracil may be used to treat hyperthyroidism because it
    a. destroys thyroid gland cells.
    b. inhibits the release of TSH.
    c. suppresses production of autoantibodies.
    d. inhibits thyroid hormone synthesis.

17. Myxedema coma is a severe condition associated with
    a. hypothyroidism.
    b. hyperthermia.
    c. acute cortisol insufficiency.
    d. pheochromocytoma.

18. Clinical manifestations of hypoparathyroidism
    a. are similar to those occurring with hypermagnesemia.
    b. result from decreased neuromuscular excitability.
    c. are similar to those occurring with hypokalemia.
    d. result from decreased serum ionized calcium.

19. The formation of active vitamin D
    a. occurs in the skin.
    b. depends on hydroxylation in the kidney.
    c. is dependent on oral intake of vitamin D.
    d. is necessary for normal potassium metabolism.

20. Adrenocortical hormones are all derived from the common precursor molecule
    a. progesterone.
    b. corticoglobulin.
    c. ACTH.
    d. cholesterol.

21. A clinical finding that is consistent with a diagnosis of adrenocortical insufficiency is
    a. hypokalemia.
    b. hypoglycemia.
    c. hypertension.
    d. moon face.

22. What effect would adrenocortical insufficiency have on an individual's response to surgical stress?
    a. more prone to hyperglycemia
    b. decreased sensitivity to anesthesia
    c. more susceptible to hypertensive crisis
    d. more prone to hypotension

23. Which response to an injection of ACTH indicates a primary adrenal insufficiency?
    a. no change in serum glucocorticoid level
    b. an increase in serum glucocorticoid level
    c. a decrease in serum glucose level
    d. an increase in serum ACTH level

24. A laboratory finding that would help confirm the diagnosis of aldosterone deficiency is
    a. hypernatremia.
    b. hyperkalemia.
    c. hypokalemia.
    d. hypoglycemia.

25. The signs and symptoms of adrenocortical hormone excess may occur from either a primary or secondary disorder. A symptom associated with primary Cushing's syndrome is
    a. hyperpigmentation.
    b. hypotension.
    c. hyperglycemia.
    d. hyperkalemia.

26. Congenital adrenal hyperplasia (adrenogenital syndrome) results from
    a. cortisol excess.
    b. testosterone-secreting tumor.
    c. exogenous androgens.
    d. blocked cortisol production.

27. The underlying pathogenic mechanism for both NIDDM and IDDM is
    a. pancreatic beta cell destruction.
    b. lack of insulin receptors.
    c. lack of exercise and chronic overeating.
    d. impaired glucose transport into cells.

28. Insulin binding to its receptor on target cells results in
    a. increased active transport of glucose into the cell.
    b. glycogen breakdown within target cells.
    c. increased facilitated diffusion of glucose into cells.
    d. gluconeogenesis.

29. A clinical finding consistent with a hypoglycemic reaction is
    a. acetone breath.
    b. warm, dry skin.
    c. tremors.
    d. hyperventilation.

30. Which of the following clinical findings is *not* usually associated with insulin-dependent diabetes mellitus?
    a. polyuria
    b. polydypsia
    c. polyphagia
    d. obesity

31. Non-insulin-dependent diabetes mellitus is often associated with
    a. nonketotic hyperosmolality.
    b. childhood.
    c. autoimmune destruction of the pancreas.
    d. ketoacidosis.

32. Which of the following indicators is most helpful in evaluating long-term blood glucose management in patients with diabetes mellitus?
    a. blood glucose levels
    b. urine glucose levels
    c. glycosylated hemoglobin levels
    d. clinical manifestations of hyperglycemia

33. Diabetic neuropathy is thought to result from
    a. elevated neuronal sorbitol levels.
    b. elevated $Hb_{A1c}$.
    c. deficient neuronal insulin receptors.
    d. neuronal demyelination.

34. Which of the following therapies would *not* be appropriate for an individual with IDDM?
    a. high carbohydrate, low fat diet
    b. daily exercise
    c. insulin
    d. oral hypoglycemic agents

35. A type of insulin that would be most appropriate for acute management of hyperglycemia is
    a. NPH.
    b. semilente.
    c. regular.
    d. ultralente.

### *Matching*

Match the clinical findings on the left with the associated disorders on the right.

| | |
|---|---|
| ____ 36. slow mentation | a. Addison's disease |
| ____ 37. hypertension | b. acromegaly |
| ____ 38. hyperglycemia | c. aldosteronism |
| ____ 39. hypotension | d. myxedema |

### *True/False*

____ 40. Oxytocin and ADH are secreted in response to hypothalamic releasing hormones.

____ 41. Thyroid-stimulating hormone passes directly through the cell membrane and binds to intracellular receptors.

____ 42. Chronic administration of glucocorticoids leads to adrenocortical atrophy.

____ 43. Secondary adrenocortical insufficiency is characterized by hyperpigmentation due to excessive secretion of melanocyte-stimulating hormones.

____ 44. Hypoglycemia is a potent stimulus for growth hormone secretion.

____ 45. Most pituitary hormones are carried in the bloodstream bound to protein carrier molecules.

## ANSWER KEY

1. c
2. b
3. a
4. c
5. b
6. d
7. a
8. b
9. c
10. b
11. a
12. d
13. b
14. a
15. b
16. d
17. a
18. d
19. b
20. d
21. b
22. d
23. a
24. b
25. c
26. d
27. d
28. c
29. c
30. d
31. a
32. c
33. a
34. d
35. c
36. d
37. c
38. b
39. a
40. F
41. F
42. T
43. F
44. T
45. F

# *Unit XII—Alterations in Neural Function*

## KEY QUESTIONS

### *Chapter 42—Neural Development and Cortical Function*

1. How do the structural components of a neuron relate to the functions of the nervous system?
2. How are action potentials initiated and propagated in nerve cells?
3. What are the synaptic mechanisms of neurotransmitter release, degradation, reuptake, and postsynaptic binding?
4. What are the common excitatory and inhibitory neurotransmitters in the CNS?
5. What is the purpose of axonal myelination?
6. What are the functions of neuroglial cells?
7. How do the central and peripheral nervous systems differ?
8. What is the general sequence of events in development of the human nervous system?
9. What are the structural components and functions of meninges?
10. What are the main routes of blood supply to CNS structures?
11. How is the somatotopic representation of sensory and motor neurons preserved in the cord and central nervous system?
12. What are the general pathways taken by afferent sensory impulses and efferent motor impulses as they are conducted from sensory receptor to sensory cortex, and motor cortex to skeletal muscle?
13. Which neurologic functions have been mapped to localized areas within the CNS?

### *Chapter 43—Acute Disorders of Brain Function*

1. What are the factors affecting intracranial pressure, and what alterations might lead to increased intracranial pressure?
2. How does the brain control its blood flow to meet its metabolic demands despite changes in blood pressure and metabolic rate?
3. How does the brain respond to ischemia?
4. How would increased intracranial pressure be clinically manifested?
5. How can assessment of level of consciousness, pupillary responses, eye movements, and vital signs be used to evaluate changes in neurologic health?
6. What are the usual causes and common manifestations of the three primary head injury types: focal, polar, and diffuse?
7. What are the proposed mechanisms and potential consequences of secondary injury?
8. What is the rationale for using each of the following therapies in the treatment of head injury: steroids, hyperventilation, free radical scavengers, head elevation, and brain dehydration?
9. How do the three most common causes of stroke (thrombi, emboli, and hemorrhage) differ in etiology, predisposing factors, and preventative measures?
10. How do clinical manifestations of stroke differ depending on the location of brain damage?
11. What treatment strategies may be used during the acute and chronic phases of stroke therapy?
12. What are the common causes of brain hemorrhage, and how are they clinically manifested?
13. What is the rationale for treating subarachnoid hemorrhage with volume expansion and elevated blood pressure?
14. What clinical manifestations indicate the presence of brain infection?
15. How do meningitis and encephalitis differ in the usual infective organisms, manifestations, and treatment strategies?

### *Chapter 44—Chronic Disorders of Neurologic Function*

1. What conditions are likely to predispose to seizures?
2. How are seizures classified?
3. What is the effect of seizure activity on brain metabolism?
4. How are seizures assessed and managed?
5. What are the organic and clinical findings that characterize Alzheimer's disease?
6. What other potentially treatable factors may mimic the clinical manifestations of organic dementia?
7. What is the proposed neurotransmitter alteration associated with Parkinson's disease, and how does this alteration lead to the usual clinical manifestations?
8. What is the rationale for using dopamine precursors, monoamine oxidase inhibitors, and anticholinergics to ameliorate the symptoms of Parkinson's disease?
9. How would the CNS demyelination characteristic of multiple sclerosis be expected to affect neurotransmission?
10. What is the rationale for using short-term steroid therapy for acute exacerbations of symptoms in patients with multiple sclerosis?

11. What characteristic clinical findings would lead to a diagnosis of amyotrophic lateral sclerosis?
12. What characteristic clinical findings would lead to a diagnosis of Guillian-Barré syndrome?
13. How does the spinal level of spinal cord injury relate to the expected degree of functional loss?
14. What are the mechanisms and manifestations of autonomic dysreflexia?
15. What changes in neurologic function signal the end of spinal shock?

### *Chapter 45—Alterations in Special Sensory Function*

1. What factors can interrupt the conductive and neural portions of the sound transmission pathway?
2. How do conductive and sensorineural mechanisms of hearing loss differ in treatment effectiveness?
3. What clinical manifestations would lead to a diagnosis of Ménière's disease?
4. How do errors of refraction and irregular corneal curvature lead to poor visual acuity?
5. Why must treatment for strabismus be initiated early to be effective?
6. What visual disturbances and clinical signs would lead to a diagnosis of cataract?
7. How do open-angle and narrow-angle glaucoma differ in structural alterations and symptoms?
8. How might disorders affecting the retina, such as retinal detachment, hypertension, and diabetes, be manifested?
9. What changes in vision are expected as a result of the aging process?
10. What are the usual causes of alterations in smell and taste sensation?

### *Chapter 46—Pain*

1. How can one determine if another individual is or is not experiencing pain?
2. How is painful stimulation of nociceptors transmitted to the CNS where it is perceived?
3. How can neurotransmission of pain signals be modulated in the spinal cord and brain?
4. How do acute and chronic pain differ in etiology and clinical and lifestyle expression?
5. Why are some painful sensations perceived at some distance from an injury (referred)?
6. What is the mechanism of neuropathic pain?
7. How is the pain of ischemia clinically manifested?
8. What treatment strategies can be used at the nociceptor, spinal cord, and brain to moderate pain transmission and perception?

## CASE EXAMPLES

M. G. is an 8-year-old boy who has been brought to the emergency department by his parents with a fever of 104°F, lethargy, headache, and stiff neck. Laboratory analysis of a spinal tap demonstrates increased white blood cells in the CSF.

### *Discussion Questions*

1. What is the most likely etiology of M. G.'s signs and symptoms?
2. What are common complications of this disorder, and how would one assess for their occurrence?
3. What is the usual treatment for this disorder?

J. S. is a 72-year-old woman with a long history of atherosclerosis (hardening of the arteries). One afternoon, her grandson found her sitting in a chair staring blankly into space. She was tilting toward the right, drooling, and had been incontinent of urine. She was able to focus her eyes on him when he spoke to her, but she was unable to verbalize a response. She was transported to the local hospital and diagnosed with CVA.

### *Discussion Questions*

1. What questions could be asked of J. S.'s family to help determine the etiology of her stroke as thrombotic, embolic, or hemorrhagic (that is, questions to assess risk factors for each type of stroke)?
2. Based on the scenario described above, which brain hemisphere (left or right) suffered the ischemic damage? What other manifestations of this stroke location would likely be apparent?
3. What medical therapies might be used to treat this CVA and/or to prevent another stroke?
4. What information might be appropriate to give J. S.'s family about the expected recovery process after stroke?

F. P. is a 66-year-old man in the hospital for surgical treatment of an enlarged prostate. His chart indicates that he has had Parkinson's disease for 5 years prior to admission, treated with a dopamine precursor (levodopa/carbodopa). He also has a seizure history, experiencing a seizure about 20 years ago as a complication of a motor vehicle accident. He has taken an antiseizure medication for many years, but stopped taking it about 3 years ago because he was "tired of taking it and hadn't had a seizure since the accident."

### *Discussion Questions*

1. What types of motor difficulties would F. P. be expected to exhibit related to his Parkinson's disease?
2. What is the rationale for treating Parkinson's disease with a dopamine precursor?
3. What safety and activities of daily living problems might F. P. have encountered while hospitalized?
4. If F. P. experienced seizure activity while in the hospital, what should have been assessed during the seizure episode? How would his seizure have been treated?

S. Y. is a 90-year-old women who is a resident of a long-term care facility. She was alert and mentally able until a year ago when she began to manifest signs and symptoms of dementia. A review of her medical records failed to document a thorough analysis of her dementia, but a diagnosis of "probable Alzheimer's disease" was recorded.

### *Discussion Questions*

1. What are the manifestations of dementia?
2. What other potentially treatable factors might have led to S. Y.'s deteriorating mental function?
3. What are the organic brain alterations that are typical of Alzheimer's disease?

## TEST ITEMS

### *Multiple Choice*

1. Neurotransmitter binding to neuronal receptors occurs primarily at the
   a. dendrite and cell body.
   b. nucleus.
   c. axon hillock.
   d. axon terminal.

2. In contrast to other cell types, nerve and muscle cells are able to conduct action potentials because they
   a. are polarized.
   b. are permeable to potassium at rest.
   c. have voltage-gated ion channels.
   d. are impermeable to sodium at rest.

3. The resting membrane potential in nerve and skeletal muscle is determined primarily by
   a. extracellular sodium ion concentration.
   b. the ratio of intra- to extracellular potassium ion.
   c. activation of voltage-gated sodium channels.
   d. activity of energy-dependent membrane ion pumps.

4. Exocytosis of neurotransmitter in response to depolarization of the presynaptic nerve membrane is mediated by
   a. neurotransmitter binding to presynaptic carrier proteins..
   b. potassium influx through voltage-gated channels.
   c. the sodium–potassium ATPase.
   d. calcium influx through voltage-gated channels.

5. Acetylcholine is cleared from the synapse by
   a. passive re-uptake of acetylcholine into the presynaptic neuron.
   b. active re-uptake of acetylcholine into the presynaptic neuron.
   c. passive diffusion into the postsynaptic membrane.
   d. degradation by acetylcholinesterase.

6. Binding of neurotransmitter to receptors on the postsynaptic neuronal membrane results in
   a. a change in ion conductance through the membrane.
   b. opening of voltage-gated calcium channels.
   c. an action potential.
   d. hyperpolarization.

7. A common inhibitory CNS neurotransmitter is
   a. acetylcholine.
   b. norepinephrine.
   c. GABA.
   d. glutamate.

8. Axonal myelination generally increases the
   a. metabolic needs of the neuron.
   b. flow of ions across the neuronal membrane.
   c. sodium permeability.
   d. speed of action potential conduction.

9. Which of the following is *not* a function of neuroglia?
   a. action potential conduction
   b. modulation of ionic composition of ECF in the brain
   c. production of cerebrospinal fluid
   d. phagocytosis of wastes within the CNS

10. One component of the peripheral nervous system is the
   a. cerebral cortex.
   b. brainstem.
   c. spinal cord.
   d. spinal nerve.

11. The entire human nervous system develops from the
    a. brainstem.
    b. neural ectoderm.
    c. mesoderm.
    d. telencephalon.

12. Which of the following is *not* considered to be part of the meninges?
    a. dura mater
    b. pia mater
    c. choroid
    d. arachnoid

13. Occlusion of which of the following arteries would interrupt bloodflow to the brain?
    a. distal aortic artery
    b. pulmonary artery
    c. vertebral artery
    d. left anterior descending artery

14. Activation of touch receptors on the left side of the body is transmitted primarily to the
    a. right somatosensory cortex.
    b. occipital cortex.
    c. left temporal cortex.
    d. right motor cortex.

15. Interruption of neuronal transmission in the lateral one-half of the spinal cord would result in loss of
    a. ipsilateral pain below the level of injury.
    b. ipsilateral touch below the level of injury.
    c. contralateral touch below the level of injury.
    d. bilateral motor control below the level of injury.

16. The language center in most individuals is located
    a. in the frontal lobe.
    b. at the junction of the parietal, temporal, and occipital lobes in the left hemisphere.
    c. in the right hemisphere near the primary sensory and motor cortex.
    d. in the hippocampal and limbic area.

17. A physiologic change most likely to lead to an increase in intracranial pressure is
    a. cerebral vasodilation.
    b. hypernatremia.
    c. respiratory hyperventilation.
    d. sleep.

18. To maintain blood flow in the face of hypotension or increased metabolism, arterioles in the brain
    a. constrict.
    b. dilate.

19. Manifestations of acute brain ischemia (Cushing's reflex) are due primarily to
    a. parasympathetic nervous system activation.
    b. sympathetic nervous system activation.
    c. autoregulation.
    d. loss of brainstem reflexes.

20. Which of the following groups of clinical findings indicates the poorest neurologic functioning?
    a. spontaneous eye opening, movement to command, oriented to self only
    b. eyes open to light touch on shoulder, pupils briskly reactive to light bilaterally
    c. assumes decorticate posture with light touch, no verbal response
    d. no eye opening, responds to painful stimulus by withdrawing

21. Acceleration–deceleration movements of the head often result in polar injuries in which
    a. injury is localized to the site of initial impact.
    b. widespread neuronal damage is incurred.
    c. bleeding from venules fills the subdural space.
    d. focal injuries occur in two places at opposite poles.

22. Secondary injury after head trauma refers to
    a. brain injury due to the initial trauma.
    b. focal areas of bleeding.
    c. brain injury due to the body's response to tissue damage.
    d. injury as a result of medical therapy.

23. An example of *in*appropriate treatment for head trauma would be
    a. head elevation.
    b. free water restriction.
    c. hypoventilation.
    d. bed rest.

24. Risk factors for hemorrhagic stroke include
    a. atherosclerosis.
    b. dysrhythmias.
    c. acute hypertension.
    d. sedentary lifestyle.

25. The most common etiology of CVA (stroke) is
    a. intracranial hemorrhage.
    b. thrombosis.
    c. embolization.
    d. cardiac arrest.

26. Clinical manifestations of a stroke within the right cerebral hemisphere include
    a. cortical blindness.
    b. right visual field blindness.
    c. expressive and receptive aphasia.
    d. left-sided muscle weakness and neglect.

27. The most important preventative measure for hemorrhagic stroke is
    a. anticoagulation.
    b. blood pressure control.
    c. thrombolytics.
    d. treatment of dysrhythmias.

28. In the acute phase of stroke, treatment is aimed at
    a. stabilization of respiratory and cardiovascular function.
    b. risk factor modification.
    c. prevention of bedsores and contractures.
    d. anticoagulation.

29. Subarachnoid hemorrhage is most often associated with
    a. head trauma.
    b. cerebral aneurysm.
    c. embolization.
    d. thrombocytosis.

30. Leakage of CSF from the nose or ears is commonly associated with
    a. epidural hematoma.
    b. temporal skull fracture.
    c. basal skull fracture.
    d. cerebral aneurysm.

31. Rupture of a cerebral aneurysm should be suspected if the patient reports
    a. ringing in the ears.
    b. transient episodes of numbness.
    c. transient episodes of vertigo.
    d. sudden, severe headache.

32. Subarachnoid hemorrhage is usually treated with volume expansion and blood pressure support to enhance cerebral perfusion. This is necessary because subarachnoid hemorrhage predisposes to
    a. cerebral vasospasm.
    b. hypotension.
    c. excessive volume loss.
    d. increased intracranial pressure.

33. Clinical manifestations of headache, stiff neck, and high fever are indicative of
    a. encephalitis.
    b. meningitis.
    c. skull fracture.
    d. cerebral ischemia.

34. Encephalitis is usually
    a. due to a bacterial infection within the CNS.
    b. fatal.
    c. due to viral infection of brain cells.
    d. asymptomatic.

35. Seizures that involve both hemispheres at the outset are termed
    a. partial.
    b. complex.
    c. focal.
    d. generalized.

36. The primary reason that prolonged seizure activity predisposes to ischemic brain damage is that
    a. respirations are lost for a time.
    b. cardiovascular regulation is impaired.
    c. the brainstem is depressed.
    d. the metabolic rate of the brain is extremely high.

37. The dementia of Alzheimer's disease is associated with structural changes in the brain, including
    a. deposition of amyloid plaques within the brain.
    b. degeneration of basal ganglia.
    c. hypertrophy of frontal lobe neurons.
    d. significant aluminum deposits in the brain.

38. Before making a diagnosis of Alzheimer's disease,
    a. a brain biopsy demonstrating organic changes is necessary.
    b. biochemical tests for aluminum toxicity must be positive.
    c. other potential causes of dementia are ruled out.
    d. a CT scan must be positive for significant brain atrophy.

39. Parkinson's disease is associated with
    a. demyelination of CNS neurons.
    b. a pyramidal nerve tract lesion.
    c. insufficient production of acetylcholine in the basal ganglia.
    d. a deficiency of dopamine in the substantia nigra.

40. Monoamine oxidase inhibitors, dopamine precursors, and anticholinergics are all used in the treatment of Parkinson's disease because they
    a. increase dopamine activity in the basal ganglia.
    b. induce regeneration of neurons in the basal ganglia.
    c. prevent the progression of the disease.
    d. produce excitation of basal ganglia structures.

41. The classic manifestations of Parkinson's disease include
    a. intention tremor and akinesia.
    b. rest tremor and skeletal muscle rigidity.
    c. ataxia and intention tremor.
    d. skeletal muscle rigidity and intention tremor.

42. What effect do demyelinating disorders such as multiple sclerosis have on neurotransmission?
    a. slower rate of action potential conduction
    b. increased rate of action potential conduction
    c. facilitation of action potential initiation
    d. faster rate of repolarization

43. Steroids may be used in the treatment of acute exacerbation of symptoms in patients with MS because
    a. viral damage can be inhibited.
    b. demyelination is mediated by immune mechanisms.
    c. steroids reverse the progression of the disease.
    d. steroids inhibit synaptic degradation of neurotransmitters.

44. Upper extremity weakness in association with degeneration of CNS neurons is characteristic of
    a. multiple sclerosis.
    b. Guillian-Barré syndrome.
    c. myasthenia gravis.
    d. amyotrophic lateral sclerosis.

45. Ascending paralysis with no loss of sensation is characteristic of
    a. multiple sclerosis.
    b. Guillian-Barré syndrome.
    c. myasthenia gravis.
    d. amyotrophic lateral sclerosis.

46. The stage of spinal shock that follows spinal cord injury is characterized by
    a. reflex urination and defecation.
    b. autonomic dysreflexia.
    c. absent spinal reflexes below the level of injury.
    d. motor spasticity and hyperreflexia below the level of injury.

47. Autonomic dysreflexia is characterized by
    a. hypertension and bradycardia.
    b. hypotension and shock.
    c. pallor and vasoconstriction above the level of injury.
    d. extreme pain below the level of injury.

48. Conductive hearing loss
    a. cannot be corrected.
    b. is due to damage to hair cells in the inner ear.
    c. usually results from chronic exposure to loud noise.
    d. is due to dysfunction of outer and middle ear structures.

49. Ménière's disease is characterized by
    a. bilateral hearing impairment.
    b. vertigo in association with hearing loss.
    c. middle ear infection.
    d. ossification of bones in the middle ear.

50. Myopia is due to an error of light refraction in which
    a. light rays are scattered as they pass through the cornea.
    b. the focal point of an image is behind the retina.
    c. near vision is impaired.
    d. accommodation is impaired.

51. Opacification of the lens is termed
    a. hyperopia.
    b. glaucoma.
    c. presbyopia.
    d. cataract.

52. A sudden onset of eye pain and impaired vision associated with pupil dilation is characteristic of
    a. narrow-angle glaucoma.
    b. open-angle glaucoma.
    c. cataract.
    d. retinal detachment.

53. Pain is
    a. a subjective experience that is difficult to measure objectively.
    b. associated with changes in vital signs reflecting the intensity of pain.
    c. experienced in the same way by all individuals.
    d. always the result of tissue damage which activates nociceptors.

54. Gate control theory of pain transmission predicts that activity in touch receptors will
    a. enhance perception of pain.
    b. decrease pain signal transmission in the cord.
    c. activate opioid receptors in the CNS.
    d. increase secretion of substance P in the spinal cord.

55. Referred pain may be perceived at some distance from the area of tissue injury but generally
    a. on the same side of the body.
    b. of less intensity.
    c. within the same dermatome.
    d. within 10–15 cm.

## ANSWER KEY

1. a
2. c
3. b
4. d
5. d
6. a
7. c
8. d
9. a
10. d
11. b
12. c
13. c
14. a
15. b
16. b
17. a
18. b
19. b
20. c
21. d
22. c
23. c
24. c
25. b
26. d
27. b
28. a
29. b
30. c
31. d
32. a
33. b
34. c
35. d
36. d
37. a
38. c
39. d
40. a
41. b
42. a
43. b
44. d
45. b
46. c
47. a
48. d
49. b
50. c
51. d
52. a
53. a
54. b
55. c

# *Unit XIII—Alterations in Neuropsychological Function*

## KEY QUESTIONS

### *Chapter 47—Neurobiology of Psychotic Illness*

1. What are the proposed roles of genetics and environment in the development of schizophrenia?
2. What are the "positive" and "negative" symptoms of schizophrenia?
3. What is the role of dopamine-1 and dopamine-2 receptors in mediating the positive and negative symptoms of schizophrenia?
4. How is schizophrenia treated?
5. What are some common themes of delusional beliefs associated with delusional disorder?
6. What alterations in brain neurotransmitter levels are thought to be associated with bipolar disorder and unipolar depression?
7. How is depression manifested and treated?
8. How is bipolar disorder manifested and treated?
9. What sleep disorders commonly occur in association with depression and mania?
10. What is the rationale for treating bipolar disorder with lithium?

### *Chapter 48—Neurobiology of Nonpsychotic Illness*

1. What are the three major categories of anxiety disorders?
2. What are the physical symptoms commonly associated with panic disorder?
3. How are panic disorder and generalized anxiety disorder different?
4. What are obsessions and compulsions?
5. How does an individual with obsessive-compulsive disorder usually react when prevented from performing compulsive rituals?
6. How do obsessive thoughts differ from schizophrenic hallucinations?
7. What types of behaviors typify borderline personality disorder?
8. What kinds of early childhood experiences are thought to contribute to development of borderline personality disorder?
9. What types of behaviors typify antisocial personality disorder?
10. How is antisocial personality disorder diagnosed?
11. What factors are thought to contribute to development of antisocial personality disorder?
12. What are the risk factors, eating abnormalities, and clinical manifestations of anorexia nervosa?
13. How does anorexia nervosa differ from bulemia nervosa?

## CASE EXAMPLE

R. B. is a 62-year-old woman who lives with her retired husband. She is an active volunteer for many church-related activities. Her five children are grown and no longer live in the same town. She has seven grandchildren who visit her frequently. R. B. has a history of periods of intense energy during which she sleeps little, cleans excessively, and makes grandiose plans for household remodeling. She also has episodes of decreased energy, difficulty initiating simple tasks, and withdrawal from social contacts. R. B. has taken lithium for many years to treat her disorder, which seems to moderate her mood swings.

### *Discussion Questions*

1. What disorder does R. B. most likely have?
2. What are the neurotransmitter abnormalities thought to be associated with this disorder?
3. What is the rationale for treating R. B.'s disorder with lithium?
4. How can the adequacy of lithium therapy be monitored?
5. What other pharmacologic measures might be helpful to treat R. B.'s depressive episodes?

## TEST ITEMS

### *Multiple Choice*

1. Schizophrenia is characterized by
   a. generalized anxiety.
   b. depression.
   c. disorganized thinking.
   d. eating disorders.

2. The usual age of onset for schizophrenia is
   a. before puberty.
   b. 15–35 years.
   c. 40–65 years.
   d. after 65 years.

3. Which of the following manifestations is characteristic of the "positive" symptoms of schizophrenia?
   a. social withdrawal
   b. flat affect
   c. lack of speech
   d. hallucinations

4. The "negative" symptoms of schizophrenia
   a. are more easily treated than the positive symptoms.
   b. are thought to be mediated by $D_1$ receptors in the brain.
   c. include rambling speech and delusional thoughts.
   d. are due to a deficiency of brain dopamine.

5. Affective disorders are characterized by
   a. disordered emotions.
   b. obsessions and compulsions.
   c. hallucinations.
   d. panic attacks.

6. Depression is thought to be associated with
   a. abnormal personality development.
   b. early childhood emotional trauma.
   c. deficient brain norepinephrine and serotonin.
   d. excessive stimulation of $D_1$ and $D_2$ receptors in the brain.

7. Mania and depression are both characterized by
   a. high energy and hyperactivity.
   b. poor appetite.
   c. hopelessness.
   d. altered decision-making ability.

8. Lithium is used to treat mania because it
   a. inhibits NE and serotonin activity in the brain.
   b. is a CNS sedative.
   c. is converted to catecholamines within the brain.
   d. blocks $D_2$ receptors in the brain.

9. Drugs that inhibit reuptake of NE or serotonin may be helpful in the treatment of
   a. schizophrenia.
   b. panic attacks.
   c. depression.
   d. delusional disorder.

10. A disorder *not* considered to be an anxiety disorder is
    a. panic disorder.
    b. generalized anxiety disorder.
    c. obsessive-compulsive disorder.
    d. borderline personality disorder.

11. Mitral valve prolapse is a common finding in people with
    a. panic attacks.
    b. generalized anxiety disorder.
    c. obsessive-compulsive disorder.
    d. bipolar disorder.

12. People with obsessive-compulsive disorder
    a. are not aware that obsessive thoughts are from their own brains.
    b. may become highly anxious if prevented from performing rituals.
    c. have disordered thinking and poor reality orientation.
    d. have a severe, untreatable psychotic illness.

13. A diagnosis of borderline personality can be made based on
    a. repeated antisocial behavior prior to age 15.
    b. repetitive threats to commit suicide.
    c. failure to secure gainful employment after age 18 years.
    d. lack of anxiety or guilt when doing harm to others.

14. Bulimia nervosa is an eating disorder characterized by
    a. episodes of binging and purging.
    b. inaccurate body image.
    c. weight loss of greater than 15%.
    d. significant malnutrition.

15. Anorexia nervosa is commonly associated with
    a. obesity.
    b. amenorrhea.
    c. psychosis.
    d. uncontrollable ingestion of large quantities of food.

## ANSWER KEY

1. c
2. b
3. d
4. b
5. a
6. c
7. d
8. a
9. c
10. d
11. a
12. b
13. b
14. a
15. b

# Unit XIV—Alterations in Musculoskeletal Support and Movement

## KEY QUESTIONS

### Chapter 49—Structure and Function of the Musculoskeletal System

1. How do the structures of compact and trabecular bone relate to bone functions?
2. What are the functions of osteoblasts and osteoclasts in bone remodeling?
3. What are the effects of increased and decreased mechanical stress on bone formation?
4. What is the relationship between joint structure and joint mobility?
5. Why is articular cartilage particularly susceptible to degenerative changes?
6. What factors determine tendon strength and compliance?
7. How does the striated structure of skeletal muscle relate to its contractile function?
8. What is the role of intracellular calcium ion in skeletal muscle contraction?
9. How does an action potential in the alpha motor neuron lead to a contraction in the muscle cells of the motor unit?
10. Why does an increase in resting muscle length (up to a point) result in a greater force of muscle contraction?
11. What is the difference among isometric, concentric, and eccentric muscle contraction?
12. What is the role of creatine phosphate in skeletal muscle energy metabolism?

### Chapter 50—Alterations in Musculoskeletal Function: Trauma, Infection, and Disease

1. How are bone fractures classified?
2. What is the process and duration of normal bone healing after a fracture?
3. How do subluxation and dislocation differ?
4. What are the clinical manifestations of scoliosis?
5. How are osteoporosis, osteomalacia, and rickets similar and how do they differ?
6. What are the clinical findings and treatment of bone infections?
7. What terminology is used to describe primary bone tumors?
8. How can clinical manifestations of soft tissue injuries be used to differentiate noncontractile and contractile injuries?
9. What are the manifestations and treatment of compartment syndrome?
10. What is the etiology and pathogenesis of muscular dystrophy?
11. What is the etiology and pathogenesis of myasthenia gravis

### Chapter 51—Alterations in Musculoskeletal Function: Rheumatic Disorders

1. How are osteoarthritis and rheumatoid arthritis differentiated on the basis of etiology, clinical findings, and treatment?
2. What are the similarities and differences among rheumatoid arthritis, lupus, and scleroderma?
3. What are the infective organisms leading to rheumatic joint disease and lyme disease?
4. What is the pathogenesis of gouty arthritis?
5. How do the two subtypes of juvenile rheumatoid arthritis—Still's disease and polyarticular arthritis—differ?

## CASE EXAMPLE

B. T. is a 22-year-old woman with complaints of increasing joint pain and stiffness in her hands, wrists, shoulders, and knees. She has been taking aspirin every 4–6 hours with little relief. Her physician suggests x-rays and blood studies to evaluate her joint dysfunction.

### Discussion Questions

1. Considering the distribution of B. T.'s joint dysfunction and her age, what is the most likely etiology of this dysfunction?
2. What laboratory tests would be helpful in confirming this diagnosis?
3. B. T.'s physician orders low dose steroid therapy (prednisolone) as part of the treatment plan. What is the rationale for using this drug?
4. What other measures would be indicated in the treatment of B. T.'s disorder?

## TEST ITEMS

### Multiple Choice

1. Osteoclast activity leads to
   a. hardening of the bones.
   b. resorption of bone.
   c. deposition of bone.
   d. arthritis.

2. Osteoblastic activity is greatest
   a. in areas of increased mechanical stress.
   b. during menopause.
   c. with vitamin D deficiency.
   d. with disuse due to immobility.

3. Diarthroses are joints that
   a. hold the skull bones together.
   b. allow little or no joint movement.
   c. contain synovial fluid.
   d. are dysfunctional.

4. Articular cartilage is avascular and
   a. incapable of regeneration.
   b. nonliving.
   c. nourished by synovial fluid.
   d. rarely damaged.

5. The primary determinant of tendon strength is
   a. collagen crosslinking.
   b. actin-myosin crossbridging.
   c. elastin composition.
   d. calcium balance.

6. Troponin is a muscle protein that
   a. binds the myosin protein to form cross-bridges.
   b. forms the noncontractile Z-lines.
   c. binds calcium and regulates tropomyosin.
   d. hydrolyzes ATP to provide energy for contraction.

7. The neurotransmitter released from the alpha motorneuron at the motor endplate is
   a. norepinephrine.
   b. epinephrine.
   c. serotonin.
   d. acetylcholine.

8. A concentric contraction results in
   a. muscle shortening.
   b. no change in muscle length.
   c. muscle lengthening.
   d. muscle damage.

9. Moderate stretching of a muscle at rest results in
   a. a more forceful contraction when stimulated.
   b. inefficient use of ATP.
   c. more rapid onset of muscle fatigue.
   d. a reduced force of contraction.

10. Creatine phosphate is
   a. an enzyme that hydrolyzes ATP for energy.
   b. a storage form of muscle energy.
   c. a waste product of muscle metabolism.
   d. a toxin that produces muscle fatigue.

11. Complete healing of a bone fracture occurs when
   a. no movement of the break is detectable.
   b. the callus has been completely replaced with mature bone.
   c. the fracture site and surrounding soft tissue are pain free.
   d. a cast is no longer required to stabilize the break.

12. Rickets is characterized by soft, weak bones resulting from
   a. poor calcium intake.
   b. estrogen deficiency.
   c. phosphate deficiency.
   d. vitamin D deficiency.

13. In older women, osteoporosis is thought to be primarily due to
   a. dietary inadequacies.
   b. estrogen deficiency.
   c. malabsorption syndrome.
   d. inactivity.

14. Pain with passive stretching of a muscle is indicative of
   a. noncontractile tissue injury.
   b. contractile tissue injury.
   c. vascular insufficiency.
   d. skeletal muscle damage.

15. Muscular dystrophy includes a number of muscle disorders that are
   a. genetically transmitted.
   b. easily prevented and treated.
   c. autoimmune diseases.
   d. demyelinating diseases.

16. Myasthenia gravis is an autoimmune disease in which
   a. neuronal demyelination disrupts nerve transmission.
   b. muscles become increasingly bulky but weakened.
   c. acetylcholine receptors are destroyed or dysfunctional.
   d. acetylcholine release from alpha motorneurons is disrupted.

17. Anticholinesterase agents may be used to treat
   a. muscular dystrophy.
   b. myasthenia gravis.
   c. fibromyalgia.
   d. rheumatoid arthritis.

18. Gouty arthritis is a complication of
   a. beta hemolytic streptococcal infection.
   b. autoimmune destruction of joint collagen.
   c. excessive production of urea.
   d. inadequate renal excretion of uric acid.

### *Case Scenarios*

J. R. is a 33-year-old lawyer who has sustained a leg fracture secondary to collision with a tree while skiing. His fracture has been diagnosed as "compound, transverse fracture of the tibia and fibula." J. R.'s leg was surgically aligned and casted. He has been admitted to the unit for observation, pain control, and antibiotic therapy. Questions 19–21 refer to J. R.

19. The type of fracture J. R. sustained is best described as bones
   a. broken in two or more pieces.
   b. cracked, but not completely separated.
   c. broken along the long axis of the bone.
   d. broken and protruding through skin.

20. Which of the following would be an *unlikely* complication of J. R.'s injury?
   a. bone infection
   b. fat emboli
   c. air emboli
   d. compartment syndrome

21. Six hours after casting of his leg, J. R. begins to complain of increasing leg pain. Assessment of the extremity demonstrates pulselessness and pallor. The appropriate action to take is to
   a. increase the adminstration of J. R.'s pain medication.
   b. initiate action to have the cast split or removed.
   c. note the increase in pain in J. R.'s chart and recheck the extremity in 30 minutes.
   d. elevate the extremity to relieve swelling.

C. S. is a 28-year-old woman diagnosed with rheumatoid arthritis 2 years previously. She has periods of relatively mild joint stiffness and pain interspersed with periods of increased symptom severity. During exacerbations of joint pain, she takes steroids. Otherwise she maintains on nonsteroidal antiinflammatory agents. Questions 22–24 refer to C. S.

22. A clinical finding consistent with C. S.'s diagnosis of rheumatoid arthritis would be
   a. systemic manifestations of inflammation.
   b. localized pain in weight-bearing joints.
   c. reduced excretion of uric acid by the kidney.
   d. firm, crystalized nodules or "tophi" at the affected joints.

23. Rheumatoid arthritis is commonly associated with the presence of rheumatoid factor (RF) autoantibodies in the bloodstream. This indicates that rheumatoid arthritis is likely to be
   a. due to bacterial infection.
   b. an autoimmune process.
   c. an infective process.
   d. due to an enzymatic defect.

24. In contrast to osteoarthritis, C. S.'s arthritis may be associated with
   a. debilitating joint pain and stiffness.
   b. improvement in symptoms with aspirin therapy.
   c. changes in activities of daily living.
   d. widespread connective tissue inflammation.

## ANSWER KEY

1. b
2. a
3. c
4. c
5. a
6. c
7. d
8. a
9. a
10. b
11. b
12. d
13. b
14. a
15. a
16. c
17. b
18. d
19. d
20. c
21. b
22. a
23. b
24. d

# Unit XV—Alterations in the Integument

## KEY QUESTIONS

### Chapter 52—Structure and Function of the Integumentary System

1. How do the epidermal and dermal layers differ in structure and function?
2. What roles do the accessory structures of the dermis—hair follicles, nails, and glands—play in skin function?
3. How do keratinocytes and melanocytes differ in function?
4. What is the composition and function of "surface film"?
5. How do various cell types in the skin function to provide the "first line of defense" against microorganisms?
6. How is skin blood flow controlled, and what is the skin's role in body temperature regulation?
7. How do the three types of glands in the skin—sebaceous, apocrine, and eccrine—differ in function?
8. How does glandular and regenerative function of the skin change with age?
9. What characteristics of skin can be assessed to detect changes associated with systemic and localized pathophysiologic disorders?

### Chapter 53—Alterations in the Integument

1. Why is it important to differentiate primary from secondary skin lesions?
2. What lesion characteristics are assessed to aid in determination of the lesion's etiology?
3. What skin manifestations are associated with fever, hypoxemia, ischemia, hyperbilirubinemia, sympathetic nervous system activation, and altered fluid balance?
4. How do systemic disorders affect nail and hair growth?
5. Which skin disorders are more likely to occur more commonly in certain age groups, including infants, children, adolescents, and the elderly?
6. What are the typical skin lesions associated with herpes, human papilloma virus, superficial fungal infections, and impetigo?
7. How are noninfectious inflammatory skin lesions usually treated?
8. What are the characteristic findings in patients with allergic dermatitis?
9. How can lesion character and distribution be used to differentiate various insect bites and infestations such as scabies, ticks, fleas, mosquitoes, and mites?
10. What are the characteristic skin changes associated with scleroderma?
11. How does ultraviolet radiation affect the skin?
12. How do superficial and deep pressure ulcers differ in presentation and etiology?
13. How can malignant melanoma be differentiated from other skin lesions?
14. How do albinism and vitiligo differ?
15. Which types of topical treatments tend to dry the skin and which tend to moisturize the skin?
16. What is the rationale for using corticosteroids to treat a variety of skin lesions?

## CASE EXAMPLE

E. S. is a 4-year-old girl brought to the clinic after her day-care provider noticed a yellowish, crusty lesion with pustules and weeping areas developing on E. S.'s face near the right nares. A diagnosis of impetigo is made, and topical Bactroban is ordered.

### Discussion Questions

1. What are the usual causative organisms associated with impetigo?
2. What precautions should be taken by the day-care provider when caring for E. S.?
3. What is the rationale for topical Bactroban therapy in this case?

## TEST ITEMS

### Multiple Choice

1. Keratinocytes are the predominant cell type of the
   a. epidermis.
   b. dermis.
   c. subcutaneous tissue.
   d. eccrine gland.

2. Melanocytes
   a. are cancerous.
   b. contain pigment.
   c. are immune cells within the skin.
   d. produce sebum.

3. Heat loss through the skin is reduced by
   a. sweating.
   b. vasodilation.
   c. vasoconstriction.
   d. hyperemia.

4. Sebaceous gland secretion is increased by
   a. androgens.
   b. sympathetic nervous system stimulation.
   c. parasympathetic nervous system stimulation.
   d. cool environmental temperature.

5. Contact dermatitis is most likely to occur in
   a. infants.
   b. children.
   c. adolescents.
   d. the elderly.

6. Atopic dermatitis (eczema) is due to
   a. parasitic infestation of the skin.
   b. superficial staph infection.
   c. superficial fungal infection.
   d. contact with skin allergens.

7. Itchy linear burrows on the hands and wrists are associated with
   a. tick bites.
   b. Rocky Mountain spotted fever.
   c. scabies.
   d. contact dermatitis.

8. Vitiligo
   a. occurs from a genetic lack of melanin production.
   b. is a depigmented patch of skin.
   c. occurs most commonly in light-skinned individuals.
   d. is a warning sign for malignant melanoma.

9. Deep pressure sores
   a. appear first as reddened areas that do not blanch.
   b. begin in the dermal and epidermal skin layers.
   c. result from thrombosis of deep vessels.
   d. are an unavoidable consequence of immobility.

10. Which of the following cancers is considered to be the most malignant?
    a. hyperkeratosis
    b. basal cell carcinoma
    c. squamous cell carcinoma
    d. melanoma

11. The presence of a widely distributed pruritic maculopapular rash and erythema is commonly associated with
    a. psoriasis.
    b. drug reaction.
    c. scleroderma.
    d. bedbug bites.

12. At puberty when sebaceous gland secretion increases, follicle obstruction and infection may occur, resulting in the condition of
    a. psoriasis.
    b. eczema.
    c. acne vulgaris.
    d. phemphigus.

13. Acute, painful inflammation along the distribution of a spinal nerve (dermatome) is characteristic of
    a. herpes zoster.
    b. herpes simplex.
    c. human papillomavirus.
    d. tinea.

14. A topical therapy that would tend to dry the skin is
    a. lotion.
    b. gel.
    c. cream.
    d. ointment.

15. Corticosteroids are commonly administered to treat skin disorders because they
    a. are analgesics.
    b. prevent infection.
    c. enhance collagen production.
    d. reduce inflammation.

## ANSWER KEY

1. a
2. b
3. c
4. a
5. a
6. d
7. c
8. b
9. c
10. d
11. b
12. c
13. a
14. b
15. d

# *Unit XVI—Selected Multisystem Alterations and Considerations in Critical Illness*

## KEY QUESTIONS

### *Chapter 54—Cardiogenic, Hypovolemic, Septic, Anaphylactic, and Neurogenic Shock*

1. What are the cellular consequences of shock?
2. What conditions are associated with each of the different types of shock?
3. How can $SvO_2$ monitoring be used to evaluate the adequacy of cardiac output and distribution of blood flow to tissues?
4. What clinical manifestations are evident during compensated shock?
5. What is the role of the SNS in compensation for low cardiac output?
6. What cellular events characterize the progressive stage of shock?
7. What hemodynamic findings and clinical manifestations typify cardiogenic shock?
8. How are cardiac contractility, preload, and afterload managed in the patient with cardiogenic shock?
9. How do the hemodynamic findings in hypovolemic shock differ from those of cardiogenic shock?
10. What is the relationship between the amount of blood loss and the severity of symptoms in hypovolemia?
11. How is hypovolemic shock managed?
12. What is the role of immune mechanisms in the development of septic shock?
13. What are the hemodynamic findings in early and late septic shock?
14. How is $SvO_2$ monitoring used to evaluate the severity of septic shock and the patient's response to therapy?
15. How is septic shock managed?
16. What is the pathogenesis of low cardiac output in anaphylactic and neurogenic shock?
17. What patients are at risk for development of neurogenic shock?
18. How is anaphylactic shock managed?
19. What is the role of immune mechanisms in development of the organ failure that is commonly associated with shock states?

### *Chapter 55—Burn Injuries*

1. What are the common causes of burn injuries?
2. Which essential skin functions are disrupted as a consequence of burn injury, predisposing the patient to serious complications?
3. How are first-degree, second-degree superficial, deep partial thickness, and third-degree burns differentiated?
4. How are the depth and extent of the burn injury correlated to burn severity?
5. What is the first priority in rescuing a burned or electrocuted individual?
6. What is *burn shock*?
7. What are the usual systemic manifestations of burn shock?
8. How do the injuries of electrical burn injury differ from thermal burn injury?
9. What are the priorities of treatment during the emergent phase of burn injury?
10. What principles guide the management of burn wounds?
11. How are nutritional requirements altered in the burned individual?
12. What is the role of skin grafting in the management of burn injury?
13. How is the *rehabilitation phase* of burn injury defined?
14. What are the priorities of care during the rehabilitation phase of burn injury?

### *Chapter 56—Nutritional Alterations in Critical Illness*

1. What information gained from a nutritional assessment would indicate potential or actual nutritional problems?
2. What anthropometric measurements are used to assess nutritional status?
3. What information about nutritional status can be gained from each of the following biochemical tests: serum albumin, transferrin, prealbumin, RBC and WBC count, BUN, serum creatinine, and urinary nitrogen excretion?
4. How is basal energy expenditure calculated?
5. How does acute physiologic stress affect body metabolism?
6. What are the metabolic changes that occur during the adaptive phase that may begin 5–7 days after acute physiologic stress?
7. How is nutritional supplementation adjusted during acute physiologic stress to avoid hyperglycemia and meet caloric needs?

8. How do kwashiorkor and marasmus differ with regard to predisposing factors, visceral and somatic protein depletion, and diagnostic findings?
9. What cardiovascular, respiratory, and immune system dysfunctions can result from malnutrition?
10. How does fever affect metabolic rate?
11. What are the usual nutritional alterations in patients suffering major trauma and major burns?
12. What factors contribute to cachexia in the person with cancer?

### *Chapter 57—Multisystem Considerations in Special Care Units*

1. What are the major factors that affect the psychosocial response to hospitalization?
2. What emotional responses commonly occur in individuals with critical illnesses?
3. How might each of the phases of grieving, shock and disbelief, awareness, restitution, and resolution be exhibited in critically ill individuals and their families?
4. What are the primary "needs" commonly expressed by families of critically ill patients?
5. What aspects of the critical care environment can lead to increased stress?
6. What factors in the critical care environment are thought to contribute to sleep deprivation?
7. What are the contributing factors and clinical manifestions of "ICU psychosis"?

## CASE EXAMPLES

C. C. is a previously healthy 27-year-old male admitted to the critical care unit after an accident in which he was hit by a car and dragged along the pavement for nearly 100 feet. He suffered a frontal contusion, fractured clavicle and ribs, and extensive abrasions on his arms, legs, side, back, and buttocks. He was tachycardic, hypotensive, unresponsive, and ventilating poorly when admitted. He was placed on a mechanical ventilator and given IV fluids to treat shock. C. C. responded well to fluids, with an increase in blood pressure and an improvement in urine output. His laboratory assessment demonstrated hyperglycemia and low serum albumin.

### *Discussion Questions*

1. Based on his case history and responsiveness to fluid therapy, what type of shock was C. C. experiencing?
2. What other clinical findings would be helpful in confirming the type of shock?
3. What is the most likely etiology of C. C.'s hyperglycemia?
4. What are the usual metabolic responses to acute physiologic stress? How might these metabolic alterations be exhibited in C. C.?
5. How does low serum albumin affect filtration of fluid from the capillaries into the interstitial spaces?
6. What factors in the ICU environment might contribute to the stress of hospitalization?

L. S. is a 2-year-old boy who suffered a scald injury on his lower extremities, buttocks, and genitals when he climbed into a bathtub of extremely hot water. His parents quickly removed him from the tub and poured cold water on his burns, wrapped him in a towel, and rushed him to the emergency department. The burn covered about 40% of the L. S.'s body and was diagnosed as a second-degree, superficial partial thickness burn. Because of the extent of injury and the involvement of the genitals, L. S. was admitted to the burn unit for observation and treatment.

1. L. S.'s parents want to know if they did the right thing in pouring cold water on the burn at home. What would be the best response?
2. Describe the type of skin injury associated with a superficial partial thickness burn.
3. How will this burn be managed?
4. Is L. S. at risk for the development of burn shock based on the extent and severity of injury? How would burn shock be clinically manifested?
5. How will this burn injury be likely to affect L. S.'s nutritional status?
6. What laboratory assessments would be helpful in evaluating L. S.'s metabolic and nutritional response to the stress of his burn injury?

## TEST ITEMS

### *Multiple Choice*

1. The early stage of hypovolemic shock is characterized by
   a. tachycardia.
   b. hypotension.
   c. lactic acidosis.
   d. cardiac failure.

2. Cardiogenic shock is characterized by
   a. hypovolemia.
   b. reduced systemic vascular resistance.
   c. reduced cardiac output.
   d. elevated $SvO_2$.

3. Low cardiac output in association with high preload is characteristic of
 a. hypovolemic shock.
 b. cardiogenic shock.
 c. anaphylactic shock.
 d. septic shock.

4. Administration of which of the following therapies would be most appropriate for hypovolemic shock?
 a. normal saline
 b. vasoconstrictor agents
 c. inotropic agents
 d. 5% dextrose in water

5. In contrast to all other types of shock, the hyperdynamic phase of septic shock is associated with
 a. high afterload.
 b. low cardiac output.
 c. high cardiac output.
 d. reduced contractility.

6. Improvement in a patient with septic shock is indicated by
 a. an increase in cardiac output.
 b. a decrease in $SvO_2$.
 c. a decrease in systemic vascular resistance.
 d. an increase in serum lactate level.

7. Hypotension associated with neurogenic and anaphylactic shock is due to
 a. hypovolemia.
 b. peripheral pooling of blood.
 c. poor cardiac contractility.
 d. high afterload.

8. Second-degree, superficial partial thickness burns
 a. are less painful than third-degree burns.
 b. involve only the epidermis.
 c. usually heal in 3–4 weeks.
 d. are rarely associated with scar formation.

9. Burns covering 25–35% of the total body surface area
 a. are often associated with burn shock.
 b. can rarely be grafted.
 c. are nearly always fatal.
 d. are classified as major burns in children but not in adults.

10. The first priority in rescuing a burned individual is
 a. establishing a patent airway.
 b. removing clothing.
 c. eliminating the source of the burn.
 d. covering the wounds.

11. Most of the manifestations of burn shock can be attributed to
 a. hypovolemia.
 b. cardiac depression.
 c. infection.
 d. increased capillary permeability.

12. Electrical shock may cause extensive damage to low resistance tissues, particularly
 a. bone and muscle.
 b. nerves and blood vessels.
 c. epidermis.
 d. dermis and subcutaneous tissue.

13. The time between the end of burn shock and closure of the burn to less than 20% of total body surface area is called the
 a. postshock phase.
 b. rehabilitation phase.
 c. critical phase.
 d. emergent phase.

14. The primary aim of burn wound management is to
 a. prevent trauma to burned tissue.
 b. prevent microbial colonization of the wound.
 c. keep the wound dry.
 d. prevent premature wound closure.

15. The treatment of choice for major burn injury is
 a. excision of the burn followed by skin grafting.
 b. frequent wound debridement to encourage wound healing.
 c. hyperbaric oxygen therapy.
 d. continuous topical antibiotic therapy.

16. Which of these laboratory tests is the best indicator of the adequacy of protein intake and utilization by the liver?
 a. serum IgG
 b. total protein
 c. prealbumin
 d. creatinine

17. Kwashiorkor is characterized by
    a. loss of somatic protein.
    b. preservation of visceral protein.
    c. body weight less than 80% of ideal.
    d. stress-induced protein catabolism.

18. Starvation is associated with
    a. loss of visceral protein.
    b. low serum albumin levels.
    c. loss of somatic fat and protein.
    d. generalized edema.

19. Which of the following patients is most at risk for severe protein malnutrition?
    a. a postsurgical patient who has been NPO for 3 days
    b. a postburn patient who has a deep partial thickness, 25 % TBSA burn
    c. a febrile patient who has had a temperature of 102.6°F for 3 days
    d. an immobile patient who has been in skeletal traction for 1 week

20. After 2–5 days in an ICU, some patients may experience "ICU psychosis," which is characterized by
    a. anger.
    b. denial.
    c. hopelessness.
    d. hallucinations.

## ANSWER KEY

1. a
2. c
3. b
4. a
5. c
6. b
7. b
8. c
9. a
10. c
11. d
12. b
13. d
14. b
15. a
16. c
17. d
18. c
19. b
20. d

# SECTION THREE

## *Sample Comprehensive Exam*

J. S. is involved in a motor vehicle accident and suffers an acceleration-deceleration head injury. His left leg is crushed, resulting in severe tissue trauma and a fractured femur. He is hospitalized after initial stabilization in the Emergency Department. Questions 1–11 refer to J. S.

1. J. S. requires frequent neurologic checks to detect any changes in intracranial pressure. An early sign of increased ICP is
   a. decreased systolic blood pressure.
   b. a change in the level of consciousness.
   c. pupillary dilation and fixation.
   d. the Cushing reflex.

2. According to J. S,'s vital signs, he seems to be hyperventilating. What is the relationship between hyperventilation and increased ICP?
   a. Respiratory alkalosis will lead to cerebral vasoconstriction and reduce ICP.
   b. Hyperventilation will increase cerebral blood flow and increase ICP.
   c. Hyperventilation will improve blood oxygenation and decrease the ischemia due to increased ICP.
   d. Intracranial pressure is not affected by $CO_2$ levels.

3. As J. S.'s brain continues to swell, increasing pressure is placed on his pituitary gland, leading to diabetes insipidus. Clinical manifestations of diabetes insipidus include
   a. polyuria, dehydration.
   b. oliguria, hypernatremia.
   c. edema, polyphagia.
   d. hyponatremia, hyperkalemia.

4. The nurse is concerned about J. S.'s fluid status and realizes that the best indicator of changes in J. S.'s extracellular volume status is
   a. serum $Na^+$.
   b. serum osmolality.
   c. neurologic symptoms.
   d. weight change.

5. Because of J. S.'s crushing leg injury, he is at risk for hyperkalemia. What signs or symptoms characterize this disorder?
   a. muscle spasm or tetany
   b. muscle weakness and cardiac dysrhythmias
   c. confusion or combativeness
   d. decreased sensitivity to pain

6. J. S. remains in skeletal traction and on bed rest for 6 weeks while his leg fracture heals. Which of the following would be appropriate to help J. S. avoid the complications of immobility-induced hypercalcemia?
   a. high calcium diet to promote bone healing
   b. antacids to bind phosphate in the gut
   c. foods and fluids that promote increased urine acidity and decrease nephrolithiasis
   d. high carbohydrate, high protein diet

7. Assessment of J. S.'s injured leg immediately after the injury reveals several signs and symptoms of inflammation. These include
   a. cool to touch.
   b. paleness.
   c. edema.
   d. paresthesia.

8. Assessment of J. S.'s leg 3 days post-trauma indicate increasing pain, pallor, and lack of pulse distal to the injury. These findings are characteristic of
   a. thrombophlebitis.
   b. compartment syndrome.
   c. venous insufficiency.
   d. post-traumatic wound healing.

9. J. S. suddenly develops severe shortness of breath and hypoxemia. Considering his history, the most likely etiology of these symptoms is
   a. status asthmaticus.
   b. pulmonary edema.
   c. hypostatic pneumonia.
   d. pulmonary embolus.

10. J. S.'s arterial blood gas sample indicate that he has an uncompensated respiratory alkalosis. Which of the following ABG's would be consistent with this diagnosis?
    a. pH 7.45, $CO_2$ 30, $HCO_3^-$ 20
    b. pH 7.56, $CO_2$ 30, $HCO_3^-$ 26
    c. pH 7.19, $CO_2$ 60, $HCO_3^-$ 22
    d. pH 7.42, $CO_2$ 35, $HCO_3^-$ 22

11. If J. S. continues to have a respiratory alkalosis, his body will try to compensate by increasing
    a. kidney excretion of $HCO_3^-$.
    b. kidney retention of $HCO_3^-$.
    c. respiratory excretion of $CO_2$.
    d. respiratory retention of $CO_2$.

Alan is an 8-year-old boy with a recent history of streptococcal throat infection. He is being followed closely because of the potential for renal involvement after an infection of this type. Questions 12–20 refer to this situation.

12. During Alan's strep throat infection, he likely experienced which of the following systemic effects of inflammation?
    a. pain
    b. fever
    c. swelling
    d. edema

13. Before Alan's body was able to combat the infection with specific antibodies, his nonspecific immunity helped fight the disease. Which is the best description of the nonspecific immune system?
    a. B-lymphocytes
    b. T-lymphocytes
    c. monocyte-macrophages
    d. memory cells

14. Glomerulonephritis following streptococcal infection is a result of
    a. prerenal ischemia.
    b. chronic postrenal urinary obstruction.
    c. bacterial destruction of glomerular vessels.
    d. immune-mediated glomerular basement membrane damage.

15. Signs and symptoms of glomerulonephritis are noted at his clinic visit. These include
    a. pyuria.
    b. mild azotemia.
    c. white cell casts.
    d. foul smelling urine.

16. Alan's physician charts that Alan is in the stage of renal insufficiency. This suggests that Alan
    a. may be unable to concentrate urine normally.
    b. has kidneys with greater than 90% of nephrons destroyed.
    c. is in end-stage renal failure.
    d. should have a high protein diet to replace protein lost in the urine.

17. Over several months, Alan's disease progresses to the uremic syndrome. Signs and symptoms of the uremic syndrome are due to
    a. dysfunction of antidiuretic hormone secretion.
    b. increased permeability of the glomerular basement membrane.
    c. inadequate numbers of functioning nephrons.
    d. increased glomerular filtration rate.

18. Alan's laboratory blood sample shows a hematocrit of 22%. Considering Alan's history, this is most likely related to
    a. insufficient kidney secretion of erythropoietin.
    b. chronic blood loss secondary to hematuria.
    c. vitamin $B_{12}$ deficiency related to lack of intrinsic factor.
    d. vitamin D deficiency.

19. Alan's arterial blood gas analysis demonstrates a compensated metabolic acidosis related to his kidneys' inability to secrete $H^+$. Which ABG is indicative of compensated metabolic acidosis?
    a. pH 7.47, $CO_2$ 60, $HCO_3^-$ 43
    b. pH 7.36, $CO_2$ 33, $HCO_3^-$ 18
    c. pH 7.45, $CO_2$ 30, $HCO_3^-$ 20
    d. pH 7.43, $CO_2$ 28, $HCO_3^-$ 18

20. Appropriate management of Alan's end-stage renal failure would include
    a. potassium supplementation.
    b. low protein diet.
    c. high phosphorus diet.
    d. liberal fluid intake.

P. K. has a history of adrenal insufficiency. She is hospitalized for a hysterectomy. Questions 21–26 refer to P. K.

21. A sign or symptom that would be consistent with P. K.'s diagnosis of adrenal insufficiency is
    a. hypokalemia.
    b. hypoglycemia.
    c. hypertension.
    d. moon face.

22. One effect that the stress of surgery would have on P. K. is
    a. exacerbation of hyperglycemia.
    b. decreased sensitivity to anesthesia.
    c. exacerbation of hypertension.
    d. increased glucocorticoid requirements.

23. P. K. has tests to determine if her adrenal insufficiency is a primary or secondary condition. A response to an injection of ACTH that indicates a primary etiology is
    a. no change in serum glucocorticoid levels.
    b. an increase in serum glucocorticoid levels.
    c. a decrease in serum glucocorticoid levels.
    d. an increase in serum ACTH levels.

24. Another clinical manifestation indicative of a primary etiology of adrenal insufficiency is
    a. low serum ACTH.
    b. high serum cortisol.
    c. hyperpigmentation.
    d. striae.

25. P. K. appears to have an associated deficiency of aldosterone secretion. Which laboratory finding would help to confirm this?
    a. hypernatremia
    b. hyperkalemia
    c. hypokalemia
    d. hypercalcemia

26. After surgery, P. K. is at risk for acute complications related to adrenal insufficiency. Which of the following findings is of greatest concern?
    a. blood pressure of 140/75 mm Hg
    b. heart rate of 135 beats/min
    c. blood glucose of 130 mg %
    d. serum potassium of 3.9 mEq/L

J. J. is a 17-year-old insulin-dependent diabetic. He learned of his diagnosis 3 months ago and has had difficulty complying with his therapeutic regime. Questions 27–33 refer to J. J.

27. Other terms that can be used to describe J. J.'s type of diabetes mellitus include
    a. type II.
    b. gestational.
    c. type I
    d. inherited.

28. J. J. neglected to take his insulin for a few days and was admitted to the hospital in diabetic ketoacidosis. What interventions would be appropriate at the time of admission?
    a. Give simple sugar per mouth or IV.
    b. Provide high protein, low fat diet.
    c. Teach the importance of regular insulin administration.
    d. Fluid and insulin administration.

29. Which of the following would indicate an effort to compensate for his ketoacidosis?
    a. hyperventilation
    b. hypoventilation
    c. excretion of $HCO_3^-$
    d. retention of $NH_3^+$

30. A serum potassium level of 5.9 mEq/L is obtained from J. J. shortly after admission to the hospital. What is the significance of this value?
    a. of little significance because it is within the normal range
    b. elevated in response to ketoacidosis
    c. low because of hyperglycemia-induced diuresis
    d. elevated in response to diabetes-induced kidney failure

31. In what way does serum potassium concentration affect the resting membrane potential (RMP) of nerve and muscle cells?
    a. Hypokalemia moves the RMP closer to the threshold.
    b. Hyperkalemia hyperpolarizes the RMP.
    c. Hyperkalemia depolarizes the RMP.
    d. Hypokalemia depolarizes the RMP.

32. The type of insulin most suitable for the immediate treatment of J. J.'s diabetic ketoacidosis is
    a. regular insulin.
    b. 70/30 NPH/regular.
    c. Lente insulin.
    d. NPH insulin.

33. An hour after J. J. is treated with subcutaneous insulin, he complains of lightheadedness and jitters. These symptoms are most likely associated with
    a. parasympathetic nervous system activation.
    b. dehydration.
    c. hyperglycemia.
    d. a drop in blood glucose level.

M. F. is a 35-year-old male hospitalized after a gastric stapling procedure for weight loss. The procedure reduced his gastric capacity to less than 10% of normal. Questions 34–38 refer to this situation.

34. Upon auscultation of M. F.'s abdomen postoperatively, an absence of bowel tones is noted. The most likely etiology of this sign is
    a. constipation or impaction.
    b. mechanical bowel obstruction related to intussusception.
    c. functional bowel obstruction related to anesthesia and bowel manipulation.
    d. intestinal adhesions.

35. M. F.'s bowel tones return on postop day 3, and he is able to eat solid food but develops nausea and vomiting after meals. Which intervention might help to decrease these symptoms?
    a. lying down for a while after meals
    b. smaller, more frequent meals
    c. increasing fluid intake with meals
    d. antacids prior to mealtime

36. Over 3 days, M. F. has a weight loss of 20 pounds. His serum sodium is 159 mEq/L. Which fluid is most appropriate to correct his fluid imbalance?
    a. normal saline
    b. 10% sodium bicarbonate
    c. blood transfusion
    d. water or 5% dextrose in water

37. M. F. experiences continued loss of gastric juices through frequent episodes of vomiting. The acid–base imbalance this is likely to cause is
    a. metabolic alkalosis.
    b. metabolic acidosis.
    c. respiratory alkalosis.
    d. combined acidosis.

38. Because of his obesity, M. F.'s abdominal wound heals poorly and appears inflamed. He is started on antibiotics and experienced anaphylaxis with moderate hypotension. What is the physiologic basis for this decrease in blood pressure?
    a. Antibiotics interfere with the baroreceptor response.
    b. The sympathetic nervous system is inhibited by inflammation.
    c. The heart is depressed due to circulating blood toxins.
    d. Histamine release leads to widespread vasodilation.

S. S. is a 76-year-old long-term care facility resident who has a history of peripheral vascular disease, two past myocardial infarctions, and severe congestive heart failure. Questions 39–45 refer to S. S.

39. S. S. complains of dyspnea during her morning assessment and has marked rales on auscultation. The most likely etiology of these findings is
    a. right heart failure.
    b. left heart failure.
    c. pneumonia.
    d. atrial septal defect.

40. What compensatory mechanism is S. S. likely to exhibit in relation to her congestive heart failure?
    a. reduced stroke volume
    b. increased blood pressure
    c. bradycardia
    d. cardiac hypertrophy

41. S. S. is treated aggressively with diuretic medications. When she sits up on the edge of the bed, she becomes tachycardic and dizzy. What is the probable physiologic explanation of these symptoms?
    a. Diuretic medications interfere with neuromuscular activity.
    b. These are signs and symptoms of another MI.
    c. The renin-angiotensin-aldosterone system has been activated.
    d. The baroreceptors are reacting to diuretic-induced hypovolemia.

42. S. S. has chronically swollen ankles, which improve somewhat when elevated. Her dependent edema is most likely a result of
    a. atherosclerotic peripheral vascular disease.
    b. right-sided heart failure.
    c. chronic hypertension.
    d. arterial insufficiency.

43. Digoxin, lasix (furosemide), and KCl are prescribed for the treatment of S. S.'s congestive heart failure. Which of the following signs would indicate a possible drug toxicity?
    a. blood pressure of 150/60 mm Hg
    b. heart rate of 128 beats/min
    c. urine output of 60 mL/hr
    d. heart rate of 64 beats/m

44. Within 1 or 2 hours of going to bed at night, S. S. usually needs to get up to urinate, even if she emptied her bladder just prior to retiring. The most likely explanation for this problem is
    a. poor bladder control and fear of incontinence.
    b. excessive evening fluid intake.
    c. poorly timed administration of her diuretics.
    d. mobilization of dependent edema fluid.

45. Inspection of S. S.'s lower extremities reveals shiny, thin, hairless skin and thickened toenails. These manifestations are consistent with
    a. arterial insufficiency
    b. venous insufficiency
    c. congestive heart failure
    d. normal aging changes

W. B. is a 64-year-old man with a long history of emphysematous COPD related to heavy cigarette use. He was recently diagnosed with lung cancer. Questions 46–55 refer to this situation.

46. W. B.'s physician writes a diagnosis of "primary oat cell carcinoma" on his chart. This terminology means that the cancer
    a. originated in the lung and is malignant.
    b. is benign and confined to the lung.
    c. poses no risk of metastasis.
    d. is due to prolonged exposure to oat dust.

47. W. B. asks what caused his lung cancer. Considering the theories of cancer causation, which statement should serve as a basis for a response?
    a. There are no known risk factors for lung carcinoma.
    b. Most lung cancers are caused by genetic factors.
    c. Most lung cancers are associated with cigarette smoke.
    d. Lung cancer is usually due to a virus.

48. Because W. B. has primarily emphysematous COPD, he would be expected to exhibit which of the following signs and symptoms?
    a. dyspnea
    b. cyanosis
    c. polycythemia
    d. major weight gain

49. Most of the signs and symptoms associated with emphysema can be attributed to
    a. decreased residual volume.
    b. decreased total lung capacity.
    c. destruction of alveolar walls and capillaries.
    d. bronchial edema and constriction.

50. An upright chest x-ray of W. B.'s lungs demonstrates a large right pleural effusion. The most likely etiology of this finding is
    a. heart failure.
    b. cancerous destruction of lung tissue.
    c. rupture of emphysematous blebs.
    d. volume overload.

51. A decision is made to aspirate the fluid from W. B.'s right pleural space (thoracentesis). Shortly after the procedure, W. B. complains of severe shortness of breath. A right tension pneumothorax is suspected. What other finding would be consistent with this diagnosis?
    a. tracheal deviation toward the right
    b. absent or diminished lung sounds on the right
    c. increased density (whiteout) on the right per x-ray
    d. decreased density (black) on the left per x-ray

52. Right tension pneumothorax is confirmed by chest x-ray and treated with a chest tube. An arterial blood gas is drawn 15 min after chest tube insertion while W. B. is breathing room air with no oxygen supplementation. Results are pH = 7.53; $PaCO_2$ = 32 mm Hg; $PaO_2$ = 50 mm Hg; $HCO_3^-$ = 26 mEq/L; $SaO_2$ = 88%. Which is the correct interpretation of W. B.'s acid–base balance?
    a. metabolic acidosis
    b. metabolic alkalosis
    c. respiratory acidosis
    d. respiratory alkalosis

53. What effect would a pH of 7.53 have on oxygen binding by hemoglobin in W. B.'s bloodstream?
    a. no effect
    b. increased hemoglobin affinity for oxygen at the lung
    c. increased hemoglobin unloading of oxygen at the tissue
    d. decreased hemoglobin affinity for oxygen at the tissue

54. Considering W. B.'s blood gas values, which statement about oxygen administration is correct?
    a. Oxygen may be effective in reducing hyperventilation and improving $PaO_2$.
    b. Oxygen is contraindicated because of W. B.'s diagnosis of COPD.
    c. Only low level oxygen (<2 L/min) can be given because of the risk of respiratory depression.
    d. Oxygen is unnecessary because ABG values are adequate.

55. When assessing the oxygen-carrying capacity of W. B.'s blood, the most important factor is
    a. arterial pH.
    b. blood volume.
    c. inspired oxygen level ($F_IO_2$)
    d. hemoglobin level.

R. J. is a 49-year-old man who came to the emergency department with complaints of crushing chest pain and shortness of breath. Questions 56–63 refer to this situation.

56. The most reliable indicator that R. J. experienced a myocardial infarction rather than angina is
   a. severe, crushing chest pain.
   b. elevated serum enzymes (MBCK).
   c. lactic acidosis.
   d. extreme anxiety or panic.

57. R. J.'s heart muscle was deprived of blood supply for a time and developed an area of necrosis. This type of necrosis is called
   a. liquefactive.
   b. gangrenous.
   c. coagulative.
   d. caseous.

58. To compensate for left ventricular dysfunction following his myocardial infarction, the filling volume of R. J.'s heart increased due to $Na^+$ and water retention. The best description of this compensatory mechanism (Frank-Starling) is
   a. increased filling volume decreases left ventricular workload.
   b. increased sympathetic activity leads to increased contractility.
   c. cardiac dilation stimulates myocardial hypertrophy.
   d. increased preload increases force of myocardial contraction.

59. R. J.'s physician prescribes a beta-blocking medication (propranolol) for him. The purpose of this medication is to
   a. decrease myocardial oxygen demands.
   b. increase contractility of the heart muscle.
   c. increase aortic resistance to flow.
   d. augment the Frank-Starling mechanism.

60. Despite aggressive therapy after his MI, R. J. progresses to congestive heart failure. Major signs and symptoms of left heart failure include
   a. hepatomegaly.
   b. oliguria.
   c. peripheral edema.
   d. jugular venous distention.

61. R. J. develops dyspnea and begins to cough up frothy pink-tinged secretions. Considering his history, the most likely etiology of these symptoms is
   a. pulmonary embolus.
   b. pneumococcal pneumonia.
   c. ruptured tricuspid valve.
   d. pulmonary edema.

62. R. J.'s physician discontinues his beta-blocking medication and orders a beta agonist. The reason for this change is to
   a. protect the myocardium from ischemia.
   b. reduce myocardial oxygen consumption.
   c. improve cardiac output.
   d. reduce left ventricular afterload.

63. The physician also wants to reduce R. J.'s preload to alleviate his congestive symptoms. An appropriate therapy to achieve this goal is
   a. supine positioning.
   b. alpha agonist administration.
   c. diuretic administration.
   d. oxygen administration.

A. L. is an 87-year-old woman admitted to the hospital for treatment of severe pneumococcal pneumonia. Questions 64–70 refer to this situation.

64. Which of the following symptoms is consistent with A. L.'s diagnosis of bacterial pneumonia rather than viral pneumonia?
   a. fever
   b. malaise
   c. dehydration
   d. productive cough

65. A. L.'s chest x-ray indicates that her pneumonia is confined to the left lower lobe. Which position would be appropriate for A. L. because it would improve her ventilation/perfusion balance?
   a. left lateral (left side down)
   b. right lateral (right side down)
   c. supine (on back)
   d. prone (on stomach)

66. What is the lungs' compensatory response to minimize ventilation/perfusion imbalance when there is an area of lung consolidation?
   a. hyperventilation
   b. hypoxic vasoconstriction
   c. polycythemia
   d. inflammation

67. A. L. is at risk for right ventricular strain because of
    a. pulmonary hypertension due to vasoconstriction.
    b. left ventricular failure due to hypoxemia.
    c. high aortic afterload.
    d. right ventricular hypertrophy.

68. An ABG analysis of A. L.'s blood is done immediately after admission. Results are pH = 7.29; $PaCO_2$ = 60 mm Hg; $HCO_3^-$ = 28 mEq/L. The acid–base disturbance is
    a. uncompensated respiratory alkalosis.
    b. partially compensated metabolic alkalosis.
    c. partially compensated respiratory acidosis.
    d. uncompensated metabolic acidosis.

69. A. L.'s pneumonia is treated with antibiotics and bronchodilators for 5 days. Another ABG is drawn to assess her respiratory status. Results are pH = 7.39; $PaCO_2$ = 42 mm Hg; $HCO_3^-$ = 25 mEq/L. The statement that best reflects her acid–base status is
    a. compensated respiratory acidosis.
    b. corrected acid–base disorder (normal).
    c. compensated respiratory alkalosis.
    d. compensated metabolic acidosis.

70. A. L.'s bronchodilator therapy consists of theophylline and a beta agonist inhaler. A common side effect of these agents is
    a. depression.
    b. hypotension.
    c. platelet dysfunction.
    d. tachycardia.

T. K. is an elderly woman living in a long-term care facility following a cerebral vascular accident (CVA). She has a long history of atherosclerotic vascular disease and hypertension. Questions 71–77 refer to T. K.

71. T. K.'s stroke is a result of platelet aggregation and clot formation in an artery perfusing her right brain hemisphere. This type of stroke is termed
    a. thrombotic.
    b. embolic.
    c. hemorrhagic.
    d. idiopathic.

72. Considering the location of brain injury, which clinical manifestation is T. K. most likely to exhibit?
    a. receptive aphasia
    b. expressive aphasia
    c. right visual field blindness
    d. left-sided weakness and neglect

73. T. K.'s blood pressure continues to be consistently elevated at about 160/100 mm Hg. Which of the following interventions for hypertension would *not* be an appropriate initial therapy?
    a. diuretic therapy
    b. sodium restriction
    c. stress reduction
    d. alpha receptor blockade

74. T. K. is given low dose subcutaneous heparin twice daily to keep her aPTT at 1.5 times control. Heparin therapy is given to
    a. aggregate platelets.
    b. activate fibrinolysis.
    c. prevent clot formation.
    d. dissolve vascular thrombi.

75. Three days after entering the long-term care facility, T. K. experiences seizure activity. Bowel and bladder control are lost, accompanied by jerking, tonic-clonic movements. T. K. has no recall of the event. This type of seizure is called
    a. grand mal.
    b. petit mal.
    c. focal.
    d. complex partial.

76. An indwelling foley catheter is inserted into T. K.'s bladder because of persistent urinary incontinence. Catheterization predisposes T. K. to development of
    a. acute tubular necrosis.
    b. nephrosis.
    c. glomerulonephritis.
    d. pyelonephritis.

77. Routine urinalysis of T. K.'s urine shows the following: specific gravity = 1.010; rare casts; protein = 1+; occasional RBC; glucose = negative; 3+ rods. Based on these results, T. K. probably has
    a. volume depletion.
    b. glomerulonephritis.
    c. a urinary tract infection.
    d. normal urine.

G. B. is a 50-year-old retired businessman. Four years ago he was diagnosed with Parkinson's disease. Questions 78–82 refer to G. B.

78. Parkinson's disease is associated with abnormalities in basal ganglia neurotransmitter levels. The primary alteration is
 a. excessive dopamine.
 b. deficient acetylcholine.
 c. an elevated acetylcholine/dopamine ratio.
 d. an elevated dopamine/acetylcholine ratio.

79. A common manifestation of Parkinson's disease is
 a. intention tremor.
 b. chorea.
 c. akinesia.
 d. ataxia.

80. Therapy for Parkinson's disease includes all the following *except*
 a. anticholinergic agents.
 b. levodopa/carbodopa.
 c. dopamine precursors.
 d. parasympathetic agonists.

81. G. B. experiences orthostatic hypotension as a side effect of his drug therapy for Parkinson's disease. In a supine position, his blood pressure is 120/78 mm Hg and his heart rate is 80 beats/min. Which of the following changes in response to sitting represents orthostatic hypotension?
 a. blood pressure = 116/80, heart rate = 82
 b. blood pressure = 130/80, heart rate = 78
 c. blood pressure = 120/90, heart rate = 80
 d. blood pressure = 118/76, heart rate = 95

82. In the 4 years after his diagnosis, G. B. experiences progressive difficulty voiding. Symptoms include difficulty initiating the urinary stream and incomplete bladder emptying. In addition to a drug side effect, a problem that could account for these symptoms is
 a. urinary tract infection.
 b. hypovolemia.
 c. acute renal failure.
 d. prostatic hyperplasia.

E. B. is a 48-year-old woman admitted to the critical care unit with acute pancreatitis. Questions 83–91 refer to E. B.

83. E. B. complains of extreme abdominal pain upon admission. Another finding helpful in confirming the diagnosis of pancreatitis is elevated
 a. erythrocyte sedimentation rate.
 b. serum amylase.
 c. SGOT, SGPT.
 d. blood glucose.

84. E. B. is immediately counseled to have nothing by mouth (NPO). Her nutritional needs were supplied parenterally. What is the rationale for this therapy?
 a. Parenteral nutrition is a more effective means of supplying nutrients than enteral nutrition.
 b. Enteral feeding stimulates the pancreas, resulting in enzymatic tissue damage.
 c. Enteral feedings will not be absorbed due to lack of pancreatic enzymes.
 d. Parenteral nutrition is less likely to stimulate pancreatic insulin secretion.

85. Within 6 hours of admission, E. B. becomes hypotensive and her urine output decreases to 15 mL/hr. She is started on intravenous fluids at 150 mL/hr. The most likely reason for E. B.'s hypotension and oliguria is
 a. acute renal failure.
 b. immune-mediated peripheral vasodilation.
 c. fluid shifting into the peritoneal cavity.
 d. cardiac failure.

86. E. B. continues to have severe hypotension and low urine output requiring large amounts of intravenous fluids. The most appropriate type of fluid would be
 a. 5% dextrose in water ($D_5W$).
 b. normal saline (0.9 NS).
 c. half normal saline (0.45 NS).
 d. whole blood.

87. Despite aggressive antibiotic therapy for her pancreatitis, E. B. develops peritonitis evidenced by a board-like abdomen, abdominal pain, and fever. Another finding characteristic of peritonitis is
 a. hyperactive bowel tones.
 b. silent abdomen.
 c. severe diarrhea.
 d. bloody stools.

88. Peritonitis may lead to sepsis because
    a. resistance to nosocomial infections is decreased.
    b. antibiotics used for peritonitis lead to superinfection.
    c. bowel flora are able to gain access to the bloodstream.
    d. the immune system is dysfunctional.

89. G. B. is at risk for developing ARDS (adult respiratory distress syndrome) because of peritonitis, sepsis, and large amounts of administered fluids. The best statement describing the pulmonary consequences of ARDS is
    a. noncardiogenic pulmonary edema, atelectasis, and fibrosis.
    b. obstructive hyperinflation with increased residual volume.
    c. calcified, necrotic lesions, and pulmonary fibrosis.
    d. bronchial constriction, mucosal edema, and hypersecretion of mucus.

90. G. B. becomes increasingly dyspneic and is placed on a mechanical ventilator. She receives supplemental oxygen to keep her $PaO_2$ above 60 mm Hg. Another therapy that is most effective in improving blood oxygenation in a patient with ARDS is
    a. hyperventilation.
    b. frequent, vigorous tracheal suctioning.
    c. fluids to liquify secretions.
    d. positive end-expiratory pressure.

91. After a week on the mechanical ventilator, G. B. continues to have sepsis and poor respiratory function. She begins to ooze from her intravenous sites, and bloody secretions are suctioned from her lungs. A coagulopathy is suspected. In view of her history, which coagulopathy is G. B. most likely experiencing?
    a. hemophilia
    b. platelet deficiency
    c. disseminated intravascular coagulation
    d. aplastic thrombocytopenia

A. Y. is a 79-year-old nursing home resident. She has multiple medical problems, including intrinsic asthma, venous insufficiency, and valvular disease. Questions 92–100 refer to this situation.

92. Because of A. Y.'s age, she is experiencing normal physiologic aging changes in her cardiovascular system. Which of the following is a normal aging change?
    a. myocardial infarction
    b. cardiomyopathy
    c. decreased blood vessel elasticity
    d. hypertension

93. An expected finding in A. Y due to normal physiologic changes of aging would be
    a. decreased cardiac reserve.
    b. atrial fibrillation.
    c. low blood pressure.
    d. generalized edema.

94. A. Y. has pitting edema of her ankles and feet as a consequence of venous insufficiency. This type of edema is best described as
    a. protein-rich edema fluid.
    b. transudate.
    c. due to decreased hydrostatic pressure.
    d. exudate.

95. A. Y. receives a beta-blocking drug (propranolol) to control her heart rate. How might this affect her asthma?
    a. Alleviate the asthma by bronchodilation.
    b. Alleviate the asthma by decreasing mucus production.
    c. Worsen the asthma by potentiating bronchoconstriction.
    d. Worsen the asthma by inhibiting phosphodiesterase.

96. When planning A. Y.'s care, it is important to realize that an asthma attack
    a. is often triggered by stress and emotion.
    b. is rarely associated with hypoxemia.
    c. should not be treated with $O_2$ of 2 liters or more.
    d. does not respond to drug therapy.

97. A. Y. has a long history of valvular disease due to age-related calcification. A heart murmur is audible during ventricular systole, which is characteristic of
    a. tricuspid stenosis.
    b. mitral stenosis.
    c. aortic regurgitation.
    d. pulmonic stenosis.

98. A cardiac catheterization procedure demonstrates an elevated left ventricular/aortic pressure gradient during systole (LV = 140 mm Hg; aortic = 90 mm Hg). This finding is consistent with a diagnosis of
    a. aortic stenosis.
    b. aortic regurgitation.
    c. mitral stenosis.
    d. mitral regurgitation.

99. Auscultation of A. Y.'s lungs reveals bilateral crackles (rales) in the bottom third of her lung fields. This finding is indicative of
    a. asthma.
    b. left heart failure.
    c. right heart failure.
    d. venous insufficiency.

100. A. Y. is treated with a diuretic (furosemide) and digitalis to reduce her lung congestion. The laboratory value most important to monitor in patients receiving these two medications is
    a. serum sodium.
    b. hemoglobin.
    c. serum potassium.
    d. serum calcium.

## *Answer Key for Comprehensive Exam*

1. b
2. a
3. a
4. d
5. b
6. c
7. c
8. b
9. d
10. b
11. a
12. b
13. c
14. d
15. b
16. a
17. c
18. a
19. b
20. b
21. b
22. d
23. a
24. c
25. b
26. b
27. c
28. d
29. a
30. b
31. c
32. a
33. d
34. c
35. b
36. d
37. a
38. d
39. b
40. d
41. d
42. b
43. b
44. d
45. a
46. a
47. c
48. a
49. c
50. b
51. b
52. d
53. b
54. a
55. d
56. b
57. c
58. d
59. a
60. b
61. d
62. c
63. c
64. d
65. b
66. b
67. a
68. c
69. b
70. d
71. a
72. d
73. d
74. c
75. a
76. d
77. c
78. c
79. c
80. d
81. d
82. d
83. b
84. b
85. c
86. b
87. b
88. c
89. a
90. d
91. c
92. c
93. a
94. b
95. c
96. a
97. d
98. a
99. b
100. c

# *SECTION FOUR*

## *Lecture Guide*

# REVIEW OF CELL PHYSIOLOGY

I. Plasma Membrane Structure

- A. Lipid bilayer
  1. Amphipathic structure
  2. Types of lipids
  3. Membrane fluidity
- B. Membrane proteins
  1. Fluid mosaic model
  2. Integral, peripheral proteins
  3. Transport
  4. Transduction
  5. Differences in cell types
  6. Tight junctions

II. Organization of Cellular Compartments

- A. The cytoskeleton
  1. Actin filaments
  2. Microtubules
  3. Intermediate filaments
- B. Nucleus
  1. DNA
  2. Nuclear envelope
  3. Functions

C. Endoplasmic reticulum (ER)

1. Synthesis of proteins and lipids

2. Rough

3. Smooth

D. Golgi apparatus

1. Cis face

2. Medial compartment

3. Trans face

E. Lysosomes and peroxisomes

1. Lysosomes

hydrolytic

phagocytic, autophagy, endocytic

lysosomal storage diseases: I-cell disease

2. Peroxisomes

oxidative

$H_2O_2$

F. Mitochondria

1. Structure

2. Matrix enzymes

3. Respiratory chain

III. Cellular Energy Metabolism

A. Biological order and energy

1. Cells obey laws of physics and chemistry

cells use energy from environment and release as heat

heat generating reactions are linked with cellular processes

first law of thermodynamics: energy cannot be created or destroyed

2. Cells use energy from oxidation of organic molecules (CH)

oxidation - removal of energy-rich electrons

energy used for cellular work

energy released from oxidation is coupled to ATP formation

ATP hydrolysis is used to drive energetically unfavorable reactions

B. Glycolysis

1. Glucose $\rightarrow$ glucose-6-P

2. Nine enzymatic steps to produce 2 pyruvate (3-carbons) uses 2 ATP, produces 4 ATP

3. No oxygen required

C. Citric acid cycle (TCA, Kreb's)

1. Pyruvate enters mitochondria

2. End products: $CO_2$ and energetic electrons. Electrons are transferred to carrier molecules.

D. Oxidative phosphorylation

1. Electrons transferred from carriers to the electron transport chain

2. Energy used to pump $H^+$ across mitochondrial membrane

3. $H^+$ gradient used to power the formation of ATP

IV. Cellular Membrane Functions

A. Membrane transport of small molecules

1. Passive transport

water

nonpolar

polar and charged

2. Active transport

against E-C gradient

3. Carriers and channel proteins

4. Common transporters

$Na^+/K^+$

Calcium

Na gradient dependent

5. Membrane channels "ion channels"

voltage gated

mechanically gated

ligand gated

leak channels

B. Membrane transport of macromolecules

1. Endocytosis

pinocytosis

phagocytosis

2. Receptor-mediated endocytosis

   example: cholesterol uptake

3. Exocytosis

C. Cellular membrane potentials

1. Principles of electrochemical gradients

   concentration gradient

   electrical gradient

   electrochemical potential

2. Nernst equation

   equilibrium potential

   can use to determine resting potential or if ion is at equilibrium

3. Resting membrane potential is a $K^+$ equilibrium potential

   a. two opposing forces on the $K^+$ ion

      (1) concentration favors flow out of cell

      (2) electrical potential favors influx

   b. at equilibrium, forces offset each other

      as $K^+$ moves out of the cell, it causes negative ions to collect on the inside of the membrane, setting up the negative resting potential

4. Effects of changes in serum $K^+$

   hyperkalemia $\rightarrow$ depolarization

   hypokalemia $\rightarrow$ hyperpolarization

6. Action potential

   threshold

ion channels

fast $Na^+$

$K^+$

$Ca^{2+}$

V. Intercellular Communication

A. Cell signaling strategies

1. Gap junctions

2. Direct cell-to-cell contact

3. Secretion of chemical mediators (ligands)

synaptic

paracrine

endocrine

autocrine

B. Receptor mechanisms

1. Cell-surface receptors

channel-linked

catalytic protein kinases

G-protein linked

2. Second messengers

cyclic AMP

$Ca^{2+}$

inositol triphosphate

3. Intracellular receptors

C. Regulation of cell growth

1. Growth factors

2. Spatial signals

3. Cell cycle

VI. Genetics

A. Molecular genetics

1. DNA structure

base pairs

sugar phosphate backbone

double helix

2. DNA replication

DNA polymerase

3. Genetic code

codons

anticodons

4. Transcription

RNA polymerases

5. Translation

B. Regulation of gene expression

1. Transcriptional controls

gene regulatory proteins

C. Tissue differentiation

1. Epithelial
2. Connective
3. Muscle
4. Nerve

D. Principles of inheritance

1. Genes and chromosomes
2. Genotype/phenotype
3. Dominant/recessive
4. Single gene/polygenic

# ALTERATIONS IN CELL FUNCTION AND GROWTH

I. Most Disease Processes Result in Changes at the Cellular Level

A. Cellular injury/death

1. Oxygen deficiency

2. Physical trauma

3. Infection

4. Chemicals

5. Radiation

6. Nutrition

B. Cellular responses to injury

1. Cell adaptation

atrophy
hypertrophy
hyperplasia
metaplasia
dysplasia

2. Reversible injury

cellular swelling
fatty changes
intracellular accumulations (e.g., bilirubin)

3. Irreversible: cell death/necrosis

permanent loss of function

foci of infection

inflammatory response

cell contents and enzymes released

C. Cellular basis of aging

1. Theories

2. Physiologic changes

## ALTERATIONS OF AGING

| System | Physiologic Changes | Assessment Findings |
|---|---|---|
| Cardiovascular | ↓Vessel elasticity due to calcification and connective tissue (↑PVR) | High blood pressure |
| | ↓No. of heart muscle fibers with ↑size of individual fibers (hypertrophy)<br>↓filling capacity<br>↓stroke volume | ↓Cardiac output and cardiac reserve |
| | ↓Sensitivity of baroreceptors | Slow response to position change (orthostatic hypotension) |
| | Degeneration of vein valves | Varicose veins |
| Respiratory | ↓Chest wall compliance due to calcification of costal cartilage | ↓$PaO_2$ (normal pH, $PaCO_2$) |
| | ↓alveolar ventilation | ↑Respiratory rate |
| | ↓Respiratory muscle strength | Shallow breathing and ↓reserve |
| | Air trapping and ↓ventilation due to degeneration of lung tissue (↓elasticity) | ↑FRC and ↓FEV1 |
| Renal/Urinary | ↓GFR due to nephron degeneration (↓1/3 to 1/2 by age 70) | Unable to excrete acute volume load |
| | ↓Ability to concentrate urine | Nocturia |
| | ↓Ability to regulate $H^+$ | Prone to acidemia |
| Gastrointestinal | Muscular contraction<br>↓esophageal emptying<br>↓bowel motility | Constipation |
| | ↓Production of HCl, enzymes and intrinsic factor | Vitamin $B_{12}$ deficiency |
| | ↓Hepatic enzyme production and metabolic capacity | Slowed drug metabolism |
| | Thinning of stomach mucosa | |
| Neuro Sensory | Nerve cells degenerate and atrophy<br>↓of 25–45% of neurons<br>↓neurotransmitters | Difficulty with recall, retrieval, memory, depression |
| | ↓rate of conduction of nerve impulses | Disturbed motility |
| | Loss of taste buds | ↓Sweet and salt taste |
| | Loss of auditory hair cells and sclerosis of ear drum | Presbycusis |
| Musculoskeletal | ↓Muscle mass | ↓Weight |
| | Bone demineralization | ↓Height, kyphosis |
| | Joint degeneration, erosion, and calcification | Osteoarthritis |
| Immune | ↓Inflammatory response | ↓Temperature with infection |
| | ↓T-cell function due to involution of thymus gland | Prone to infection |
| Integumentary | ↓Subcutaneous fat | ↓Skin turgor |
| | ↓Elastin | ↑Wrinkles |
| | Atrophy of sweat glands | Dryness |
| | Atrophy of epidermal arterioles causing altered temperature regulation | Cold |

II. Genetic and Congenital Disorders

Congenital defect: abnormal development diagnosed prior to or shortly after birth

Causes: 1. hereditary

2. environmental (teratogens)

Hereditary (single gene, polygenic, chromosomal)

A. Single gene

1. Autosomal dominant (Marfan's, Huntington's)

2. Autosomal recessive (PKU, albinism)

3. Sex-linked (hemophilia)

B. Polygenic—two or more genes interact to produce trait: e.g., allergy, cleft lip, diabetes, hypertension

C. Chromosomal—defect in chromosome number or structure due to a problem during meiosis

1. Monosomy: only one chromosome instead of normal pair

Turner's syndrome

2. Polysomy: more than two chromosomes to a set

Trisomy 21 (Down syndrome)

Polysomy 47 (Kleinfelter's)

D. Teratogenic agents

1. Vulnerable periods

2. Irradiation

3. Drugs: thalidomide

alcohol

4. Infections: toxoplasmosis, rubella, CMV, herpes (TORCH)

III. Alterations in Cell Differentiation: Neoplasia

Cancer is second leading cause of death in U.S., one in four will get cancer

A. Carcinogenesis: What causes cancer?

Heredity and environment both involved, no single cause

1. Majority of cancer is associated with environmental carcinogens (80–85%)

2. Rare hereditary cancers

3. Cancer "runs in families"

B. Cellular defects in cancer

1. Uncontrolled growth

2. Poorly differentiated growth

C. Theories of cancer causation

1. Genetic basis

a. oncogenes (proto-oncogenes)

b. antioncogenes

c. cellular alterations

growth factors

receptors

second messengers

DNA

2. Multistep nature

a. initiation

b. promotion

c. progression

D. Role of immune system in cancer surveillance.

1. Mutant cells are constantly formed, but destroyed by immune cells. Immune system can distinguish between cancerous and normal cells.

2. People with depressed immune systems have much higher incidence of cancer.

3. Current research is assessing the use of normal immune products to treat patients with cancer (interleukin II, interferon, etc.).

E. Benign vs. malignant tumors

| | **Benign** | **Malignant** |
|---|---|---|
| Character | not called "cancer"<br>slowly growing<br>well-defined border<br>strictly local | termed cancerous<br>rapidly growing<br>invades surrounding tissue<br>can spread (metastasis) |
| Problems | space occupying<br>site of necrosis/ infection<br>compress vessels | same as benign plus<br>destroys local tissue<br>compete for nutrients |
| Treatment | surgical removal | surgical removal plus radiation/chemotherapy |
| Terminology | ends in "oma" | ends in "carcinoma" (epithelial) or "sarcoma" (connective) |
| | adenoma: gland<br>lipoma: fat<br>osteoma: bone | adenocarcinoma<br>liposarcorna<br>osteosarcoma |

EXCEPTION: Lymphoma and leukemia are not benign.

F. Why does cancer kill?

1. Loss of function

2. Hemorrhage

3. Necrosis

4. Obstruction

5. Nutrient trapping

6. Produce toxins and enzymes

7. Untreated cancer will eventually kill the host.

G. Cancer therapy

1. Surgery

2. Radiation

3. Chemotherapy

4. Immunotherapy

# ALTERATIONS IN DEFENSE

I. The Stress Response

A. General adaptation syndrome

B. Neuro-endocrine-immune response

C. Stressors

D. Coping strategies and adaptation

II. Immunology

A. Immune cell differentiation

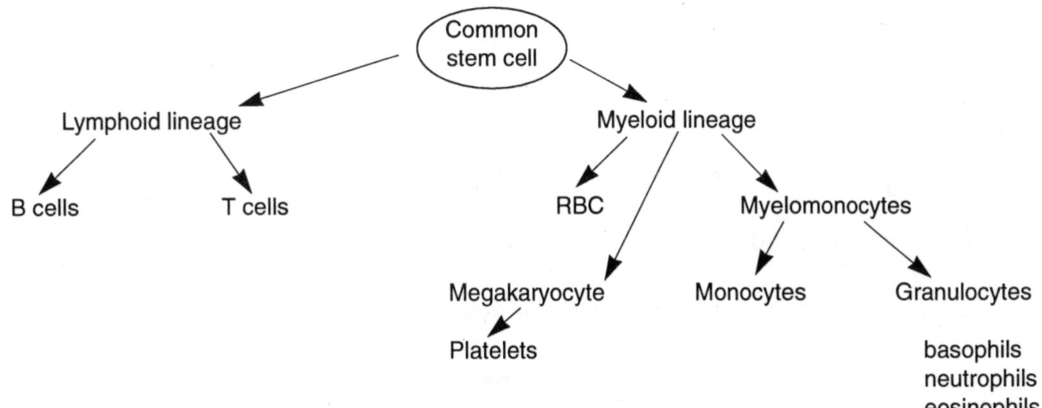


B. Nonspecific response cells

1. Monocyte/macrophage

large, phagocytic, sentinal

2. Neutrophils

90% of circulating granulocytes, phagocytic, early responder

3. Eosinophils (2-5%)

degranulate → degrade inflammatory mediators → inhibit inflammation

4. Basophils and mast cells (<0.2%)

degranulation releases inflammatory mediators (histamine, PGE, enzymes)

bind IgE to surface receptors

C. Specific response cells

1. T cells

$CD_4^+$—helper T cells

$CD_8^+$—cytotoxic T cells

$CD_8^+$—suppressor T cells

natural killer cells

2. B cells

plasma cells secrete antibodies

D. Nonspecific immunity: inflammation

1. Monocyte—macrophage system

widespread locations

initiate immune response

2. Inflammatory process

a. localization

vasodilation

↑capillary permeability

clotting

migration

macrophages release chemotactic signals

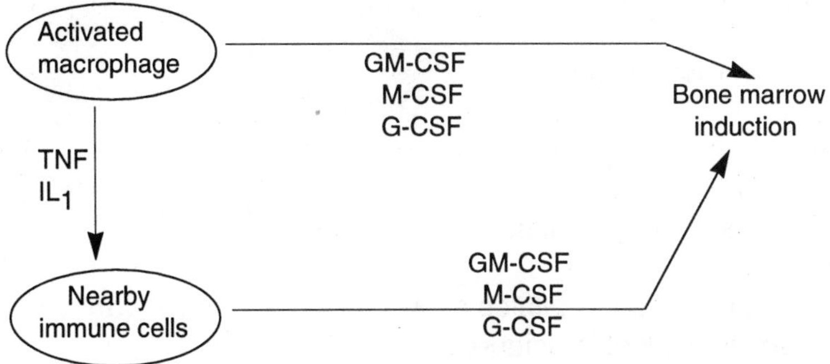


b. Recognition

cell surface abnormalities

foreign structures

c. Phagocytosis

enzymatic digestion by macrophages, neutrophils

3. Complement activation:

a. inactive proteins (proenzymes)circulate in bloodstream

b. activation results in cascade effect

classic pathway: Ag-Ab complex

alternate pathway: no Ab required

c. mechanism of action

$C_{3b}$ + $C_{5b}$—inflammation

$C_{5b6789}$—membrane attack complex

(MAC) → ↑ cell permeability → cell lysis

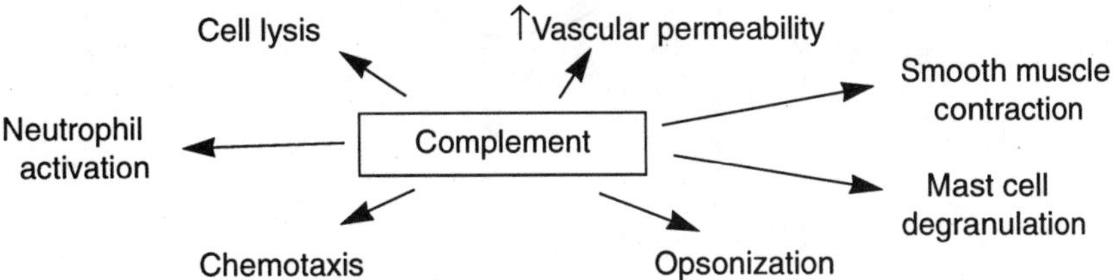

4. Cardinal S & S of inflammation

E. Basis of self vs. foreign recognition

1. MHC genes

a. MHC genes code for cell surface markers

b. Large number of MHC alleles allows for huge genetic variability. Each individual is unique.

c. MHC class I glycoproteins are present on all nucleated cells

d. MHC class II glycoproteins are present on certain immune cells (macrophages, monocytes)

2. Immune tolerance theory

a. clonal deletion/anergy

b. T suppressor cells

c. antiidiotype suppression

F. Cell-mediated immunity

1. T lymphocyte development

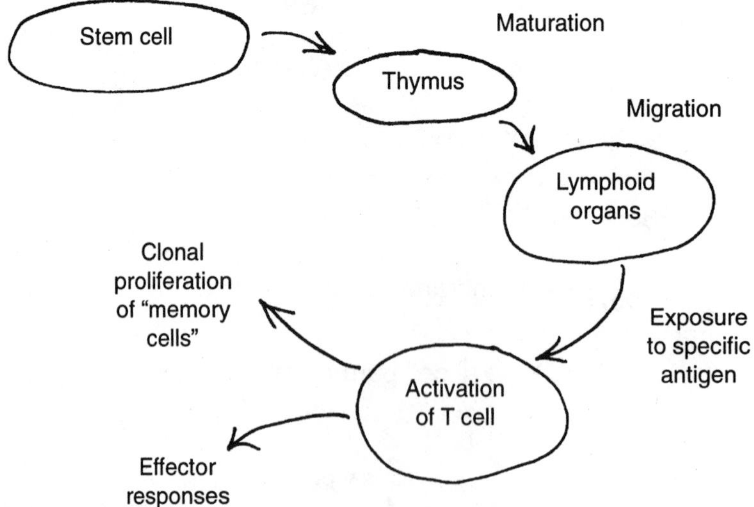

2. Helper T cells bind to antigen presented by B cells and macrophages

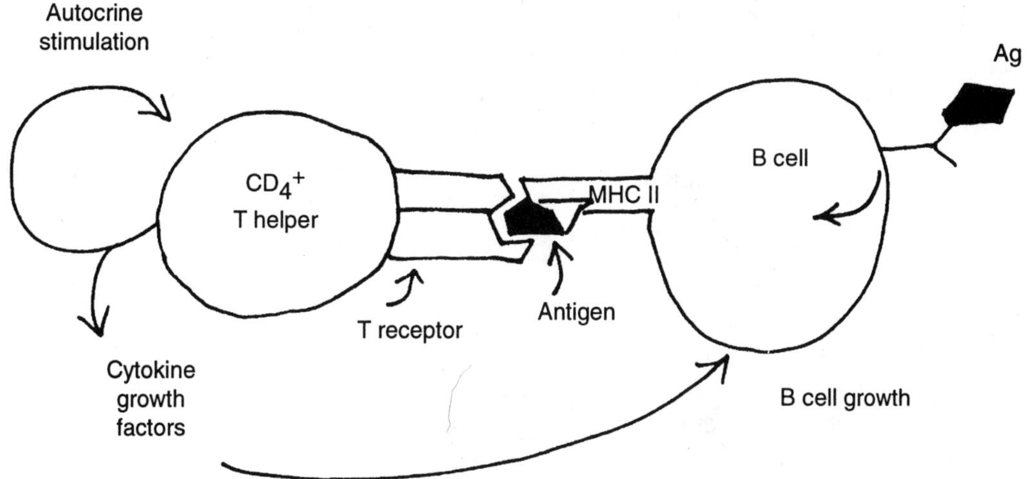


3. Cytotoxic T cells bind to antigen associated with MHC I

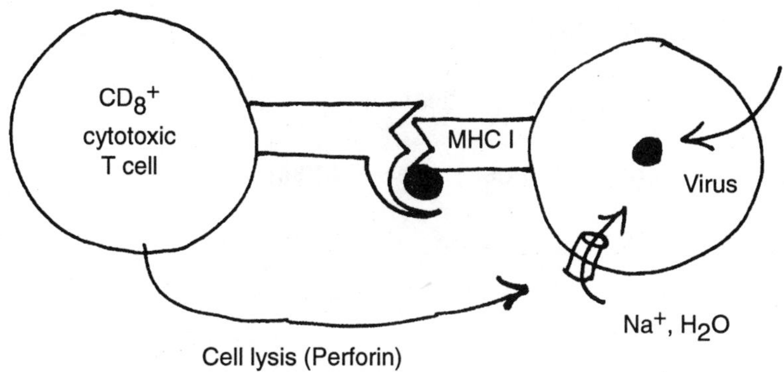


G. Antibody-mediated immunity

1. B lymphocyte development

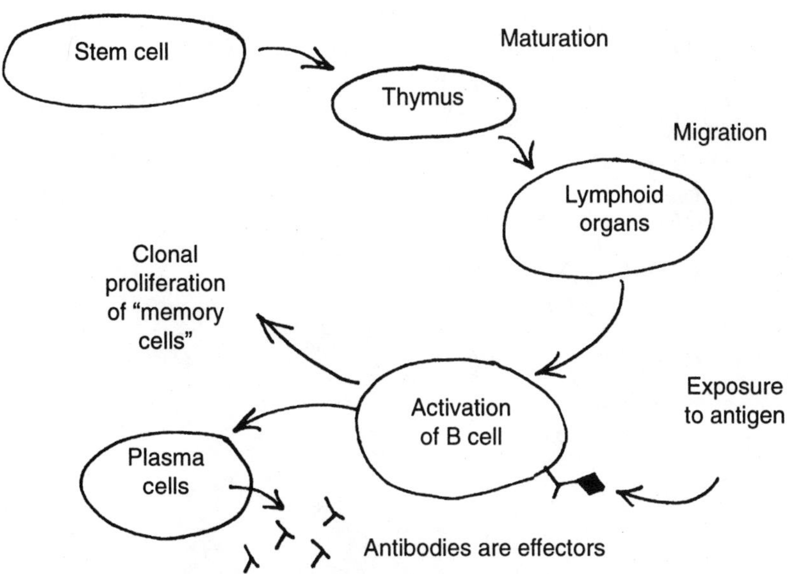

2. Antibody class

IgG, IgD, IgE

IgM pentamer

IgA dimer

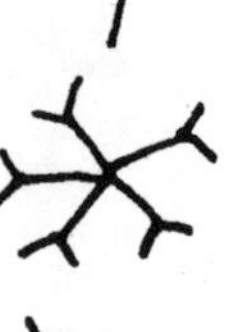

3. Antibody functions

a. agglutination

b. precipitation

c. neutralization

d. lysis

e. opsonization

f. complement activation

H. Cytokines: chemical messengers of the immune system

1. Stimulators of hematopoiesis

$IL_3$

$IL_7$

GM-CSF, G-CSF, M-CSF

2. Mediators of inflammation

TNF

$IL_1$

$IL_6$

$IL_8$

interferon

3. Lymphocyte growth factors

$IL_1$

$IL_2$

$IL_4$

$IL_5$

$IL_6$

I. Role of memory cells in active immunity

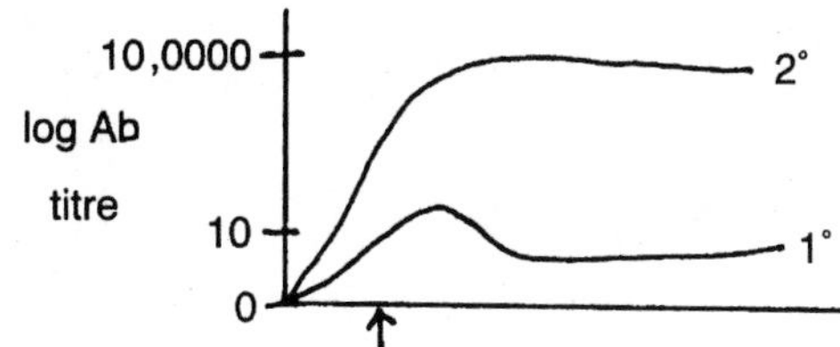


J. Active vs. passive immunity

III. Dysfunction of the Immune System: Over and Under Reactions

A. Hypersensitivity reactions: etiology usually unknown

1. B-cell reactions

a. anaphylactic "allergic" histamine release

b. cytotoxic: antibodies fix to cell and lyse it

transfusion reaction

erythroblastosis fetalis

c. immune-complex reaction: antigen and antibody

stick together, may lodge in small capillaries

glomerulonephritis

lupus

2. T-cell reactions “delayed hypersensitivity”

skin or tissue is recognized as foreign and attacked

contact dermatitis

TB test

transplant rejection

3. Treatment for hypersensitivity

drugs: antihistamines

steroids

epinephrine

desensitization therapy

B. Immunodeficiency disorders

1. Congenital agammaglobulinemia

2. Acquired immune deficiency

a. Chemotherapy

b. AIDS

Etiology: Human immunodeficiency virus (HIV)

Transmission: AIDS virus has been found in body fluids including blood, semen, tears, urine, saliva, sputum. Known to be transmitted through contact with blood and semen. Other routes not yet shown. Not transmitted by casual contact.

High risk groups: IV drug abusers and people sexually active with many partners

Pathology: HIV attacks lymphocytes. Causes a decrease especially in T-helper cells. Unable to fight off invading organisms.

Not all infected individuals develop immune deficiency (AIDS). It is not known if they will eventually develop AIDS.

Prognosis: Rarely survive more than 2 years after AIDS diagnosis. Death due to opportunistic infections, not the HIV itself.

(i) *Pneumocystis carinii* pneumonia

(ii) Kaposi's sarcoma

(iii) others: herpes, CMV, candida

Treatment: No effective treatment for HIV. Treatment focuses on the opportunistic infections. (AZT?)

C. Autoimmune disorders: failure of immune system to recognize self

1. Theories of autoimmunity

a. sequestered tissue

b. decreased T-suppressor activity

c. altered self

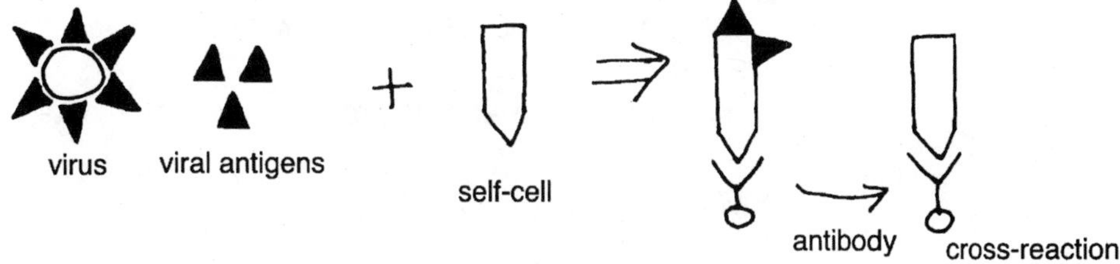


2. Genetic predisposition and viral stimulus

3. Examples: rheumatoid arthritis, lupus, multiple sclerosis, myasthenia gravis, scleroderma, idiopathic thrombocytopenia

4. Therapy: chemo

steroids

plasmapheresis

D. Lymphoproliferative disorders: excessive, abnormal growth of a type of WBC

1. Infectious mononucleosis: Epstein-Barr virus (EBV)

EBV attacks B lymphocytes. Infected B cells are recognized as foreign by T killer cells. Have large number of T killer cells.

Care: symptomatic

2. Leukemias: malignant proliferation of a type of WBC; usually involves lymphocytes or granulocytes

<u>Types:</u> acute lymphocytic (ALL)

acute nonlymphocytic (ANLL)

chronic lymphocytic (CLL)

chronic nonlymphocytic (CNLL)

acute: children, rapid progression

chronic: adults, gradual onset

<u>Etiology:</u> unknown (radiation?, viral)

<u>Pathology</u>: WBC proliferate

WBCs are immature, low immune competence

WBCs crowd out other marrow cells

WBCs infiltrate and destroy tissues (brain, kidney)

<u>Signs/Symptoms:</u>

infection

anemia

hemorrhage/thrombocytopenia

pain

increased WBC "shift to left" (15–500 K)

organ dysfunction

Treatment:

protective isolation

activity restriction

transfusion

chemotherapy

Prognosis with treatment:

ANLL 1 1/2 yr

CNNL 3 yr

ALL 50% 5 yr

CLL 10 yr

3. Multiple myeloma: malignant proliferation of activated B cells (plasma cells) invade bone tissue

   Etiology: unknown

   Pathology: excessive plasma cells invade bone tissue and destroy.

   Signs/Symptoms: similar to leukemia plus bone destruction, pathologic fractures, spinal compression

   Treatment: symptomatic, chemo?

   Prognosis: poor, 1 1/2 to 2 yr

4. Malignant lymphoma: cancerous proliferation of cells in the lymph node tissue

   Hodgkin's if certain cell type is cancerous (Reed-Sternberg)

   Non-Hodgkin's if other lymph node cells are involved

   Hodgkin's:

   Etiology: unknown

<u>Pathology:</u> cell in lymph node proliferates. Nodes are swollen, necrotic, fibrotic. The spread of Hodgkins disease is usually predictable and contiguous.

<u>Treatment:</u> surgery, chemo

<u>Prognosis:</u> stage I or II, 95% cure
later stages 70% cure

IV. Wound Healing

A. Primary intention

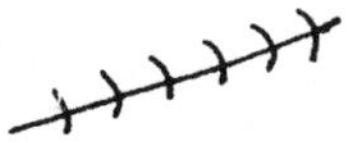

B. Secondary intention

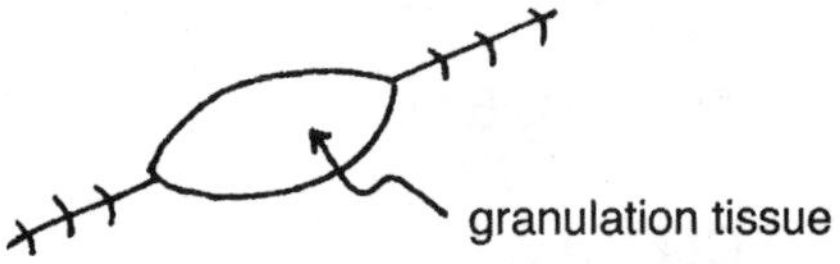

granulation tissue

C. Factors affecting healing

1. Obesity
2. Nutrition
3. Circulation
4. Diabetes

# ALTERATIONS IN TISSUE PERFUSION AND OXYGENATION: THE BLOOD

I. Red Blood Cell Production

A. Production of normal RBCs (erythrocytes) depends on:

1. Adequate iron for hemoglobin

2. Erythropoietin

3. Functional bone marrow stem cells

B. Red cell production must equal red cell destruction. If it doesn't:

1. Anemia

2. Polycythemia

C. Diagnostic lab tests for RBC abnormalities

1. Hematocrit

2. RBC count

3. Hemoglobin

4. Red cell indices

a. MCV (mean corpuscular volume)

normocytic

microcytic

macrocytic

b. MCHC (mean corpuscular hemoglobin concentration)

normochromic

hypochromic

II. The Anemias

A. Decreased Hgb, Hct, and RBC count

B. Signs and symptoms due to decreased oxygen-carrying capacity

1. Restlessness/confusion/fatigue

2. Increased respiratory rate/dyspnea

3. Increased heart rate/palpitations/angina

C. Causes of anemia (see following table)

1. Blood loss

2. Impaired production

3. Increased destruction

III. The Polycythemias

A. Elevated Hbg, Hct, and RBC count

B. Signs and symptoms due to increased blood viscosity

1. May be none

2. Thrombosis

C. Causes of polycythemia (see following table)

1. Idiopathic—polycythemia vera

2. Hypoxia—secondary polycythemia

3. Dehydration—relative polycythemia

**Anemia: $\downarrow$ Hbg $\downarrow$ Hct $\downarrow$ RBC**

(Signs and Symptoms of Hypoxemia: Fatigue, Dyspnea, Pallor, $\uparrow$ HR, Palpitations, Angina)

| Type | Causes | Lab | Signs & Symptoms | Treatment |
|---|---|---|---|---|
| LOSS/DESTRUCTION<br>Blood Loss | | | | |
| Acute | Trauma/surgery | Normochromic<br>Normocytic | Volume depletion<br>$\downarrow$ bp $\uparrow$ hr $\rightarrow$ shock | Hemostasis<br>$O_2$<br>Transfusion |
| Chronic | GI bleed (ulcer)<br>Menstruation | Microcytic<br>Hypochromic | S/S hypoxemia | Treat cause<br>Iron therapy |
| Hemolytic (inherited)*<br>Spherocytosis<br>Sickle cell<br>Thalassemia<br>$G_6$PD deficiency | Inherited | Variable | S/S hypoxemia<br>Jaundice<br>Splenomegaly<br>Hepatomegaly<br>Organ damage:<br>esp. kidney due<br>to vascular obstruction<br>from RBC debris | Eliminate cause<br>$\uparrow$ fluids<br>Steroids<br>Splenectomy<br>$O_2$ |
| Hemolytic (acquired) | Drugs, infection,<br>transfusion re-<br>action, erythro-<br>blastosis fetalis | + Coombs'<br>Usually normocytic,<br>normochromic,<br>often $\uparrow$ bilirubin | | |
| IMPAIRED PRODUCTION<br>Aplastic | Ideopathic<br>Radiation<br>Chemotherapy | Normocytic<br>Normochromic | Due to $\downarrow$ bone marrow<br>Infections<br>Bleeding<br>S/S hypoxemia | Stop drugs<br>Transfusions<br>Bone marrow<br>transplant |
| Nutritional<br>Iron deficiency | $\downarrow$ intake, absorption<br>Chronic blood loss | Microcytic<br>Hypochromic | S/S hypoxemia | iron—diet,<br>supplement,<br>parenteral iron |

<u>Nutritional</u> *(continued)*

| Type | Causes | Lab | Signs & Symptoms | Treatment |
|---|---|---|---|---|
| Vitamin $B_{12}$ deficiency | ↓ intake<br>↓ intrinsic factor<br>↑ ETOH use | Macrocytic<br>Normochromic | S/S hypoxemia<br>Neurologic symptoms: paresthesias | ↑ Vitamin $B_{12}$ in diet<br>Parenteral $B_{12}$ |
| Folic acid deficiency | ↓ intake<br>↑ ETOH use | Macrocytic<br>Normochromic | S/S hypoxemia<br>0 neuro symptoms | ↑ intake: diet, supplements |
| | | POLYCYTHEMIA: ↑ Hct ↑ Hbg ↑ RBC | | |
| Vera | Ideopathic | Normocytic<br>Normochromic | ↑ blood viscocity<br>↓ | Phlebotomy |
| Secondary | Hypoxia | | ↑ risk thrombosis | Correct hypoxia |
| Relative | Dehydration | | | Hydration |

***Specific examples of inherited hemolytic anemias:**

1. Sickle cell anemia: autosomal recessive. Have abnormal hemoglobin that polymerizes easily at low oxygen tension and with hemoconcentration. Must avoid hypoxemia and dehydration.
2. G6PD deficiency: sex linked recessive. Have a defect of a metabolic pathway for glucose that results in increased susceptibility to oxidant injury. Must avoid foods/drugs that are oxidative.
3. Thalassemias: absent or diminished synthesis of one of the hemoglobin A chains. May have compensatory increase in synthesis of other chain types, HbF, $HbA_2$. Main therapy is transfusion.
4. Spherocytosis: autosomal dominant. Have defective cell membrane with inefficient Na/K pumping. Na accumulates in the cell resulting in cell swelling. Cells become round and inflexible and are trapped and hemolyze within the spleen. Treated by splenectomy.

IV. Disorders of Coagulation

A. Normal hemostasis involves several steps

1. Vessel spasm
2. Platelet plug
3. Activation of clotting cascade
4. Clot retraction
5. Clot dissolution (fibrinolysis)

B. Blood clotting cascade

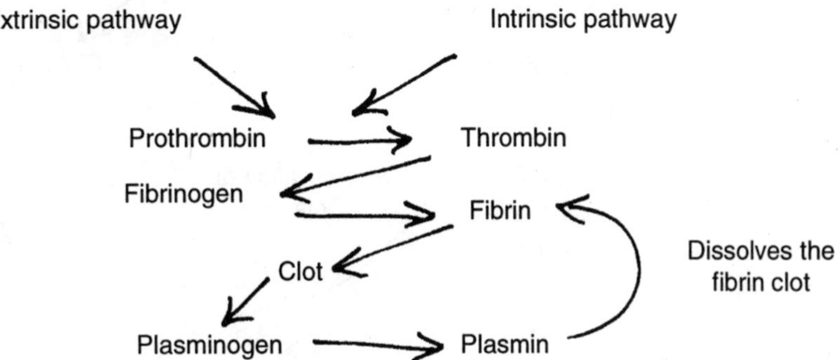


C. Tests to evaluate clotting function

1. Platelet count
2. Bleeding time
3. PT
4. aPTT
5. FDP

C. Clotting abnormalities

1. Thrombocytopenia: normally 150–400K/mm$^3$
   <50K → bleeding tendencies

   a. aplastic anemia
   b. idiopathic
   c. chemotherapy

2. Hemophilia—hereditary defect

   a. factor VIII or IX deficiency

3. DIC (disseminated intravascular coagulation): There is diffuse, inappropriate clotting, which leads to clotting factor consumption and results in bleeding

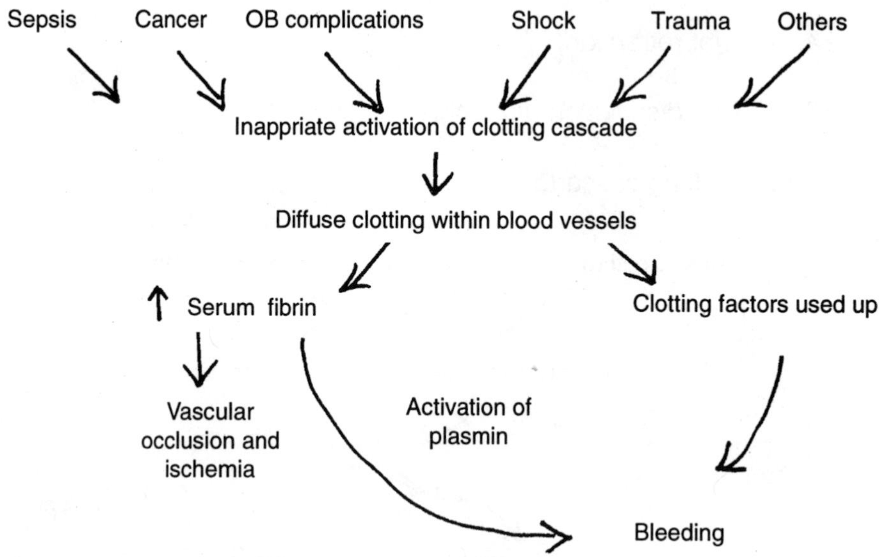


Treatment: heparin

# CARDIOVASCULAR PHYSIOLOGY

## A. CARDIAC ELECTROPHYSIOLOGY

### I. Cardiac Membrane Potentials

A. Phase 0

B. Phase 1

C. Phase 2

D. Phase 3

E. Phase 4

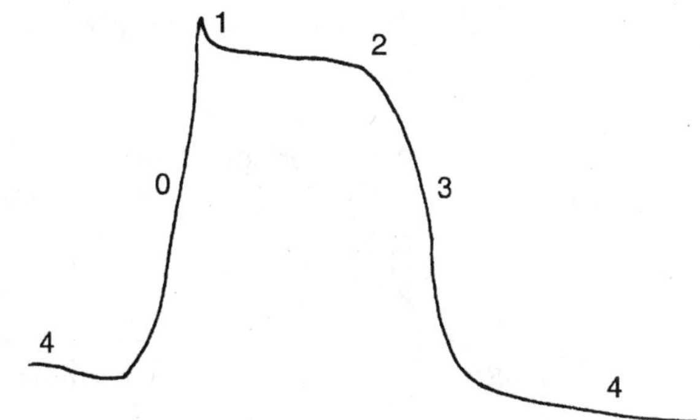


Refractoriness: absolute, relative

### II. Automaticity: Spontaneous Depolarization

A. Leak channels → spontaneous phase 4 depolarization

B. Slow $Ca_2^+$ channels → action potential

C. $K^+$ efflux via voltage gated → repolarization

D. Autonomic influences

SNS: ↑ rate of spontaneous depolarization

↑ $Na^+/Ca^{2+}$ conductance (& $K^+$)

PSNS: ↓ rate

↑ $K^+$ conductance (hyperpolarizing)

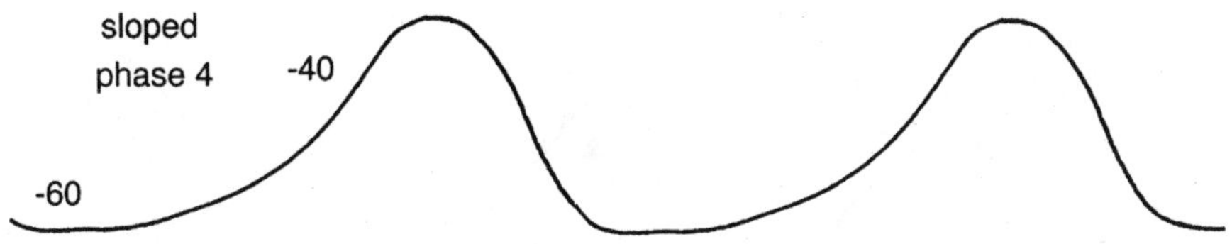

## III. Conduction Pathways

Atrial SA → Atria
Bachmann's Bundle

Internodal pathways (3)

AV Node

Regions
A-N (principal delay)
N (area of ANS influence)
N-H

His - Purkinje System — R & L Bundles branch into network of Purkinje fibers

Ventricular Muscle Cells
1. Septum L → R
2. Apex endo → epi
3. Base of heart

## IV. Normal ECG

Q =

R =

S =

T =

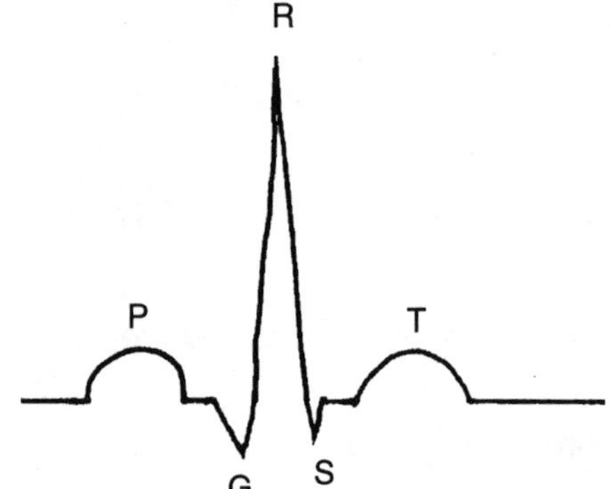


## V. Re-Entry

A, Unidirectional block

1. Prolonged conduction time/distance

2. Altered refractory time

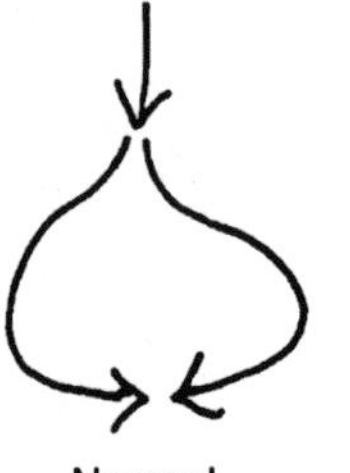

Normal

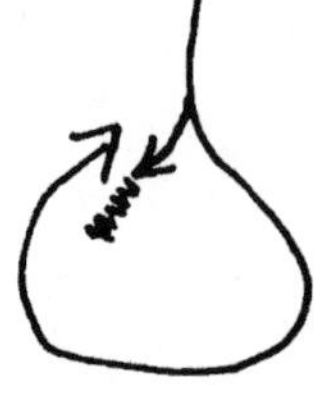

Unidirectional block

## B. AUTONOMIC NERVOUS SYSTEM CONTROL OF CV FUNCTION

I. Effector Organs

  A. Smooth muscle

  B. Cardiac muscle

  C. Glands

  D. Enteric nervous system

II. Differences Between Two Branches

  A. Location of preganglionic cell bodies

  B. Preganglionic NT

  C. Location of postganglionic cell bodies

  D. Postganglionic NT

III. Architecture of SNS

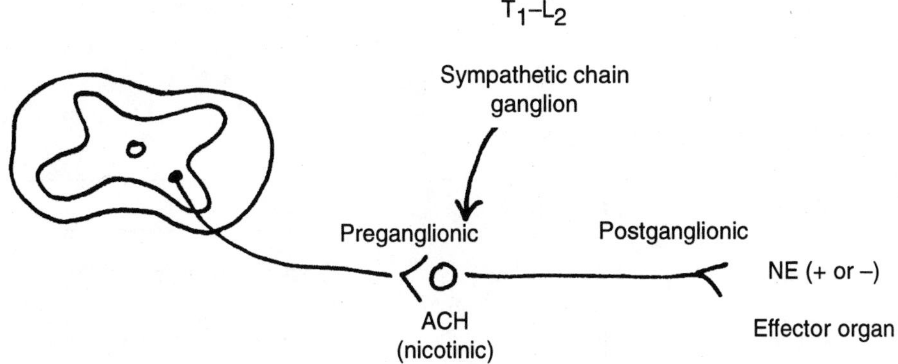


IV. Architecture of PSNS: CN III, V, VII, IX, X ($S_{2-4}$)

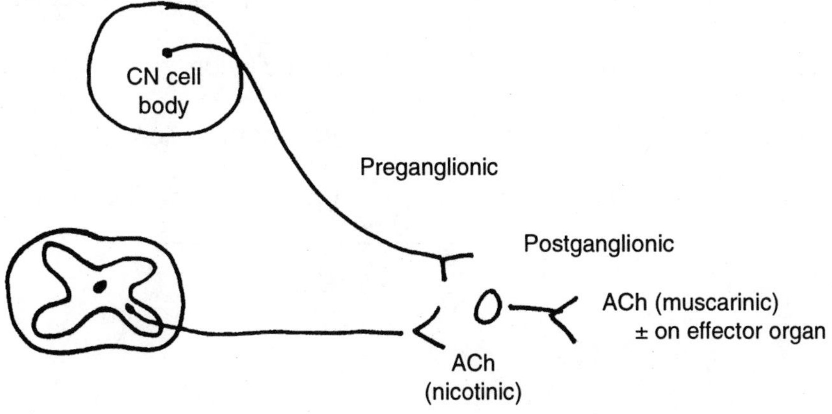

# V. Receptors and Pharmacology

## A. Neurotransmitters and receptors

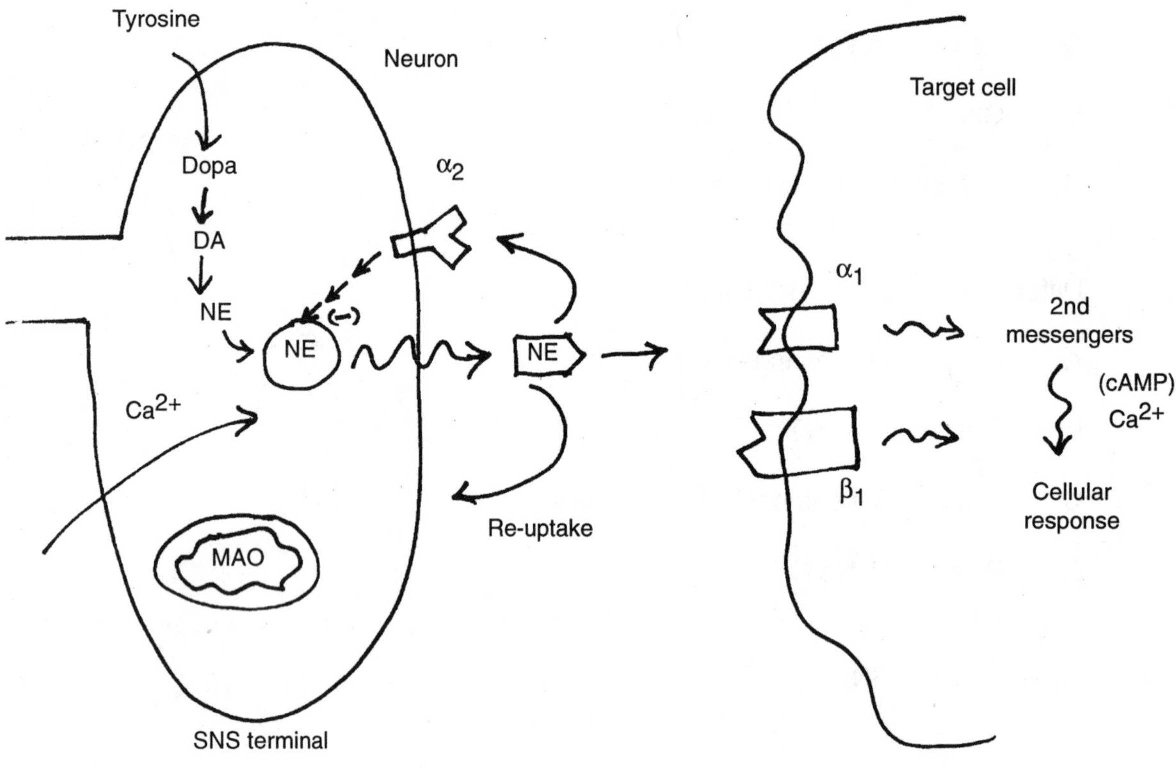


| NT | Site | Receptor | Effect |
|---|---|---|---|
| NE | Heart | $\beta_1$ | ↑ rate, ↑ contractility |
| | Bronchi | $\beta_2$ | Bronchodilitation |
| | Arterioles | $\alpha_1$ | Vasoconstrict |
| | SNS ending | α2 | ↓ release of NE ⟶ ↓effect |
| Epi | Arterioles | $\beta_2$ | Vasodilation |
| NE | Venules | $\alpha_1$ | Venoconstriction |
| Epi | Venules | $\beta_2$ | Venodilation |

B. Mechanisms of parasympathetic activity

1. Mechanisms of action

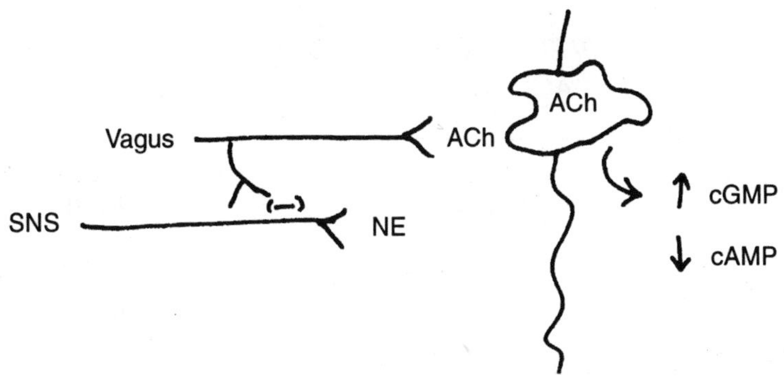


a. ACh release inhibits NE release from SNS nerve

b. ACh increases cGMP

c. ACh inhibits cAMP production

2. Effects on the system

| NT | Site | Effect |
|---|---|---|
| ACh | Heart | ↓ rate, ↓ contractility |
| | Bronchioles | Constriction |
| | Arterioles | 0 |
| | Venules | 0 |

VI. Autonomic Reflexes: Baroreceptor Response for Increased Blood Pressure

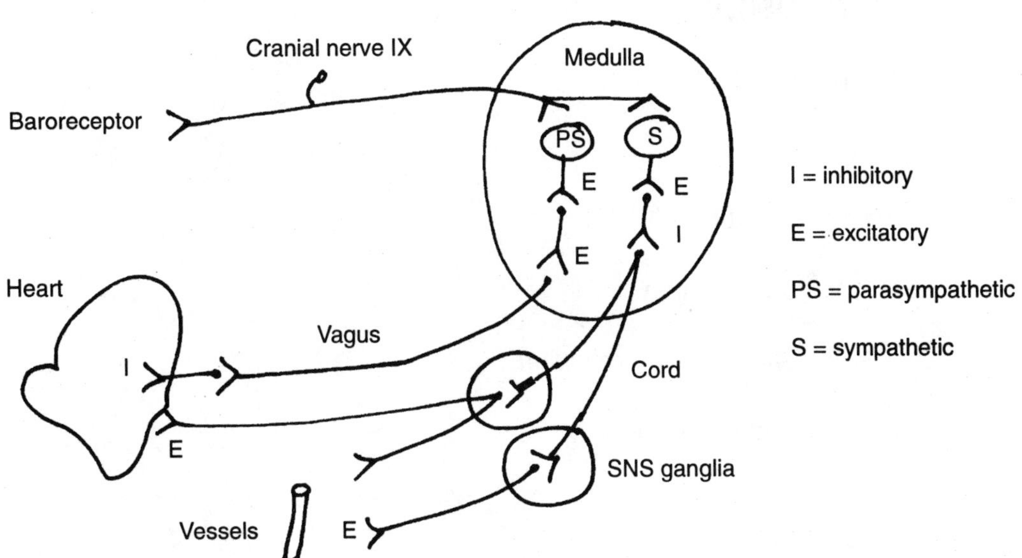

VII. Effects of Parasympathetic and Sympathetic Innervation on Some of the Important Effector Organs

| EFFECTOR | PARASYMPATHETIC (ACh throughout) | SYMPATHETIC | |
|---|---|---|---|
| | | Receptor | Result |
| Eye | | | |
| Pupils | Constrict | Alpha | Dilate |
| Heart | | | |
| Heart rate and contractility | Decrease | Beta | Increase |
| Arterioles | | | |
| Skeletal muscle | — | ACh | Dilate |
| Intestines | Dilate | Alpha | Constrict |
| Almost everywhere else | — | Alpha | Constrict |
| Lungs | | | |
| Bronchial muscle | Contract | Beta | Relax |
| GI | | | |
| Motility and secretion | Increase | Beta | Decrease |
| Sweat glands | — | ACh | Secretion |
| Adrenal medulla | — | ACh | Secretion |

## C. CARDIAC MUSCLE

I. Cardiac Muscle Contraction

A. Structure

1. Striated

2. Sarcolemma

3. Sarcoplasmic reticulum

4. Gap junctions

B. Contractile Unit: Sarcomere

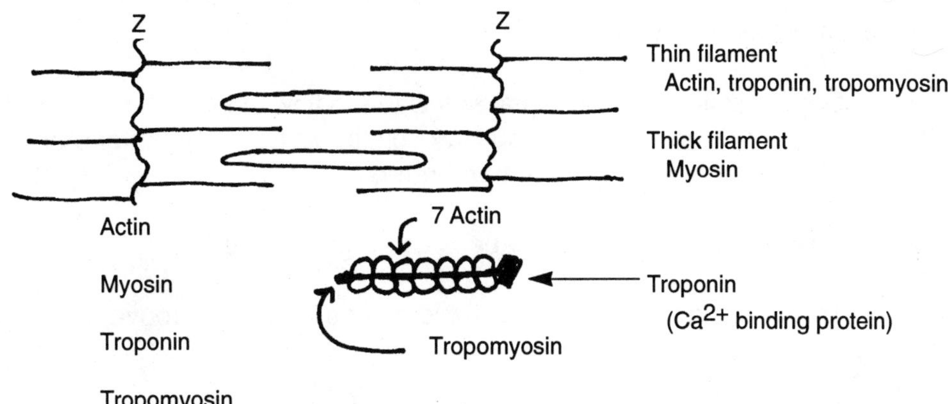


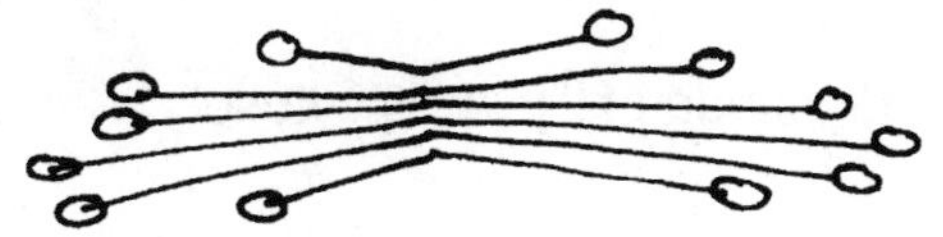

Myosin head binds actin, hydrolysis ATP

C. Cross-bridge Mechanism

1. Myosin heads bind actin, pull and release causing filaments to slide together and shorten

2. Two states of myosin:

   a. High affinity (ADP + $P_i$ bound)

   b. Low affinity (ATP bound)

   Cycles between these two states

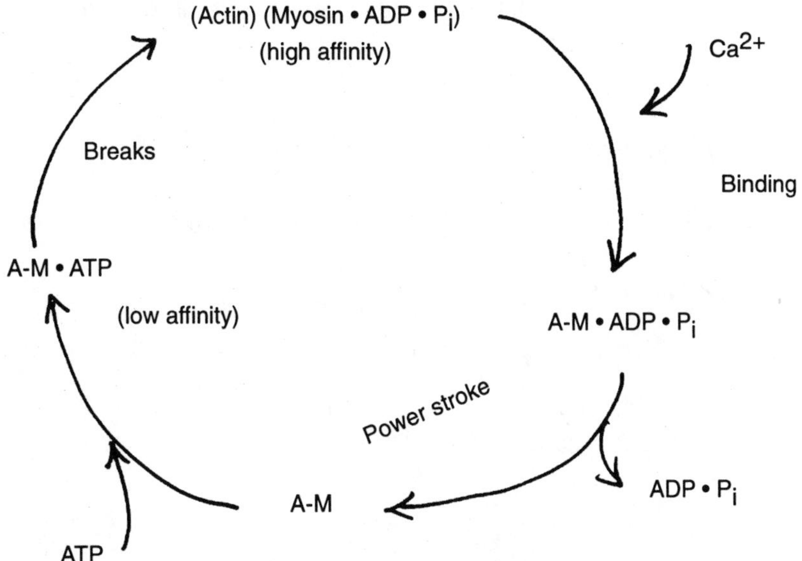

D. Electromechanical Coupling

1. Depolarization of muscle causes $Ca^{2+}$ to flow out of SR into sarcoplasm via voltage-gated $Ca^{2+}$ channels in SR membrane and in across plasma membrane.

2. $Ca^{2+}$ binds troponin and causes conformational change.

3. Troponin tugs on tropomyosin and moves it into the groove between actin strands.

4. Actin sites are now exposed and myosin can bind and form cross-bridge.

5. Cardiac contraction force depends on

    a. Length and magnitude of $\uparrow[Ca^{2+}]$ cytosol

    *Anything that $\uparrow Ca^{2+}$ entry into cell or $\downarrow Ca^{2+}$ extrusion will $\uparrow$ force of contraction

E. Length-Tension Rules (Law of Frank Starling)

"$\uparrow$ Stretch $\rightarrow$ $\uparrow$ tension developed on subsequent contraction"

1. Prestretch to > 3.7 µm $\rightarrow$ no force, no xbridging

2. At short length - less force - actin fibers overlap, interfere with bridging

3. Optimal stretch - $\uparrow$ force with $\uparrow$ stretch (up to a point)

    When A & M are disengaged - no stretch

4. In the heart $\rightarrow\uparrow$filling of chamber $\rightarrow\uparrow$stretch of sarcomere $\rightarrow\uparrow$stroke volume

F. ATP Consumption

1. ATP provided by glycolysis and oxidative phosphorylation

2. Direct phosphorylation

$$\text{ADP} + \text{CrP} \rightleftarrows \text{ATP} + \text{Cr}$$

Storage pool (↗ CrP)

3. Energy used for:

    a. maintenance—ion pumps, etc.

    b. contraction—rate, tension, inotropy

    c. relaxation—lusitropy

G. Energy substrates

1. Fasting: 85% fatty acids

    15% glucose

2. After eating: 50/50

H. Structure of heart muscle layers

1. Contraction → squeezing

2. Layers

    a. epicardium

    b. myocardium

    c. endocardium

I. Blood supply to heart

1. Coronary arteries

    areas supplied

2. Determinants of coronary flow ($Q = \Delta P/R$)

    a. driving pressure = aortic – RA

    b. Vascular resistance

        artery dilation

            ANS

            autoregulation

        external compression

            systole → ↑compression

## D. THE HEART AS A PUMP

### I. The Cardiac Cycle

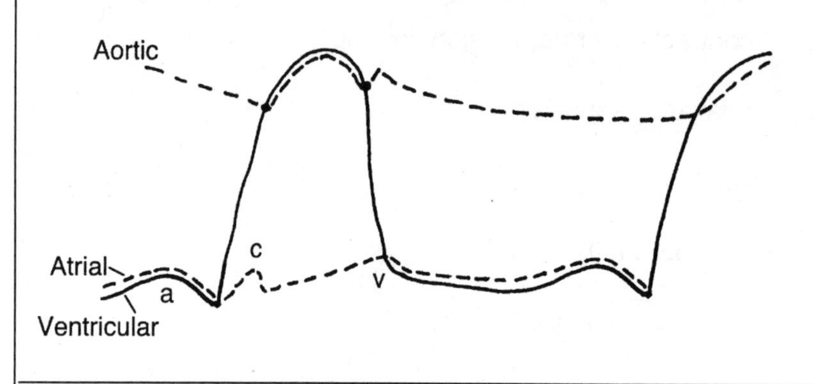


A. Artrial contraction and pressure changes

1. a wave

2. c wave

3. v wave

B. Ventricular contraction and pressure changes

1. Isovolumic contraction

2. Ventricular ejection

3. Isovolumic relaxation

4. Ventricular filling/diastasis

C. Aortic pressure/flow

D. Normal right and left heart pressures

1. All values in figure are in mmHg (TORR)

2. When the valve between two chambers is open, the pressures become equal.

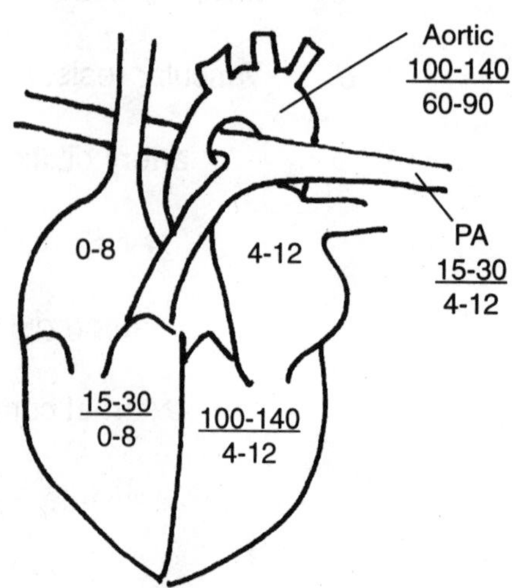

II. Regulation of Cardiac Output

CO = HR X SV

A. Heart rate (↑HR → ↑CO)
mostly regulated by ANS

1. Baroreceptor

2. Chemoreceptor (complex)

Carotid bodies —direct effect→ ↓HR

→ ↑Respiration ——→ ↑HR

3. Stretch (Bainbridge reflex)

↑atrial filling → stretch receptors → ↑HR

B. Stroke volume (↑SV → ↑CO)

1. Length/force relationship (Frank-Starling Law)

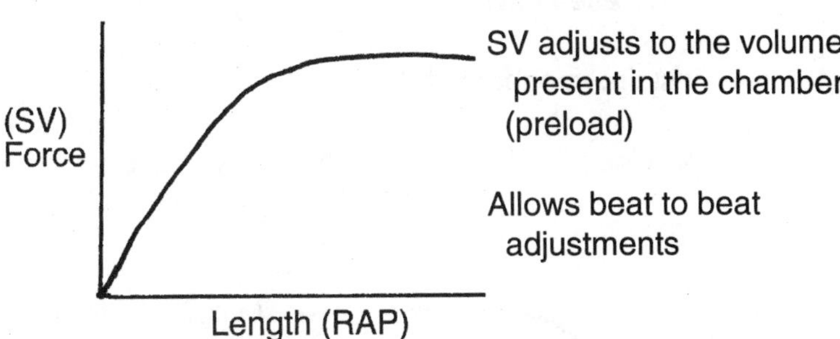


↑ Preload → lengthening of sarcomere → greater crossbridge potential → greater shortening

2. Afterload: ↑ afterload → reduced SV (If no change in preload or contractility)

3. Contractility (inotropy)

independent of preload

depends on intracellular [$CA^{2+}$]

↑contractility

↑release from internal sites

↑entry from extracellular fluid

↓extrusion/sequestration

e.g., a. frequency induced ↑ in contractility

↑HR → ↑$Ca^{2+}$ in → ↑force

b. post-extrasystolic potentiation

pause → $Ca^{2+}$ in release pool → ↑[$Ca^{2+}$]

c. SNS → ↑cAMP → augments $Ca^{2+}$ channel opening → ↑dp/dt; also ↑rate of relaxation (lusitropy)

d. glucagon: similar effect as catecholamines

e. thyroid → affects myosin synthesis → type that has ↑ATPase activity

f. insulin: mechanism?

g. peptides

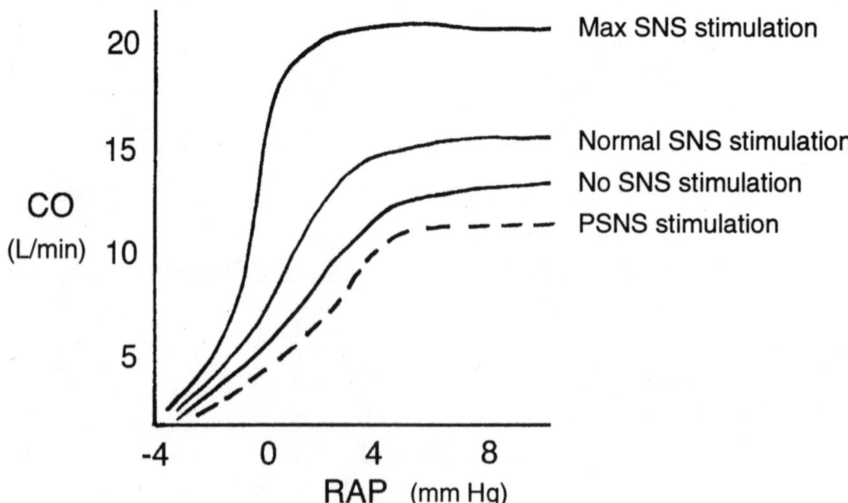

## E. THE VASCULAR SYSTEM AND HEMODYNAMICS

### I. The Circulatory System

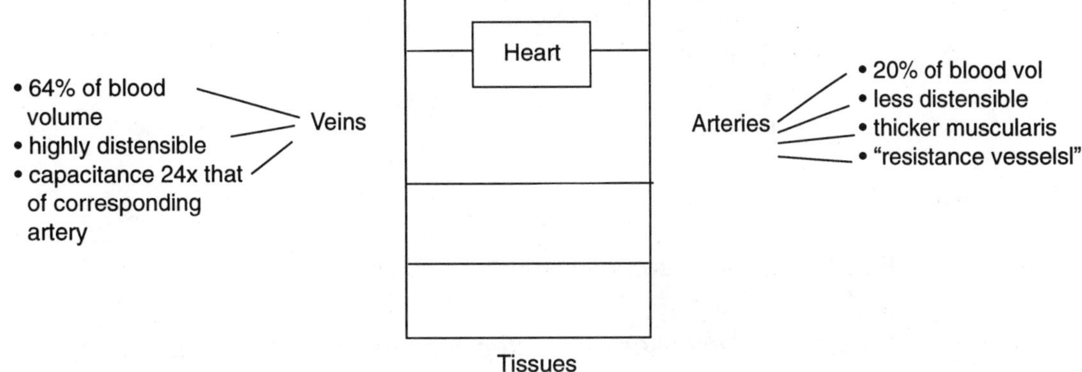


### II. Blood Pressure—A Reflection of the Blood Ejected from Heart.

A. BP = CO x SVR

B. Blood flow lags significantly behind blood pulsation

C. Effects of gravity cause a pressure to be exerted by a column of fluid—positional effects

### III. Physics of Blood Flow and Pressure (Hemodynamics)

A. Ohm's Law: $\text{Flow (Q)} = \dfrac{\text{Driving pressure } (\Delta P)}{\text{Resistance (R)}}$

$$Q = \frac{\Delta P}{R}$$

$$P = Q \cdot R$$

$$R = \frac{\Delta P}{Q}$$

So,

1. Decreased $\Delta P$ (MAP-CVP) = decreased flow

2. Increased R = decreased flow

B. Poiseuille's Law: $Q = \frac{\pi P r^4}{8nL}$ and $R = \frac{8nL}{\pi r^4}$

where
$Q$ = flow
$\Delta P$ = change in pressure
n = viscosity
L = length
r = radius

So,

1. Resistance increases with length, viscosity.

2. Resistance decreases with increasing radius by $r^4$—a small change in vessel radius → huge change in resistance

3. Flow is inversely proportional to resistance (same as Ohm's)

C. Laminar flow vs. turbulent flow

1. Turbulent flow—higher resistance, must develop higher pressure to maintain flow

2. Factors causing turbulence

↑ vessel size

↑ velocity of flow

pulsatile flow

branch points

↓ viscosity

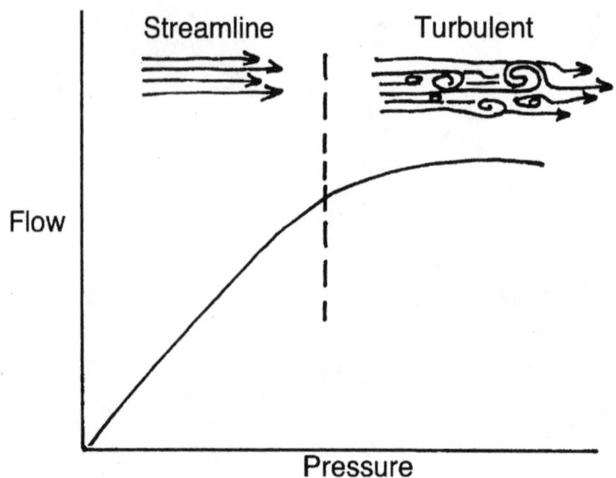

D. Distending pressure (Law of Laplace)

$$\text{Tension} = \frac{P_{distending} \times \text{radius}}{\text{wall thickness}}$$

So,

1. ↑radius = ↑wall tension

2. ↑wall thickness → ↓radius → ↓wall tension

E. Flow/velocity relationship

$$\text{velocity} = \frac{\text{flow}}{\text{cross-sectional area}}$$

So,

1. At a constant flow (CO), velocity is slower for large areas

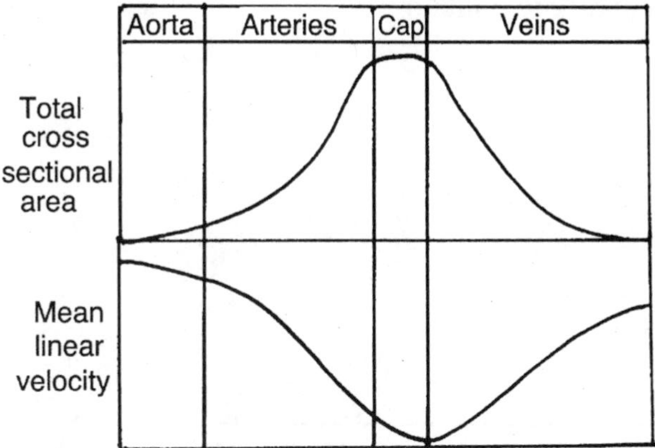


IV. Local Control of Blood Flow—"Autoregulation"

A. Importance of blood flow to local areas

1. Delivery of $O_2$

2. Delivery of nutrients (glucose, FA, AA)

3. Removal of $CO_2$

4. Removal of metabolites ($H^+$, adenosine)

5. Maintenance of ion concentration ($K^+$)

6. Transport of hormones to and from

B. Importance of local flow regulation

1. Provide adequate flow

2. Keep workload on heart to a minimum

C. Structure of vascular bed

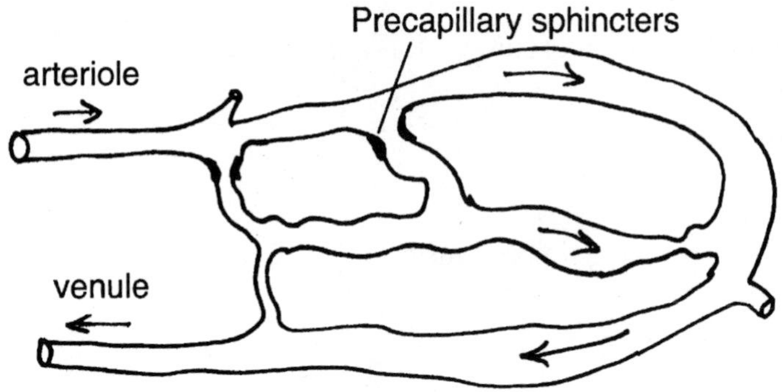


D. Mechanisms of autoregulation

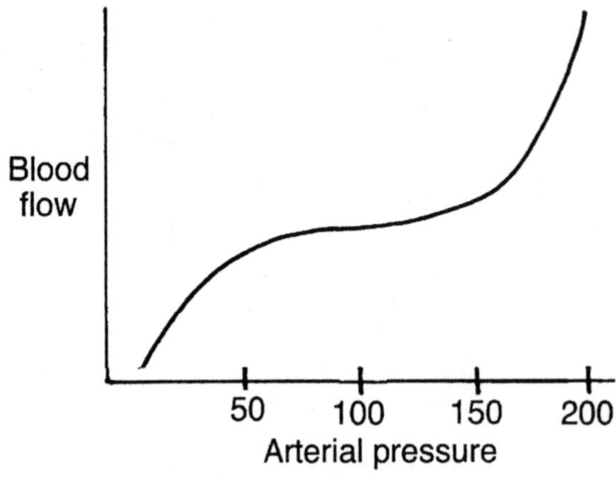


1. Metabolic hypothesis

a. inadequate $O_2$ $\rightarrow$ release of vasodilators

b. ↑vasodilators due to ↓flow or ↑metabolism

c. ↓vasodilators due to ↑flow or ↓metabolism

2. Examples

a. active hyperemia

b. reactive hyperemia

V. Central Control of Blood Flow

A. SNS

1. Resistance vessels

2. Capacitance vessels—venoconstriction causes major mobilization of volume

3. NE versus EPi

B. PSNS—minimal innervation of most vascular beds

VI. Microcirculation and Lymphatics

A. Capillary structure—thin walled, no smooth muscle, narrow lumen

B. Transcapillary exchange

1. Diffusion (major exchange route)

$$J = PS\,(C_o - C_i)$$

where $J$ = flux
$P$ = capillary permeability
$S$ = surface area
$(C_o - C_i)$ = concentration gradient

So, diffusion increases with ↑concentration gradient

↑surface area

↑capillary permeability

2. Filtration—determined by the algebraic sum of hydrostatic and oncotic forces across the capillary membrane

$$\text{Fluid movement} = K\,[\underbrace{(P_c + \pi_i)}_{\text{Filtration}} - \underbrace{(P_i + \pi_p)}_{\text{Reabsorption}}]$$

where $K$ = filtration constant
$P_c$ = capillary hydrostatic pressure
$\pi_i$ = interstitial oncotic pressure
$P_i$ = interstitial hydrostatic pressure
$\pi_p$ = plasma oncotic pressure

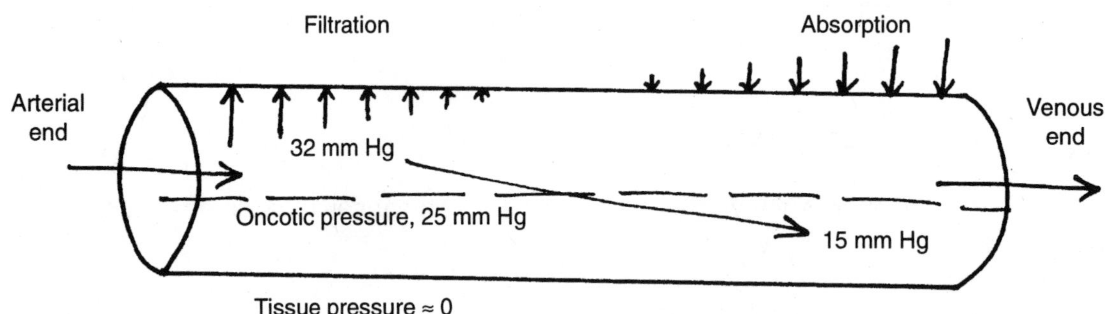


3. Pinocytosis—vesicle transport

C. Lymphatics

1. Volume transported per day approx. equals total plasma volume

2. Returns about 25–50% of the total blood circulating proteins per day

3. Lymphedema

VII. Control of Blood Pressure

A. Baroreceptors—acute, short-term regulation

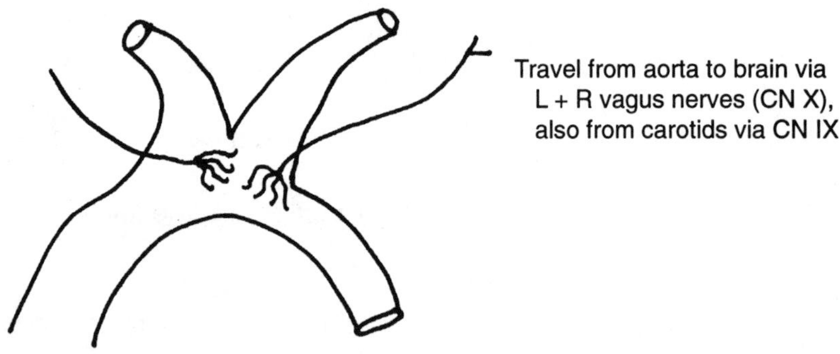


B. Hormonal Control

1. Renin - angiotensin - aldosterone axis

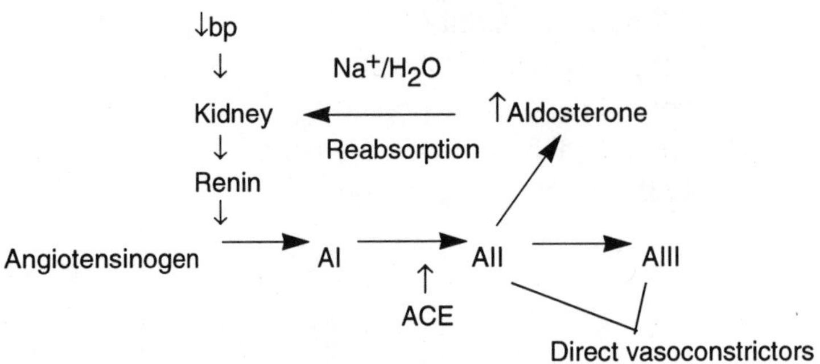

2. Nitric oxide

3. Antidiuretic hormone

4. Endothelin

5. Adrenal catecholamines

6. Atrial natriurectic peptide

C. Renal control

**F.** CIRCULATORY REGULATION: INTERDEPENDENT FUNCTION OF HEART AND VESSELS

I. Venous Pressure Curve: CO determines CVP

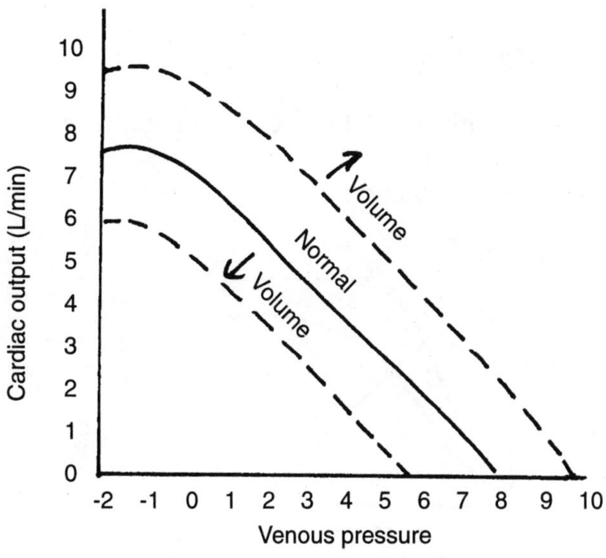


A. If CO is zero, mean circ pressure at normal volume is 7 mm Hg. As CO is increased, circ pressure falls toward zero.

B. A sudden ↑ in CO → ↓CVP

II. Cardiac Function Curve (Starling)

A. As CVP ↓, so does CO

B. Equilibrium point

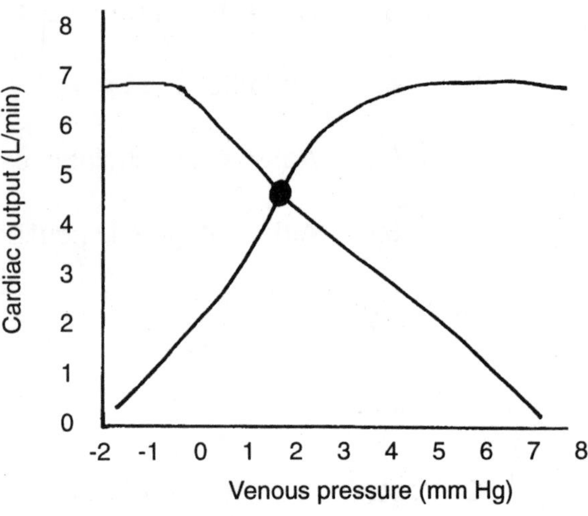


III. Coupling of Heart and Vessels: CO

A. Cardiac factors: HR and contractility

B. Coupling factors: preload and afterload

System functions at equilibrium: over time, CO must equal venous return

Effect of sympathetic stimulation of heart

No change in vascular curve

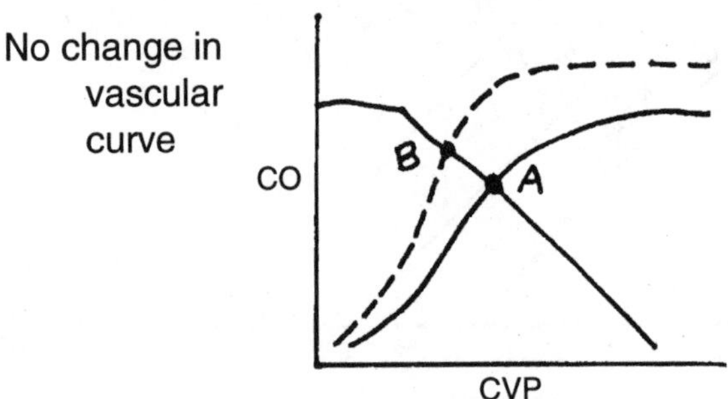


Effect of blood transfusion

No change in cardiac curve

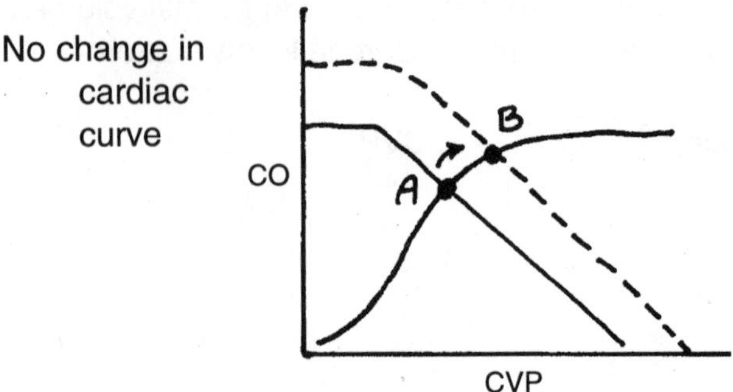


Real life—more complex!!

# CARDIAC PATHOPHYSIOLOGY

I. Ischemic Heart Disease

A. Pathogenesis of cardiac ischemia

1. Atherosclerosis
2. Thrombus
3. Vasospasm
4. Hemodynamics

B. Theories of atherosclerosis

1. Response to injury
2. Monoclonal
3. Lipid infiltration
4. Intimal cell mass
5. Evidence implicating hyperlipidemia in atherosclerotic heart disease

a. Atherosclerotic plaques are rich in cholesterol, which is derived primarily from serum lipoproteins.

b. Atherosclerosis can be produced in experimental animals by feeding diets that increase plasma cholesterol levels.

c. Genetic disorders causing severe hypercholesterolemia lead to early severe atherosclerosis.

d. Acquired diseases such as hypothyrodism and nephrotic syndrome which cause hyperlipidemia are associated with increased incidence of ischemic heart disease.

e. Populations having higher blood cholesterol levels have higher mortality from ischemic heart disease.

f. Recent prospective studies have shown that treatment with diet and cholesterol-lowering drugs reduces cardiovascular mortality in selected patients with hypercholesterolemia.

C. Ischemic syndromes

1. Angina

2. MI

3. Chronic ischemic heart disease

4. Sudden death

D. Supply/demand imbalances

1. Transient imbalance between myocardial oxygen demands and oxygen supplied by coronary arteries

| ↑ Demand | ↓ Supply |
|---|---|
| Exercise | >75% occlusion |
| Hypertrophy | Spasm (Prinzmetal's) |
| Preload | Stenosis and inability to dilate |
| Afterload | Decreased perfusion pressure (DBP - RAP) |
| Stress (SNS) | "Steal phenomenon" |
| REM sleep | |

2. Consequences of demand > supply

a. ischemic pain—8th cervical and 1–4 thoracic dorsal root ganglia

mechanisms: bradykinins, serotonin?

referred pain: jaw, neck, arm

b. Metabolic events

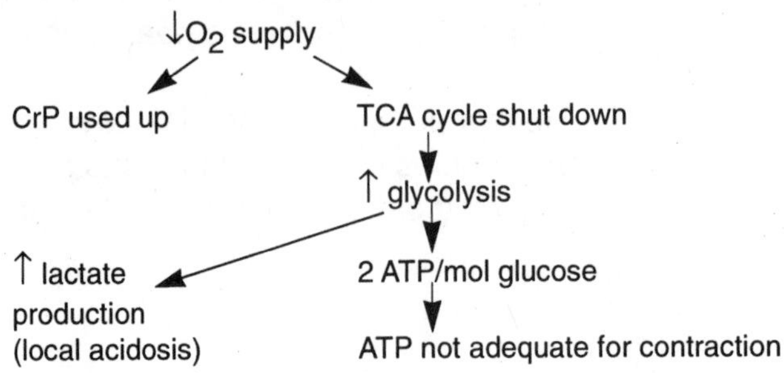

3. Sequela of MI

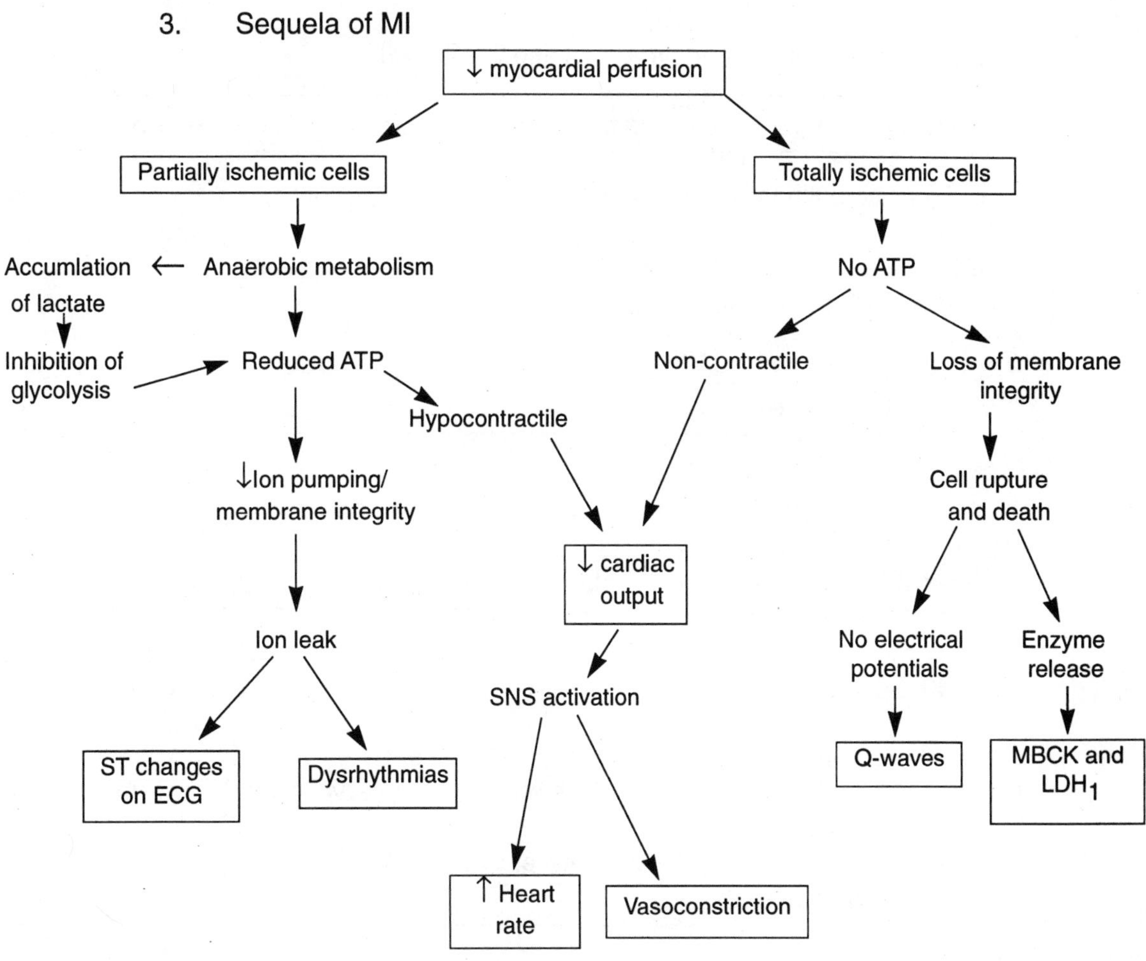


E. Differentiation of angina and MI

| | Angina | MI |
|---|---|---|
| Pain | 3–5 min usually relieved by rest or NTG; generally less intense | >15–30 min, not relieved by NTG or rest; crushing, "elephant on chest" |
| ECG | ST elevation (depression) | ST changes<br>Q waves<br>T-wave inversion |
| Enzymes | Not elevated | Increased $CK_{MB}$ (peak 24°)<br><br>$LDH_1$ > $LDH_2$ (2–3 days) |

F. Time course of enzyme elevations after MI

| Enzyme | Initial Rise | Peak | Return to Normal |
|---|---|---|---|
| CK (creatine kinase) | 4–6 hours | 24 hours | 2–4 days |
| GOT (glutamine oxalo-acetic transaminase) | 8–12 hours | 24–48 hours | 4–6 days |
| LDH (lactic - dehydrogenase) | 12–24 hours | 3–6 days | 8–14 days |

G. Location of MI according to coronary artery affected

| Arterial Obstruction | Location of Infarct |
|---|---|
| Left anterior descending (40–50% of infarcts) | Anterior wall of LV near apex<br>Anterior 2/3 of interventricular septum |
| Right coronary (30–40% of infarcts) | Posterior wall of LV<br>Posterior 1/3 of interventricular septum |
| Left circumflex (15–20% of infarcts) | Lateral wall of LV |

H. Hemodynamic response to MI

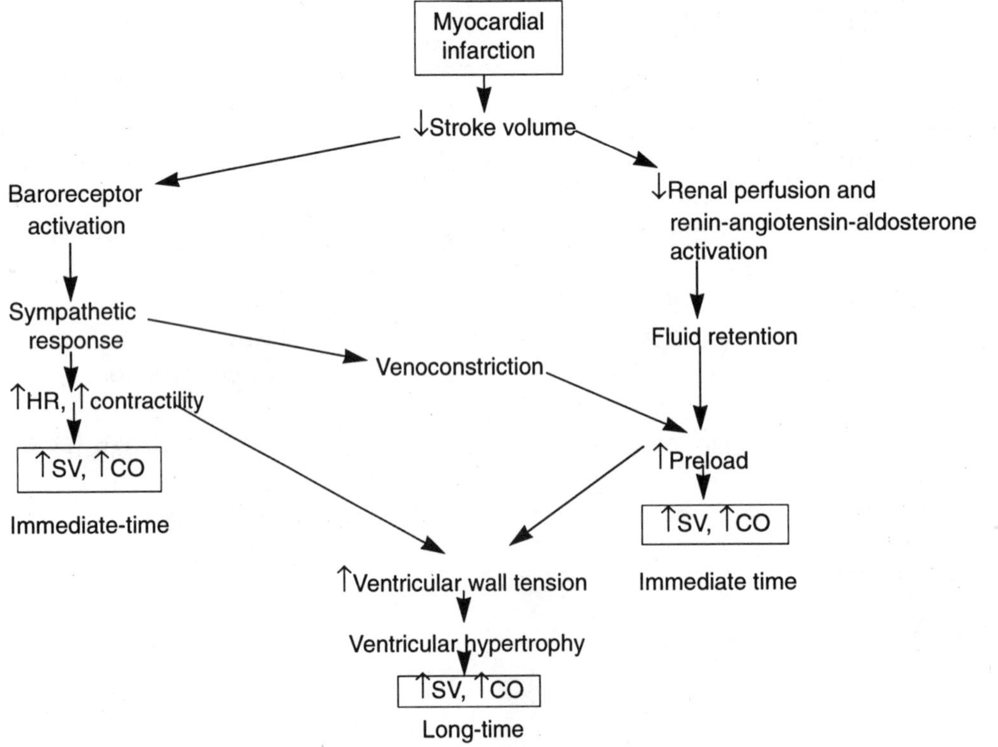

II. Heart Failure

A. Etiology of heart failure

1. Diminished contractility

2. Increased workload

B. Compensatory mechanisms

1. SNS

2. Preload

3. Hypertrophy

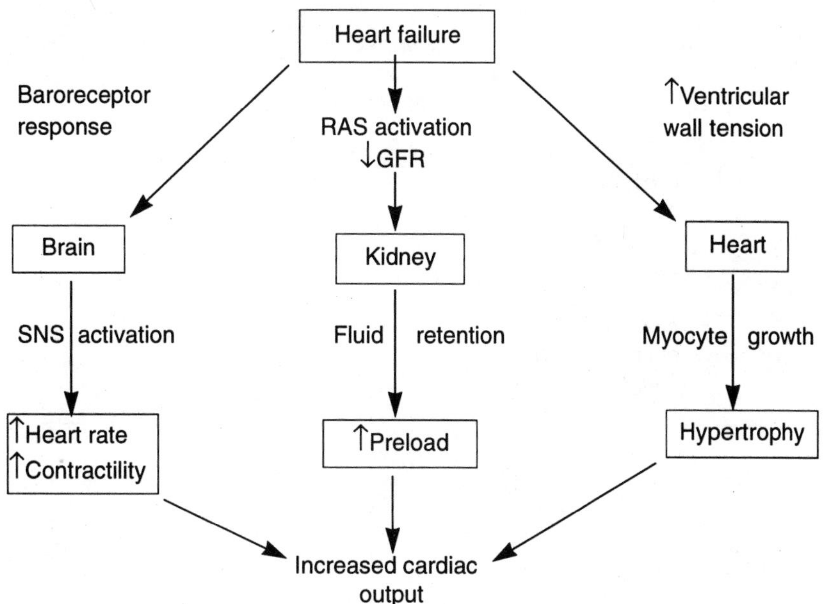


Compensatory responses in heart failure

C. Pathophysiology of heart failure

1. Left

2. Right

3. Biventricular

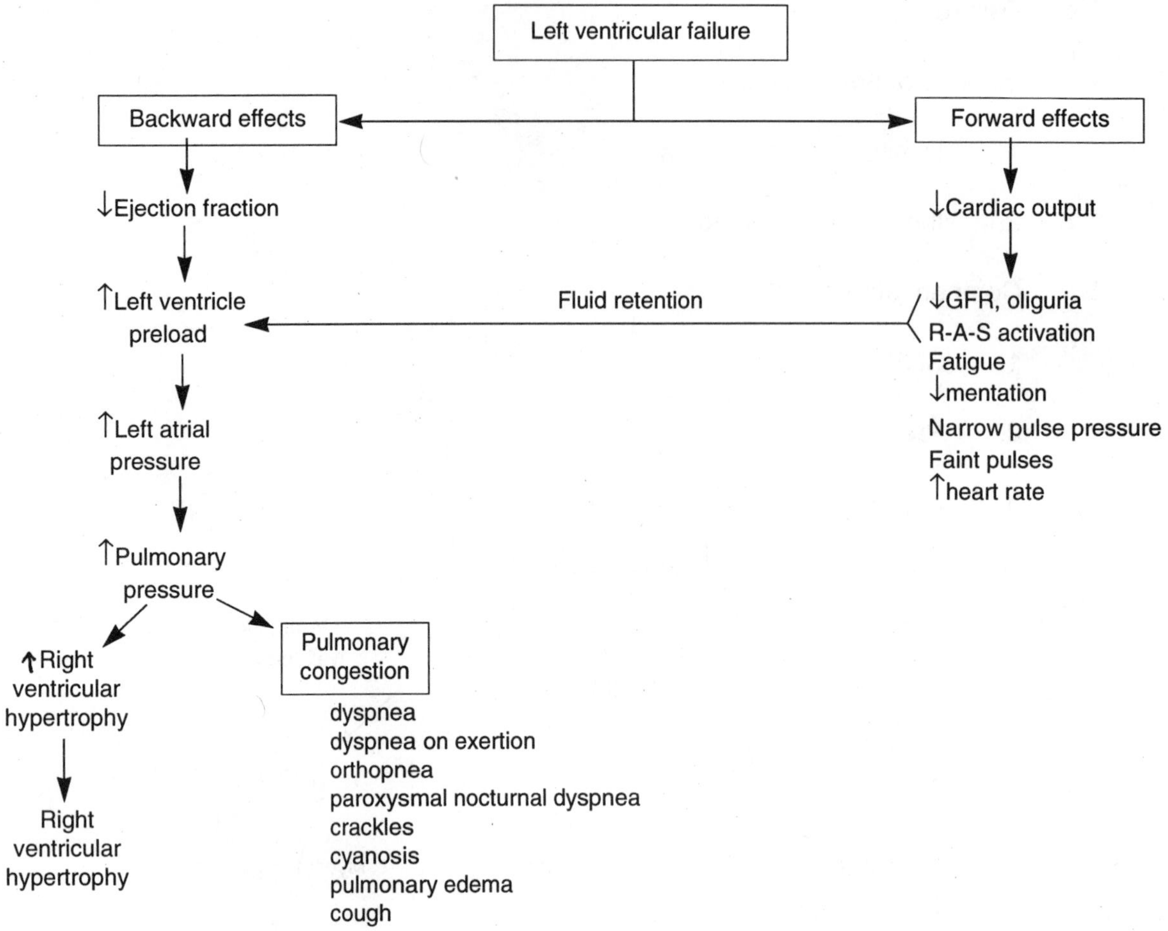

Left ventricular failure
Backward effects
Forward effects
↓Ejection fraction
↑Left ventricle preload
↑Left atrial pressure
↑Pulmonary pressure
↑Right ventricular hypertrophy
Right ventricular hypertrophy
Pulmonary congestion
dyspnea
dyspnea on exertion
orthopnea
paroxysmal nocturnal dyspnea
crackles
cyanosis
pulmonary edema
cough
↓Cardiac output
Fluid retention
↓GFR, oliguria
R-A-S activation
Fatigue
↓mentation
Narrow pulse pressure
Faint pulses
↑heart rate

Right ventricular failure
Backward effects
Forward effects
↓Ejection fraction
↑Right ventricular preload
↑Right atrial pressure
Systemic congestion
hepatomegaly
splenomegaly
anorexia
peripheral edema
jugular vein distention
↓Output to left ventricle
↓Left ventricle cardiac output
Fluid retention
↓GFR, oliguria
R-A-S activation
Fatigue
↓mentation
Narrow pulse pressure
Faint pulses
↑heart rate

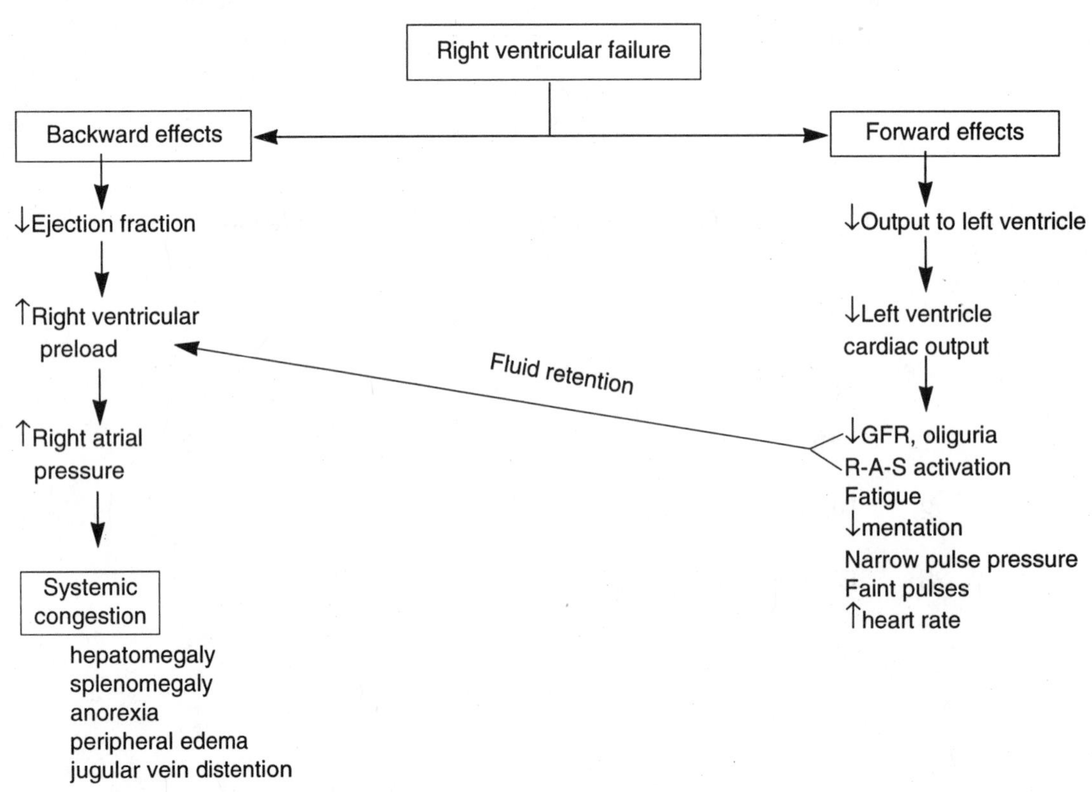

D. Principles of treatment

1. Management of preload

2. Management of afterload

3, Management of contractility

E. Commonly used drugs for treatment of heart failure

| Category | Drug generic name (Brand Name) |
|---|---|
| PRELOAD REDUCING DRUGS | |
| Diuretics | |
| Loop diuretics | furosemide (Lasix)<br>ethacrynic acid (Edecrine)<br>bumetanide (Bumex) |
| Thiazide and thiazide-like | chlorothiazide (Diuril)<br>hydrochlorothiazide (HCTZ)<br>metolazone (Diulo)<br>chlorthalidone (Hygroton)<br>inadapamide (Lozol) |
| Osmotic diuretic | mannitol (Osmitrol) |
| Venodilators | |
| Narcotic | morphine |
| Nitrates | erythrityl trinitrate<br>isosorbide dinitrate (Isordil)<br>nitroglycerine (Nitrobid) |
| Angiotensin converting enzyme inhibitors | captopril (Capoten)<br>enalapril (Vasotec)<br>lisinopril (Zestril) |
| AFTERLOAD REDUCING DRUGS | |
| Angiotensin converting enzyme inhibitors | as above |
| Calcium channel blockers | diltiazem (Cardizem)<br>nicardipine (Cardene)<br>nifedipine (Procardia)<br>verapamil (Calan) |
| Centrally acting anti-adrenergics | clonidine (Catapress)<br>guanabenz (Wytensin)<br>methyldopa (Aldomet) |

Commonly used drugs for treatment of heart failure *(continued)*

| Category | Drug generic name (Brand Name) |
|---|---|
| Peripherally acting anti-adrenergics | guanethedine<br>reserpine |
| Direct vasodilators | hydralazine (Apresoline)<br>nitroprusside (Nipride)<br>prazosin (Minipress)<br>minoxidil (Rogaine) |
| INOTROPIC DRUGS (INCREASE CONTRACTILITY) | |
| Cardiac Glycosides | digitoxin<br>digoxin (Lanoxin)<br>deslanoside |
| Beta adrenergics | dobutamine (Dobutrex)<br>dopamine (Inotropin)<br>isoproterenol (Isuprel) |
| Phosphodiesterase inhibitor | amrinone (Inocor) |

III. Valvular Disorders

A. Principles of valve function

B. Etiology

1. Congenital
2. Rheumatic
3. Degenerative
4. Infective

C. Mitral stenosis

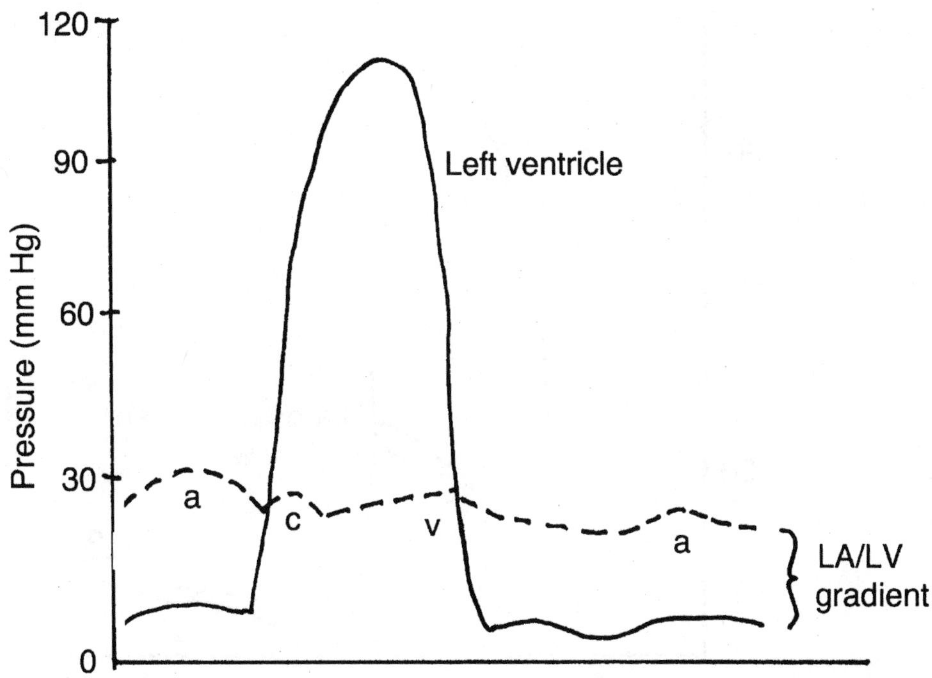


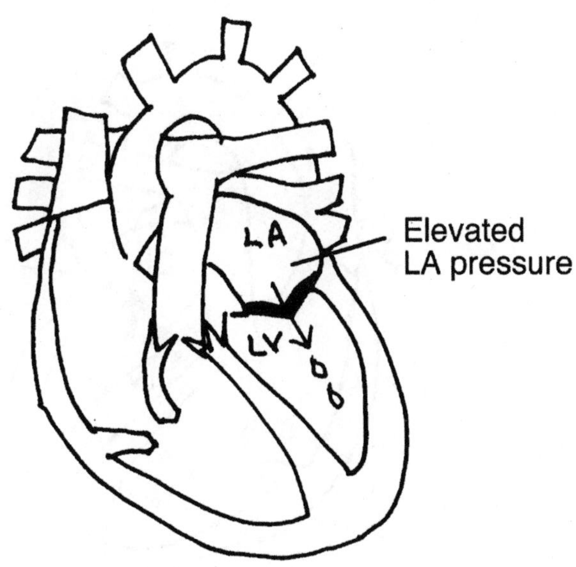

D. Mitral regurgitation

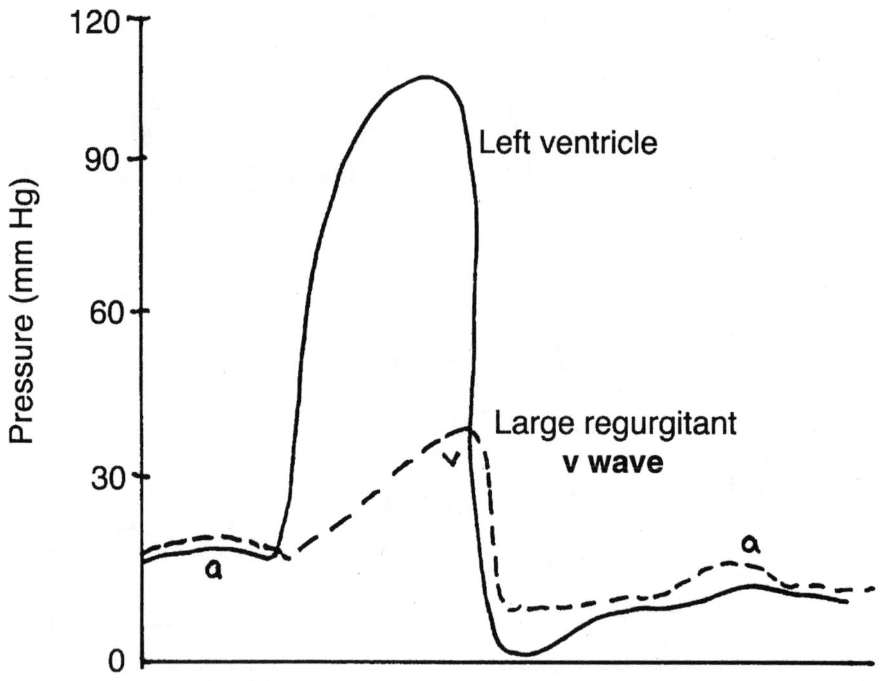


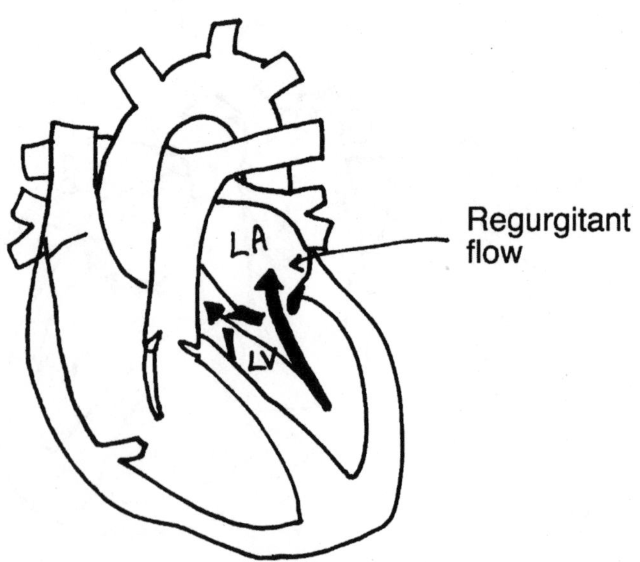

E. Aortic stenosis

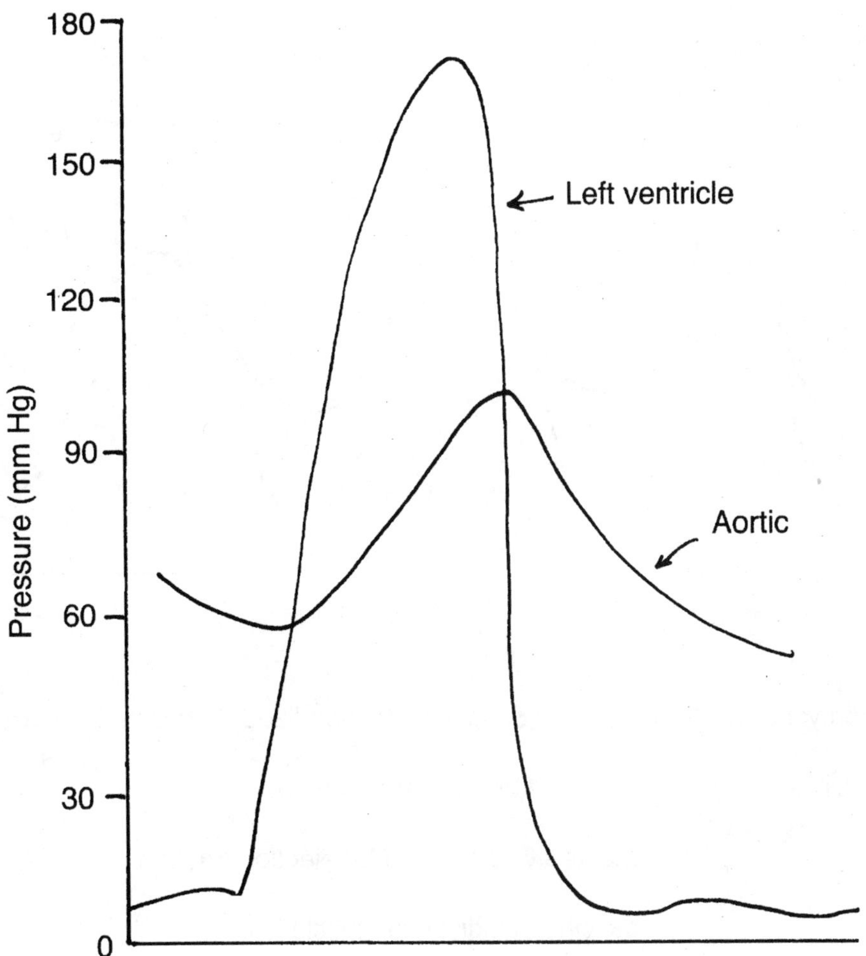


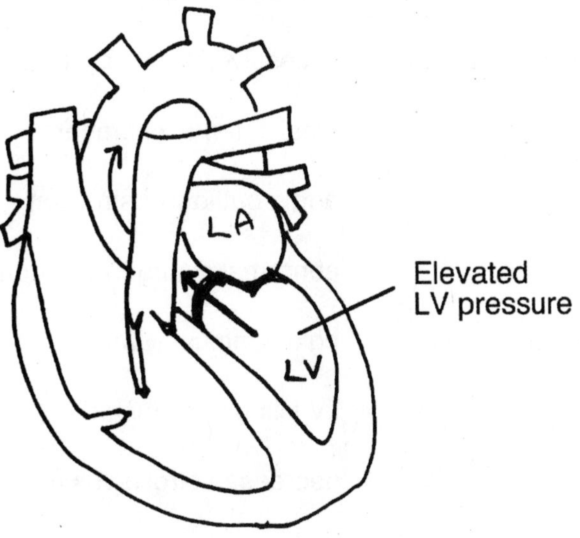

F. Aortic regurgitation

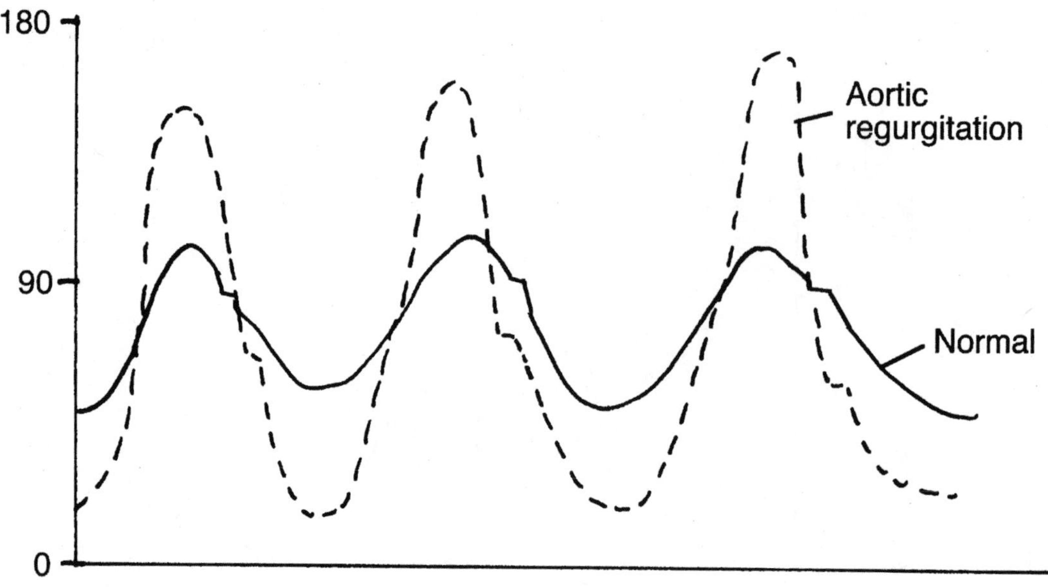


IV. Cardiomyopathy: Primary Cardiopathies—Generalized Disorders of Heart Muscle

A. Dilated:
- enlarged heart chambers
- markedly decreased LV ejection fraction
- atrophy of individual muscle fibers
- associated with ETOH, viral
- poor prognosis (biventricular failure)

B. Hypertrophic:
- excessive LV muscle mass
- small internal chamber
- aortic outflow obstruction
- abnormal disorganized muscle fibrils

C. Restrictive:
- rigid ventricular walls
- LV filling is restricted
- decreased stroke volume

V. Congenital Heart Defects

A. Acyanotic defects (left to right shunt)

1. Atrial septal defect (ASD)

2. Ventricular septal defect (VSD)

3. Patent ductus arteriosis

4. Coarctation of the aorta

B. Cyanotic defects (right to left shunt)

1. Transposition of the great vessels

2. Tetrology of Fallot

a. pulmonic valve stenosis

b. VSD

c. overriding aorta

d. RV hypertrophy

C. General signs and symptoms of heart defects

1. Dyspnea

2. Failure to thrive

3. Tachycardia

4. Murmurs

5. Cyanosis

6. Poor activity tolerance

7. Squatting

8. Clubbing of fingers and toes

VI. Shock

A. $O_2$ below basal consumption → shock and organ system failure

B. Classification of global shock states

1. Low perfusion

a. hypovolemic

(i) fluid loss

(ii) dilatory

b. cardiogenic

(i) electrical

(ii) mechanical

c. obstructive

(i) intravascular occlusion

thrombotic

embolic

(ii) extravascular pressure

tension pneumothorax

edema accumulation

2. Low oxygen content

a. pulmonary failure

b. ↓Hb

c. carboxy Hb

C. Manifestations

1. Low perfusion—SNS activation, ↑RAS, ↑ADH

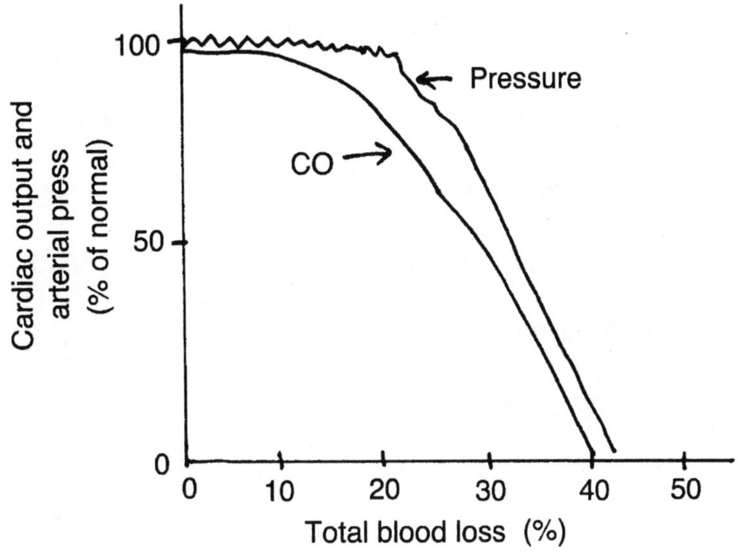


2. Low $O_2$—S/S are subtle. Often first manifestation is organ failure

D. Pathophysiology—initiation of the dying processes

1. Calcium entry into cytosol
   ↓
   Activation of phospholipases
   ↓
   Activation of FFA cascades
   ↙ ↘
   Prostanoids (Vasoconstrictors) | Free radicals (↑vascular permeability)

2. Circulating lipases—autodigestion

3. Hypercoagulability

4. Activation of clotting cascades

<u>Conclusions:</u> Shock is global inflammation?

Shock is initiation of dying process?

E. Therapy

1. Restoration of volume

   Even with septic shock, there appears to be volume deficit.

   ↑volume → ↓[lactate] and ↑$O_2$ consumption

2. Keep patients warm

   Except maybe with focal ischemia (pack head in ice)

3. Hemodilution to ↓viscosity

4. Free-radical scavengers

5. Anti-inflammatory agents

6. Antibodies

7. Calcium blockers

8. Cardiogenic

   manage preload

   inotrops

   IABP (intra-aortic balloon pump)

   VADS (ventricular assist devices)

# VASCULAR PATHOPHYSIOLOGY

I. Arterial Aneurysm

A. Complications: rupture, dissection

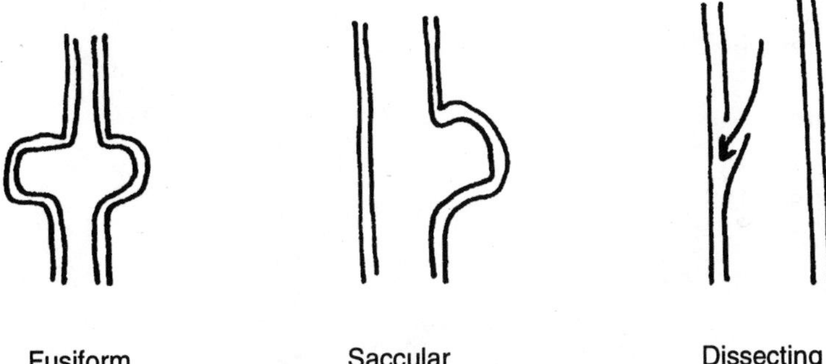


B. Treatment: surgical insertion of graft

II. Vascular Obstruction

A. Factors that can lead to obstruction

1. Thrombus
2. Embolus
3. Compression
4. Vasospasm
5. Structural changes—atherosclerosis

B. Pathophysiology of obstruction

1. Arterial

↓flow downstream → Ischemia → Pain; Atrophy, loss of hair, thin skin

2. Venous

↑pressure upstream → Edema, stasis → Pain; Color changes

C. The six classic "P's" of acute arterial obstruction

1. pain

2. pallor

3. pulselessness

4. paresis

5. paralysis

6. poikilothermy (cool)

D. Chronic arterial insufficiency

1. Peripheral atherosclerosis

a. pathophysiology: progressive occlusion of artery, decreased responsiveness (cannot dilate)

b. signs and symptoms: often affects legs

intermittent claudication

reduced pulses

cool to touch

postural color changes

elevation, pallor
dependent, red, cyanotic

chronic changes, atrophic

c. treatment

mild exercise

position with legs dependent (not elevated)

endarterectomy, grafting

2. Raynaud's disease: affects mainly young women

a. pathophysiology: transient, functional arterial insufficiency. Probably due to intermittent arterial spasms. Usually no permanent ischemic changes.

b. signs and symptoms: precipitated by cold, anxiety usually affects hands.

spasm: cold, pale, ischemic pain

after spasm: hyperemia, cyanosis, throbbing pain

c. treatment: stress management

3. Buerger's disease: affects mainly males 20–45 years old, severe arterial insufficiency related to tobacco use.

a. pathophysiology: Chronic arterial inflammation leads to sclerosis and occlusion. There is often severe, chronic ischemia that leads to ulcers, gangrene, amputation.

b. signs and symptoms: similar to severe arterial insufficiency due to atherosclerosis

c. treatment: stop smoking

amputation often necessary

E. Venous insufficiency

1. Causes of venous obstruction/incompetent valves

pregnancy

obesity

prolonged standing

leg crossing

bed rest (no muscle-pump)

right heart failure

congenital defective venous valves

2. Consequences of venous insufficiency

a. varicose veins

stasis

b. edema formation: Increased venous pressure or obstruction causes a net movement of fluid into interstitial space (transudation)

Edema interferes with $O_2$ transport to tissues

Transudate:

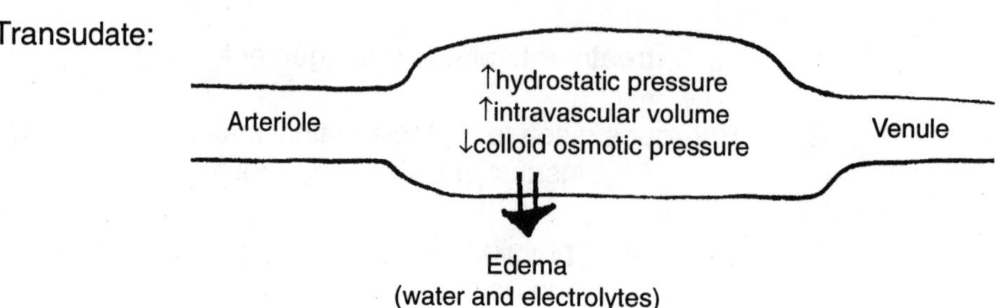


Exudate: Inflammatory

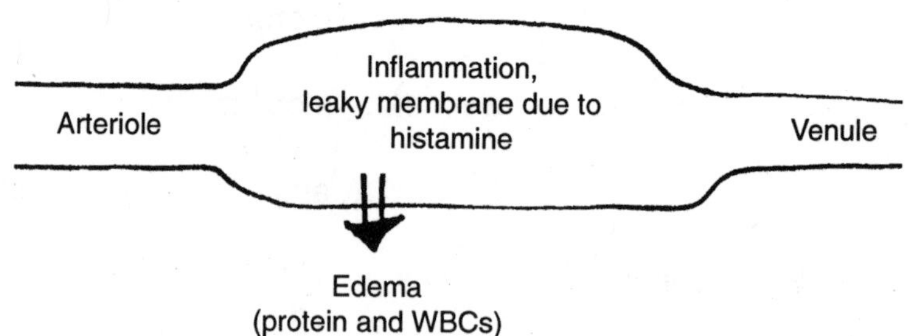


F. Thrombophlebitis: thrombus formation in a vein with associated inflammation

1. Predisposing factors: stasis—bed rest, immobility, pregnancy, varicose veins, hypercoagulation, endothelial injury

2. Signs and symptoms:

| Deep vein (DVT) | versus | Superficial vein thrombosis |
|---|---|---|
| Generalized leg edema<br>Generalized leg pain<br>Fever<br>More serious risk of emboli | | Superficial inflammation<br>(red, hot, tender, swollen)<br>Collateral veins minimize edema |

3. Treatment: elevate extremity

   immobilize

   anticoagulation

   monitor for S/S of emboli

   prevention: muscle activity

G. Lymphedema: insufficiency of lymphatic drainage

1. Pathology: blockage by tumor or infection

   congenital incompetence of lymph valves

2. Signs and symptoms: may be massive extremity edema "Elephantiasis"

3. Treatment: pneumatic pumping

   coumadin (dissolves proteins)

   surgery

H. Compare and contrast arterial and venous obstruction

| | Arterial | Venous |
|---|---|---|
| Site | | |
| Causes | | |
| Signs and symptoms | | |
| Positioning | | |

III. High and Low Blood Pressure

A. Low blood pressure (hypotension)

1. Orthostatic hypotension (↓blood volume)

2. Cardiogenic (↓CO)

B. High blood pressure (hypertension)

1. Secondary: known causes (e.g., kidney disease, endocrine disorders) (5%)

2. Essential hypertension: idiopathic (90–95%), affects 25% of U.S. population

   a. definition: Systolic > 140 mm Hg and/or diastolic > 90 mm Hg

b. pathogenesis: not well understood

inappropriate $Na^+$ and $H_2O$ retention

altered baroreceptors (desensitized)

excess renin secretion

abnormally constricted arterioles

c. signs and symptoms: may be none

headache

blurred vision

retinal changes

3. Treatment

a. weight reduction

b. sodium and fat restriction

c. relaxation therapy

d. drugs to decrease vascular resistance

ACE inhibitors

adrenergic inhibitors

calcium antagonists

direct vasodilators

e. drugs to decrease blood volume

diuretics

# THE RESPIRATORY SYSTEM

I. General Concepts of Respiratory Physiology and Pathophysiology

A. Interdependence of cardiovascular and respiratory systems

1. Cyanosis: indicates desaturation of hemoglobin, indicates hypoxemia, but very unreliable—Hgb must be about 1/3 reduced

2. Central versus peripheral cyanosis

a. central—due to lungs not oxygenating the blood

b. peripheral—blood is oxygenated by lungs but does not reach the tissues

artery occlusion

low cardiac output

3. Poor tissue oxygenation can result from either failure of lungs to oxygenate or failure of heart to perfuse

B. Control of ventilation

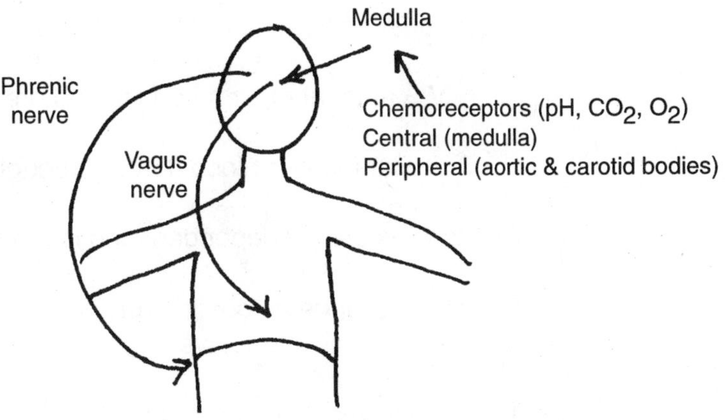


1. An increase in $CO_2$ or decrease in $O_2$, pH $\rightarrow$ $\uparrow$ respiration

2. A decrease in $CO_2$ or increase in pH $\rightarrow$ $\downarrow$ respiration

C. Terminology for respiratory rate/rhythm

1. Apnea

2. Bradypnea

3. Tachypnea

4. Hyperventilation

5. Hypoventilation

6. Dyspnea

D. Factors that may contribute to rate/rhythm problems

1. Drugs

2. ↓Level of consciousness

3. Resp muscle weakness

4. Temperature

5. Anxiety

6. "$CO_2$ narcosis"

II. Ventilation and Perfusion of the Lungs

A. There must be adequate $\dot{V}/\dot{Q}$ matching to oxygenate the blood

$\dot{V}$ = amount of air moved in and out of the lungs

$\dot{Q}$ = amount of blood flowing through the lungs

Perfusion is gravity dependent and is greatest in dependent lung areas.

B. For gas exchange across the alveolus, must have

Air

Blood →

1. Good ventilation to alveolus

2. Adequate blood flow past alveolus

3. Minimal barriers for gas to diffuse across

C. Ventilation/perfusion imbalance

1. Poor ventilation: unoxygenated blood is shunted past lung

a. causes: Airway obstruction, mucus, edema, restrictive diseases, atelectasis

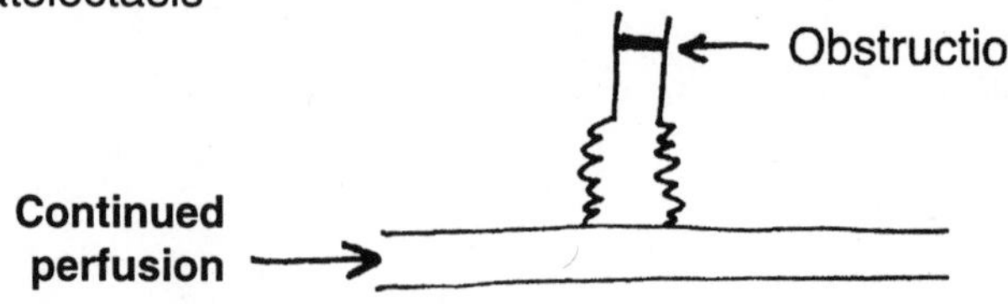

b. compensatory response: hypoxemic vasoconstriction

2. Poor perfusion: ventilation is wasted. If large vessel or multiple areas are obstructed, may cause pulmonary hypertension.

   a. causes: pulmonary emboli

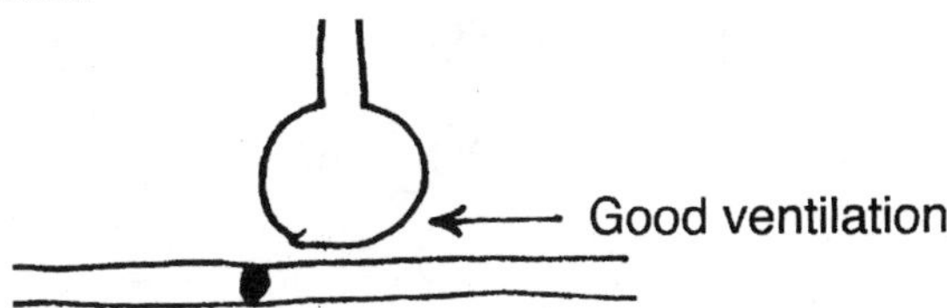


   b. pathogenesis: usually secondary to DVT or fat emboli. Sudden onset of dyspnea. May have severe hypoxemia.

3. Impaired diffusion: Ventilation and perfusion may be adequate, but there is a barrier to diffusion across alveolar membrane.

   a. causes: pulmonary edema

      pulmonary fibrosis

Fluid or scar tissue

D. Positioning for unilateral lung dysfunction: Maximize vent/perf matching. Position with well-ventilated lung down (dependent). Then blood will flow past good lung.

E. Calculating A-a $DO_2$ and $CaO_2$

F. Oxyhemoglobin saturation curve

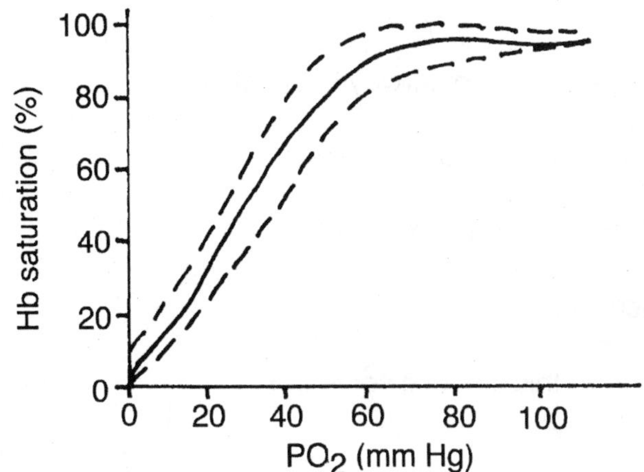

1. Shifts in curve

   a. shift to right: $\downarrow O_2$–Hb affinity

   b. Shift to left: $\uparrow O_2$–Hb affinity

2. At $PO_2 < 60$ mm Hg, saturation falls sharply

3. At $PO_2 > 80$ mm Hg, little increase in saturation

## III. Obstructive Pulmonary Diseases

### A. General concepts

1. Radial traction

2. Airways open wider on inspiration and get narrower on expiration

3. Autonomic effects on the airways ($\beta_2$)

   sympathetic: bronchodilation

   parasympathetic: bronchoconstriction

4. Obstructive diseases are characterized by air trapping hyperinflation. Cannot get air out. There is increased lung compliance.

5. Three major forms of obstructive disease

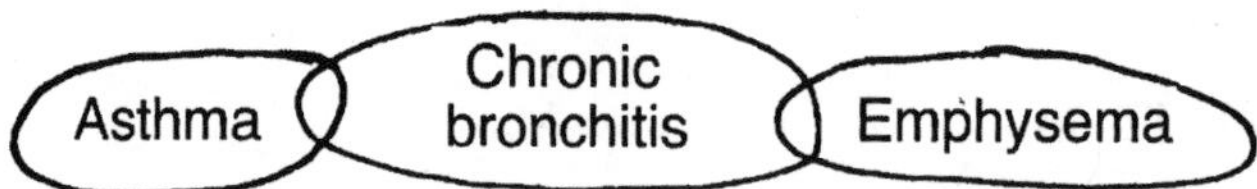


### B. Asthma: reversible episodes of airway obstruction

1. Three major problems during attack

   smooth muscle spasm

   bronchial mucosa edema

   excessive thick mucus secretion

2. Characteristic signs and symptoms

   wheezing on expiration

   low $PaO_2$

   severe dyspnea

   air trapping—hyperinflated lungs

3. Etiology

   a. extrinsic—"allergic" inflammatory reaction to specific irritants

   b. intrinsic—cannot identify specific cause, may occur with anxiety, cold exposure, exercise

      may have overly sensitive airways to parasympathetic stimulation

4. Treatment: beta adrenergic drugs, parasympathetic antagonists

5. Status asthmaticus

6. Asthma not usually classified as COPD unless it is associated with chronic structural damage

C. Chronic bronchitis: chronic airway inflammation

1. Definition: cough for more than 3 months per year for 2 consecutive years

2. Characteristic signs and symptoms

   productive cough

   chronic airway obstruction

3. Etiology: associated with cigarette smoking and air pollution

4. Pathology: chronic airway inflammation with hypertrophied mucous glands, WBC infiltration. Bronchial walls may become scarred, fibrotic.

5. Treatment: stop smoking

   antibiotics

6. Bronchiectasis: may be a complication of chronic bronchitis and other causes of chronic coughing strain. Develop weak spots in bronchial wall with pouches that trap mucus. Mucus is medium for bacterial growth. Have very productive cough, foul-smelling secretions.

D. Emphysema

1. Irreversible destruction of alveolar walls resulting in

   a. loss of radial traction → airway collapse → air trapping

   b. decreased surface area for gas exchange

2. Etiology

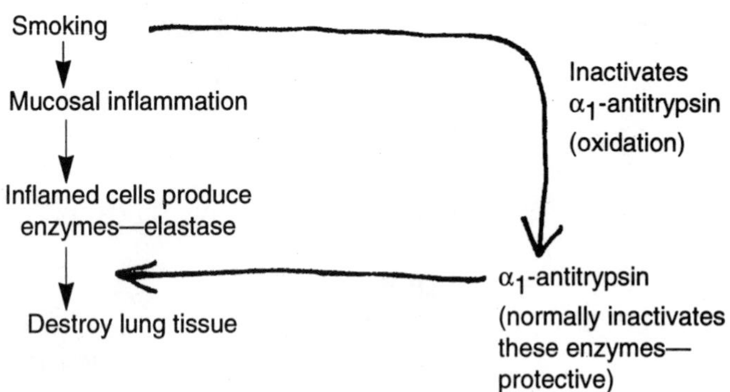


3. Signs and symptoms

   a. barrel chest

   b. decreased gas exchange ↓$PaO_2$

   c. flat diaphragm

   d. dyspnea

   e. blebs and bullae that may rupture

4. Treatment

   a. stop smoking

   b. $O_2$

   c. bronchodilators

E. Chronic obstructive pulmonary disease (COPD) is usually a combination of emphysema and chronic bronchitis. The obstructive changes are chronic and irreversible. There are two common clinical presentations of COPD.

1. Primarily emphysematous, "pink puffer"

2. Primarily bronchitic, "blue bloater"

IV. Restrictive Pulmonary Diseases

A. General concepts:

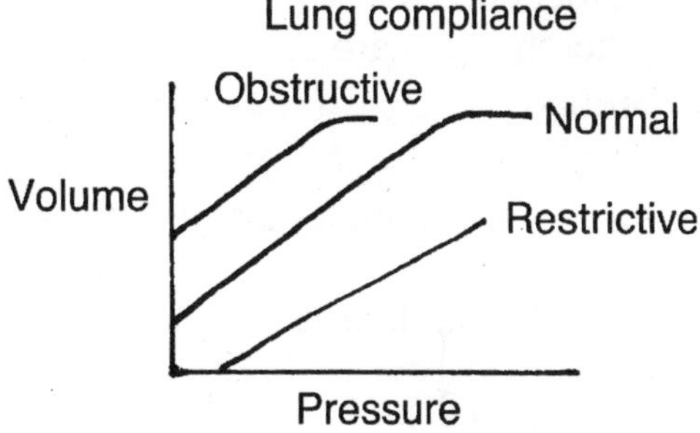


1. Restrictive diseases are characterized by difficulty getting the air in

2. There is decreased lung or chest wall compliance, i.e., increased stiffness

3. Breathing tends to be shallow and rapid. There is alveolar hypoventilation and increased dead space air

4. Restrictive processes may occur in the pleural space, thoracic cage, or lung tissue itself

B. Pleural cavity: Pleural space is normally only a potential space. If space is filled lung expansion may be prevented causing compression atelectasis.

1. Pleural effusion

   a. transudate

   b. exudate

   c. empyema

2. Hemothorax

3. Pneumothorax

   simple
   tension

C. Thoracic cage disorders

1. kyphoscoliosis

2. congenital malformations of chest wall

3. flail chest

4. Pickwickian syndrome

D. Pneumoconioses: "dust diseases," e.g., black lung, silicosis, asbestosis

1. Pathogenesis: inert particles in lung cause inflammatory response, but macrophages are unable to degrade the material. Fibrotic nodules form around particles. Lung fibrosis $\rightarrow \downarrow$elasticity.

a. decreased lung compliance

b. barrier to diffusion

2. Signs and symptoms

a. progressive dyspnea and hypoxemia

b. late: problems with $CO_2$ excretion

3. Treatment: prevention

E. ARDS (adult respiratory distress syndrome)

1. Etiology: Triggered by many factors:

a. shock

b. sepsis

c. trauma

d. fluid resuscitation

e. oxygen toxicity

2. Pathogenesis: widespread alveolar collapse and lack of surfactant associated with inflammation

a. atelectasis

b. pulmonary edema (non-cardiogenic)

c. pulmonary fibrosis and scarring

3. Signs and symptoms
    a. dyspnea
    b. severe hypoxemia
    c. 50% mortality
4. Treatment
    a. correct underlying cause
    b. PEEP
    c. $O_2$
    d. surfactant replacement

V. Lung Infection and Inflammation

A. Pneumonia

1. Causes

2. Viral pneumonia: less severe

3. Bacterial pneumonia: more severe
    a. Pneumococcal pneumonia
    b. Progression of bacterial pneumonia
        exudation
        consolidation
        resolution

B. Tuberculosis (mycobacterium tuberculosis)

1. Transmission

2. Pathogenesis "Ghon tubercule"

3. Signs and symptoms

4. Treatment

   Rifampin

   INH

5. TB testing

   a. Negative test: 1. never exposed

      2. exposed but not infected

   b. Positive test: 1. infected but no disease

      2. active TB disease

VI. Respiratory Insufficiency and Respiratory Failure

A. Insufficiency: cannot maintain normal ABGs under conditions of increased demand

B. Failure: $PaO_2 < 50$ mm Hg and/or $PaCO_2 > 50$ mm Hg

VII. Cor Pulmonale: Right Ventricular Hypertrophy Due to Respiratory Disease

A. Cause: pulmonary hypertension

B. Path: decreased cross-sectional area of pulmonary capillary bed

1. Destroyed lung tissue (COPD)

2. Restricted with fibrosis

3. Emboli

4. Hypoxic vasoconstriction

# ALTERATIONS IN ACID–BASE BALANCE

I. Basis of Acid–Base Problems

Occur when there is too much or too little acid in relation to base

II. Principles of Acid–Base Regulation

A. The body tightly regulates pH as enzyme function is impaired with large shifts, which are not compatible with life.

B. The $PaO_2$ and $SaO_2$ are important but are not a part of acid–base balance.

C. A fairly fixed ratio of $HCO_3^-$ to $H_2CO_3$ in the body maintains pH in the normal range. An increase in one is followed by an increase in other as the body tries to compensate and bring pH to normal.

$$\frac{HCO_3^-}{H_2CO_3} = \frac{20}{1}$$

D. Three main regulators of pH

1. buffers
2. lungs: regulate $H_2CO_3$
3. kidneys: regulate $HCO_3^-$ and $H^+$

E. Compensation vs. correction

F. The body will not normally overcompensate; e.g., if you start out with acidemia ($pH < 7.35$), the body will not overcompensate and get the pH back to $>7.40$.

G. Normal values

pH: 7.35–7.45

$PaCO_2$: 35–45 mm Hg

$PaO_2$: 80–100 mm Hg

$HCO_3^-$: 22–26 mEq/L

$SaO_2$: >95%

## III. Lab Tests Related to Acid–Base Disturbances

A. Serum K+

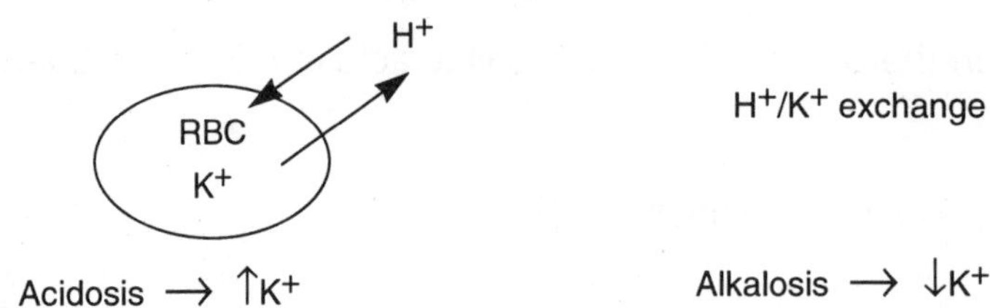


B. Chloride shift: To maintain electrical neutrality, the $Cl^-$ may change with changes in $HCO_3^-$

↑ $HCO_3^-$ ↔ ↓ $Cl^-$ (alkalosis)

↓ $HCO_3^-$ ↔ ↑ $Cl^-$ (acidosis)

C. Anion gap: difference between positive ions ($Na^+$, $K^+$) and negative ions ($Cl^-$, $HCO_3^-$)

1. Normal gap = 15
2. A large anion gap means there are some unmeasured ions, usually indicating metabolic acidosis.

## IV. Interpreting ABGs

| | Acidosis ← | | → Alkalosis |
|---|---|---|---|
| pH | 7.2 | 7.40 | 7.6 |
| (Resp) $CO_2$ | 60 | 40 | 20 |
| (Metabolic) $HCO_3^-$ | 18 | 24 | 30 |

A. Plot the pH: determines if acidosis or alkalosis

B. Plot the $CO_2$ and $HCO_3$. The value that is on the same side as the pH is the primary event.

C. The value that is either normal (not compensating) or on the opposite side is the secondary, compensatory event.

D. If both $CO_2$ and $HCO_3^-$ are on the same side as pH: mixed disorder.

V. Example Problems

A. pH 7.30, $CO_2$ 60, $HCO_3^-$ 28.6

B. pH 7.49, $CO_2$ 30, $HCO_3^-$ 22.2

C. pH 7.31, $CO_2$ 32, $HCO_3^-$ 15.6

D. pH 7.20, $CO_2$ 60, $HCO_3^-$ 22.7

VI. Examples of Specific Acid–Base Imbalances

A. Respiratory acidosis: $H_2CO_3$ excess

1. Cause: decreased alveolar ventilation

2. Signs and symptoms

headache

tachycardia

CNS depression

cardiac arrhythmias

3. Compensatory mechanisms: Kidneys retain $HCO_3^-$

4. Example

| Uncompensated | Partially Compensated | Compensated |
|---|---|---|
| pH: 7.26 | pH: 7.34 | pH: 7.37 |
| $PaCO_2$: 50 | $PaCO_2$: 50 | $PaCO_2$: 50 |
| $HCO_3^-$: 22 | $HCO_3^-$: 26.2 | $HCO_3^-$: 28 |

B. Respiratory alkalosis: $H_2CO_3$ deficit

1. Cause: increased alveolar ventilation (hyperventilation)

2. Signs and symptoms

   lightheadedness

   CNS irritability: tingling, tetany

   cardiac arrhythmias

3. Compensatory mechanisms: Kidneys excrete $HCO_3^-$

4. Example

| Uncompensated | Partially Compensated | Compensated |
|---|---|---|
| pH: 7.55 | pH: 7.48 | pH: 7.43 |
| $PaCO_2$: 30 | $PaCO_2$: 30 | $PaCO_2$: 30 |
| $HCO_3^-$: 24 | $HCO_3^-$: 21.7 | $HCO_3^-$: 19.3 |

C. Metabolic acidosis: noncarbonic acid excess

1. Causes

   acid accumulation: poisoning, abnormal metabolism, shock

   loss of base ($HCO_3^-$): diarrhea, pancreatic fistula

2. Signs and symptoms

   headache

   CNS depression

3. Compensatory mechanisms: Lungs excrete more $H_2CO_3$ ($H_2O + CO_2$)

4. Example

| Uncompensated | Partially Compensated | Compensated |
|---|---|---|
| pH: 7.28 | pH: 7.33 | pH: 7.37 |
| $PaCO_2$: 40 | $PaCO_2$: 35 | $PaCO_2$: 32 |
| $HCO_3^-$: 18 | $HCO_3^-$: 18 | $HCO_3^-$: 18 |

D. Metabolic alkalosis: noncarbonic acid deficit

1. Causes

base accumulation: excessive $NaHCO_3$ intake, blood transfusions

loss of acid: vomiting, gastric suction

2. Signs and symptoms:

CNS irritability → eventual CNS depression

3. Compensatory mechanisms: lungs retain $H_2CO_3$ ($H_2O + CO_2$)

4. Example

| Uncompensated | Partially Compensated | Compensated |
|---|---|---|
| pH: 7.64 | pH: 7.52 | pH: 7.45 |
| $PaCO_2$: 43 | $PaCO_2$: 57 | $PaCO_2$: 66 |
| $HCO_3^-$: 45 | $HCO_3^-$: 45 | $HCO_3^-$: 45 |

VII. Therapy for Acid–Base Disorders

A. Respiratory acidosis: artificial ventilation

measures to improve ventilation

B. Respiratory alkalosis: anti-anxiety measures

$O_2$ if due to hypoxemia

$CO_2$ rebreathing

C. Metabolic acidosis: give $NaHCO_3$

correct underlying cause (ketoacidosis)

improve tissue oxygenation (lactic acid)

D. Metabolic alkalosis: stop cause—antacids, ↓$Cl^-$, ↓$K^+$, vomiting

almost never give acid (HCl)

# ALTERATIONS IN FLUID AND ELECTROLYTE BALANCE

I. Water Imbalance Versus Saline Imbalance

A. Distribution of body water and electrolytes

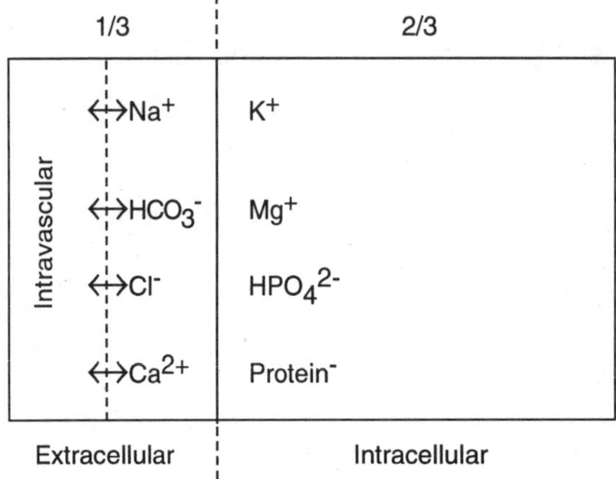


Two-thirds of the body's water is in the intracellular compartment. The extracellular compartment contains 1/3 of the total body water, which is distributed between the interstitial and intravascular spaces.

B. Saline is confined to extracellular body compartments

1. Sodium is osmotically active, i.e., it pulls water. Since sodium is an extracellular ion, saline (0.9% NaCl) will remain in the extracellular compartment.

2. Gain or loss of saline (iso-osmotic) is associated with increases and decreases in extracellular volume. Since the concentration of sodium in saline is the same as in the blood, gaining or losing saline will not change the serum $Na^+$ level.

3. History and signs and symptoms of fluid volume excess or deficit indicate saline disorders.

a. saline deficit (serum [Na+] → normal)

low blood pressure

orthostatic hypotension

weight loss

tachycardia

loss of skin turgor

low urine output

b. saline excess (serum [$Na^+$] $\rightarrow$ normal)

hypertension

weight gain

edema

signs and symptoms of congestive heart failure

increased urine output

C. Water distributes throughout both extracellular and intracellular compartments.

1. Water excess or deficit causes a change in concentration of solutes in the blood, which is reflected in the serum $Na^+$ level.

2. The main signs and symptoms are due to changes in osmolality, which cause cells to swell or shrink.

3. There may be associated hyper- or hypovolemia, but this must be determined by signs and symptoms.

4. Hypernatremia and hyponatremia

sodium: normal range is 135–145 mEq/L

| | Excess (Hypernatremia) | Deficit (Hyponatremia) |
|---|---|---|
| Causes | | |
| | Chronic diarrhea | Excess hypotonic IV fluid |
| | No access to water or ↓thirst | Excess ADH secretion |
| | High solute load (tube feeds) | Excess $H_2O$ intake |
| | | Tap water enemas |
| | | NG irrigation with $H_2O$ |
| | Diabetes insipidus | Psychogenic polydipsia |
| | Diabetes mellitus | |
| | ↑Resp rates | |
| Signs &symptoms | | |
| | Due to water deficit and increased osmolality | Due to a water excess and decreased osmolality |
| | Cells shrink | Cells swell |
| | Confusion, lethargy, muscle weakness, convulsions | Confusion, lethargy, nausea, coma |
| Treatment | | |
| | Prevent | Don't treat unless <130 mEq/L |
| | ↑Free water intake | Fluid restriction |
| | Treat slowly | Don't usually give hypertonic fluid |

5. Pathophysiology of hyper- and hyponatremia

a. hypernatremia

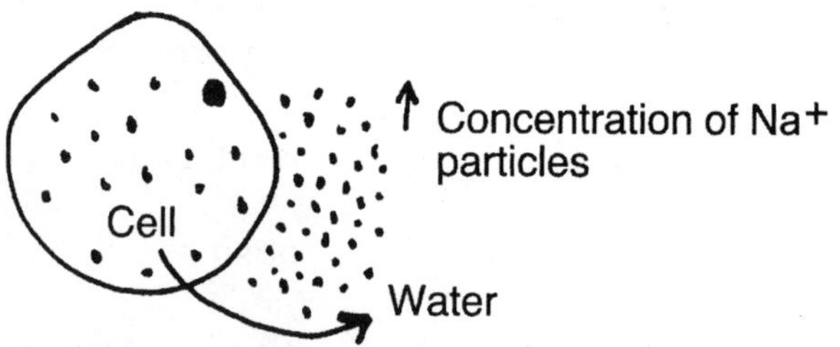


pathophysiology: Water moves out of cell according to concentration gradients, leading to cell shrinkage.

b. hyponatremia

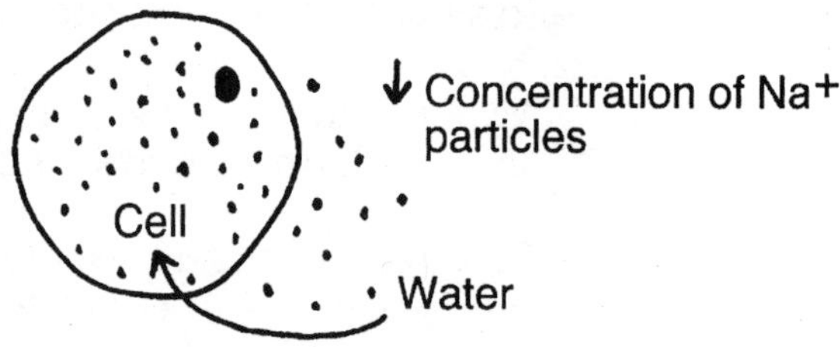


pathophysiology: Water moves into cells according to concentration gradients leading to cell swelling.

II. Changes in Many Electrolyte Levels are Due to

A. Changes in intake

B. Changes in output

C. Shifts between intracellular and extracellular compartments

III. Disorders of Potassium Balance

A. $K^+$ is responsible for the resting membrane potential of cells

B. Hyperkalemia: makes resting potential less negative. Nerve and muscle depolarize more easily. May not be able to repolarize normally.

1. muscle weakness and cardiac arrhythmias

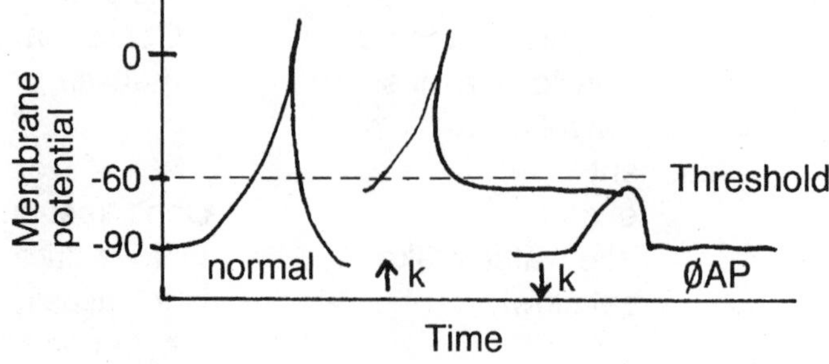

C. Hypokalemia: hyperpolarizes membrane potential making it more difficult to reach threshold and create an action potential.

1. Muscle weakness and cardiac arrhythmias

D. Potassium excess and deficit

potassium: normal range is 3.5–5.0 mEq/L

| | Excess (Hyperkalemia) | Deficit (Hypokalemia) |
|---|---|---|
| Causes | | |
| | Increased intake | Decreased intake |
| | Accidental IV bolus | NPO |
| | Salt substitute in children | Anorexia |
| | Administration of old blood | Increased excretion |
| | | Diuretics |
| | | ↑aldosterone (Conn's) |
| | Decreased excretion | Diarrhea/vomiting/NG suction |
| | Oliguric renal failure | Shift into cells |
| | ↓aldosterone secretion | Alkalosis |
| | Shift from body cells | |
| | Crushing injuries | |
| | Acidosis | |
| | Chemotherapy | |
| Signs and symptoms | | |
| | Due to decrease (less negative) in resting potential | Due to increased resting potential (more negative) |
| | Muscle weakness | Muscle weakness |
| | Ascending paralysis | Paralytic ileus |
| | Cardiac arrhythmias | Cardiac arrhythmias |
| Treatment | | |
| | Dialysis | $K^+$ rich foods/fluids |
| | Kayexalate | Oral/IV KCL |
| | Insulin/glucose | Correct alkalosis |
| | Correct acidosis | |

IV. Disorders of Calcium Balance

A. Only ionized calcium is physiologically active. Bound calcium is not.

B. Calcium affects membrane permeability and the threshold potential.

C. Hypercalcemia: Decreased membrane permeability and higher threshold makes it more difficult to excite nerve/muscle cells.

D. Hypocalcemia: Increased permeability and lower threshold make nerve/muscle cells easier to stimulate.

E. Calcium excess and deficit

calcium: normal ranges are 9–11 mg/100 mL (total) or 4.5–6 mEq/L (ionized)

| | Excess (Hypercalcemia) | Deficit (Hypocalcemia) |
|---|---|---|
| Causes | | |
| | Increased intake | Decreased intake |
| | Excessive antacids | Malabsorption |
| | Excessive vitamin D | Milk intolerance |
| | Decreased excretion | Increased excretion |
| | Hyperparathyroidism | Chronic renal insufficiency |
| | Shift from cells | Hypoparathyroidism |
| | Immobility | Shift out of blood |
| | Hyperparathyroidism | Massive blood transfusion (citrate) |
| | Some malignancies | Hypoalbuminemia |
| Signs and syptoms | | |
| | Due to ↓cell membrane permeability and ↓neuromuscular excitability | Due to ↑membrane permeability and ↑ neuromuscular excitability |
| | Constipation | Twitching, cramping |
| | Muscle weakness | + Chvostek's sign |
| | CNS depression | + Trousseau's sign |
| | | Convulsions, laryngospasm |
| Treatment | | |
| | ↑Fluid intake | Calcium supplement IV/po |
| | Treat cause | |
| | Parathyroidectomy | |

V. Disorders of Magnesium Balance

A. Magnesium interferes with the release of acetylcholine from the neuromuscular junction. Actions on neuromuscular excitability are clinically similar to calcium.

B. Hypermagnesemia: decreased excitability

C. Hypomagnesemia: increased excitability

D. Magnesium excess and deficit

magnesium: normal range is 1.5-2.5 mEq/L

| | Excess (Hypermagnesemia) | Deficit (Hypomagnesemia) |
|---|---|---|
| Causes | | |
| | ↑ Antacid intake | Malabsorption |
| | IV infusion (for PIH) | Alcoholism |
| | Renal failure | Diuretics |
| Signs and symptoms | | |
| | Due to ↓ release of acetylcholine | Due to ↑ excitability |
| | Hypotonic, floppy muscles | Hypertonic muscles |
| | Similar to hypercalcemia | Similar to hypocalcemia |
| Treatment | | |
| | ↑ Fluid intake | $MgSO_4$ supplement IV/po |
| | Diuretics | |

VI. Review

A. Floppy, weak muscles

1. ↑ or ↓ $K^+$

2. ↑ $Mg^{2+}$

3. ↑ $Ca^{2+}$

B. Twitchy easily stimulated muscles

1. ↓ $Ca^{2+}$

2. ↓ $Mg^{2+}$

## ALTERATIONS IN RENAL FUNCTION

I. Hormonal Control of Urine Output

   A. Antidiuretic hormone (ADH)

   B. Angiotensin II

   C. Aldosterone

   D. Atrial Natriuretic Peptide (ANP)

II. Mechanisms of Urine Concentration

   A. Purpose: concentrate urine and conserve body fluids

   B. Site: occurs in juxtamedullary nephrons

   C. Dysfunction: polyuria, nocturia, fixed specific gravity

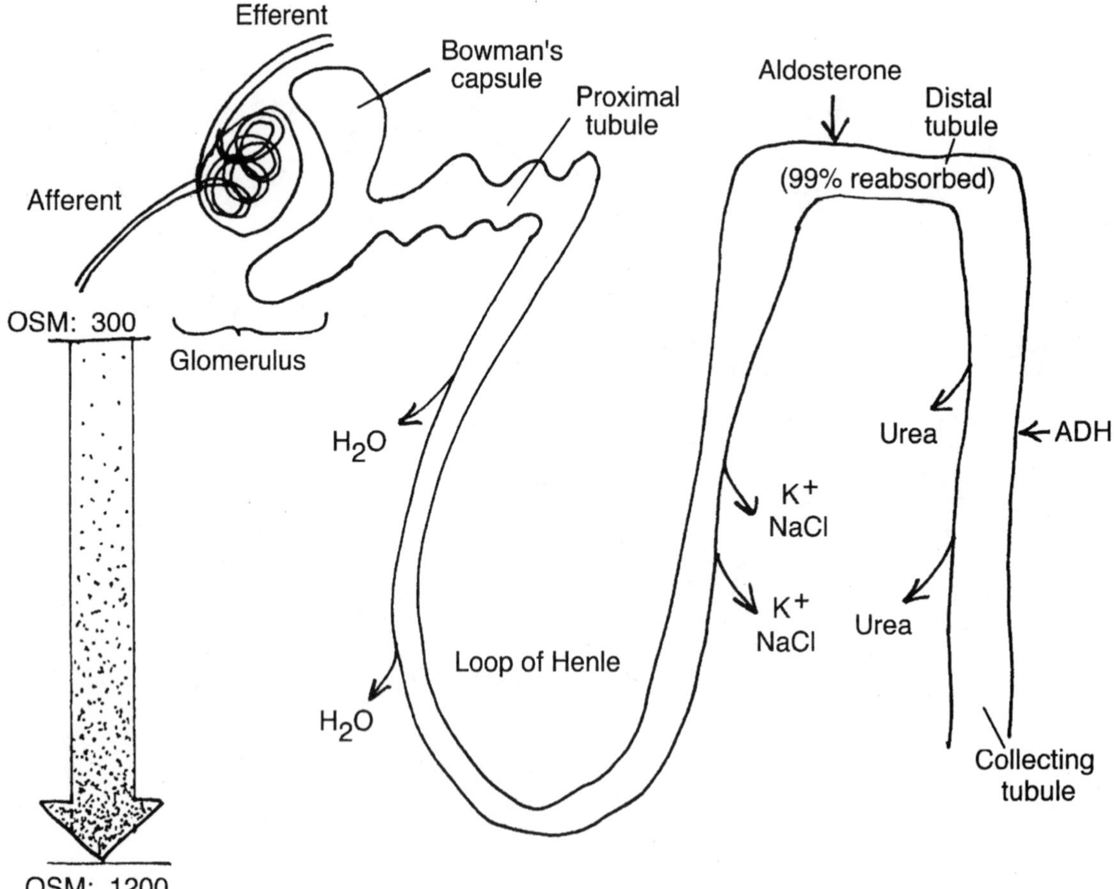

III. Congenital/Hereditary Defects of Renal System

A. Horseshoe

B. Supernumerary

C. Renal agenesis

D. Polycystic kidney disease

1. Newborn: autosomal recessive

2. Adult: autosomal dominant—third leading cause of chronic renal failure

IV. Obstructive Disorders of the Urinary Tract

A. Benign prostatic hyperplasia

B. Prostate cancer

C. Bladder tumors

D. Urinary calculi; nephrolithiasis

E. Plugged urinary catheter

V. Infections of the Urinary Tract

A. Cystitis and/or urethritis (lower UTI)

1. Signs and symptoms

2. Predisposing factors

a. female

b. stasis of urine

c. catheterization

3. Organism: *E.coli*

4. Treatment/prevention

B. Pyelonephritis (upper UTI) kidney infected

1. Signs and symptoms

a. Acute: CVA tenderness

chills/fever

pyuria

white blood cell casts in urine

b. Chronic: May be asymptomatic

2. Predisposing factors

a. complication of cystitis

b. malimplanation of ureters

c. vesico-ureteral reflux

d. hydroureter, hydronephrosis

3. Organism: *E.coli*

4. Treatment: Antibiotics—Usually no residual kidney damage. Inadequately treated or recurrent pyelonephritis may lead to chronic pyelonephritis.

5. Chronic pyelonephritis: 2nd leading cause of RF

a. Signs and symptoms: vague, inability to concentrate urine

b. IVP: small, scarred kidneys

VI. Inflammatory Renal Disease: Glomerulonephritis (#1 cause of renal failure)

A. Causes of GN

1. Immune complex reaction after strep infection

2. Autoimmune destruction of glomerular basement membrane e.g., Goodpasture's

3. Ideopathic

B. Pathology: inflammation of glomerulus (not infection)

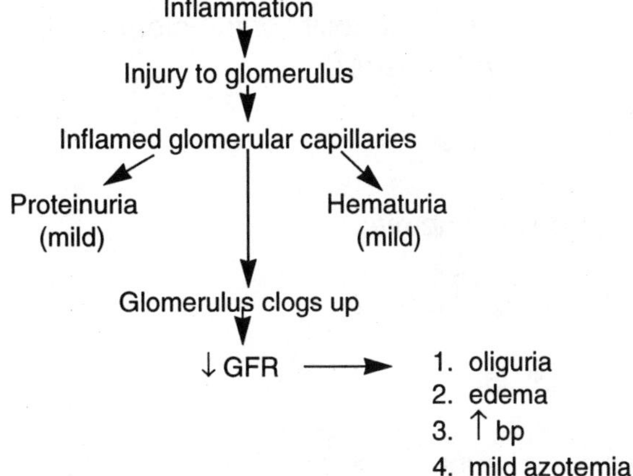


C. Types of glomerulonephritis

1. Acute GN (usually post-strep infection)

   children
   90% complete recovery
   treat strep with antibiotics to avoid

2. Rapidly progressing GN (unknown cause)

   rapid kidney destruction
   progress to renal failure (2 months to 2 years)

3. Chronic GN (autoimmune, unknown)

   chronic inflammation of glomerulus
   leads to (1) chronic renal failure or (2) nephrosis

VII. Compare and Contrast Pyelonephritis (PN) and Glomerulonephritis (GN)

| | PN | GN |
|---|---|---|
| Cause | | |
| S/S | | |
| Prognosis | | |
| Treatment | | |

## VIII. Nephrotic Syndrome (Nephrosis)

A. Due to increased permeability of the glomerular membrane secondary to GN or unknown causes

1. Proteinuria
2. Hypoalbuminemia
3. Generalized edema
4. Hyperlipidemia

B. Management: supportive/symptomatic, no cure

1. Steroids
2. Chemotherapy
3. High protein diet
4. Adequate fluid intake
5. Albumin?

C. Prognosis

1. May spontaneously resolve
2. May progress to renal failure

## IX. Vascular Kidney Disorders

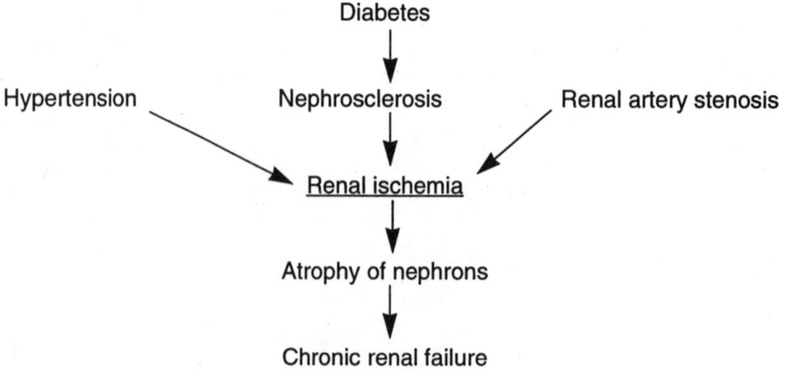

X. Chronic Renal Failure

A.

| Cause | Example |
|---|---|
| Inflammatory | |
| Infection | |
| Toxins | |
| Obstructive nephropathy | |
| Congenital/hereditary | |
| Renal vascular disease | |

B. Stages of CRF (clinical course) may progress slowly over many years or rapidly over a few weeks

1. Decreased renal reserve: Up to 75% of nephrons are destroyed. Can still function well on 25% of nephrons.

   no signs or symptoms

   BUN/creatine normal

   not usually diagnosed

2. Renal insufficiency >75%, <90% nephrons destroyed. Concentrating mechanism begins to fail. Unable to concentrate urine normally.

   polyuria, nocturia

   modest increase BUN, creatinine

   may be diet controlled

3. End-stage renal failure > 90% nephrons destroyed. Make very little urine, unable to excrete waste products.

   oliguria → anuria

   fixed specific gravity

   uremia, "urine in the blood"

XI. Uremic Syndrome (Uremia)

A. Definition: complex of symptoms due to failure of kidneys to excrete wastes, fluids, and electrolytes and perform other metabolic functions

B. Pathology

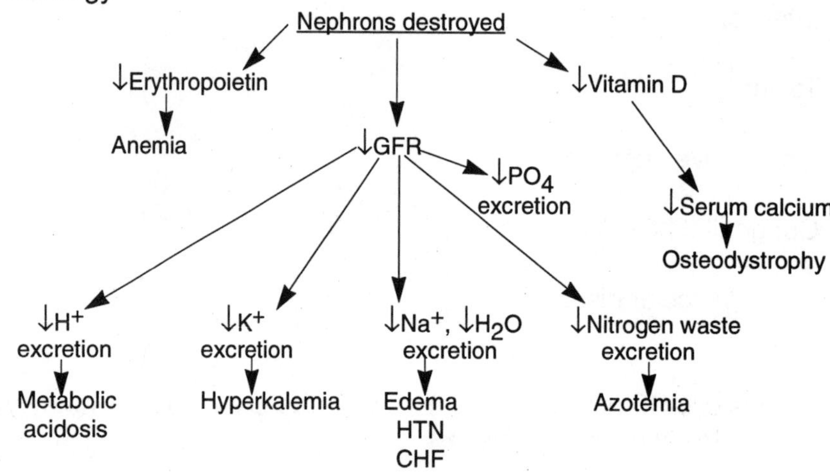


1. Azotemia: ↑BUN and serum creatine and uric acid

   BUN: 10–20 mg/100 mL (normal range)

   creatinine: 0.7–1.5 mg/100 ml (normal range)

   uric acid: excreted through skin → "uremic frost"

2. Osteodystrophy

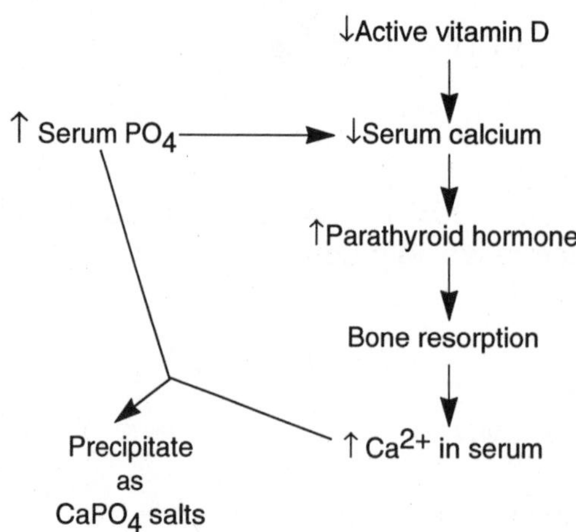

C. Management of renal failure

1. Restrict fluids, $Na^+$, $K^+$, $PO_4$

2. Low protein diet

3. Antacids for $PO_4$ binding

4. Vitamin D

5. Dialysis → renal transplant

XII. Compare and Contrast Nephrotic and Uremic Syndromes

| | Nephrotic | Uremic |
|---|---|---|
| Anemia | | |
| Proteinuria | | |
| Metabolic acidosis | | |
| Azotemia | | |
| Serum K | | |
| Serum protein | | |
| Oliguria | | |
| Edema | | |
| Diet | | |

XIII. Acute Renal Failure (ARF)

A. Sudden severe decrease in renal function caused by

1. Prerenal

2. Intrarenal

3. Postrenal

B. Most ARF is due to prerenal causes. There is inadequate blood flow to the kidney, which results in ischemia and ↓GFR.

1. Related to: shock
trauma
sepsis
hemorrhage
dehydration
massive hemolysis

2. Stages of ARF

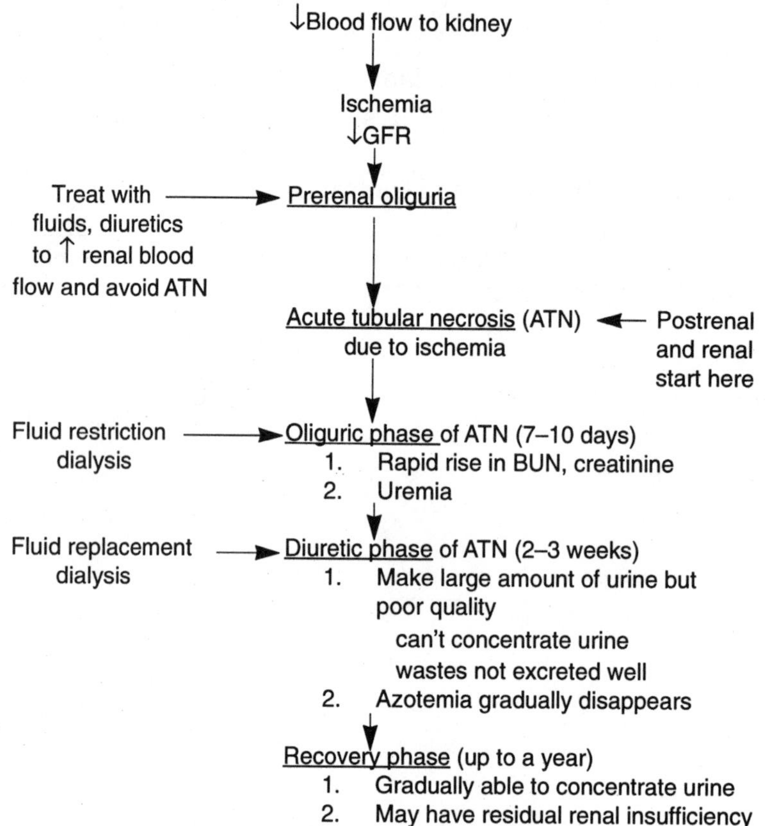


3. Prognosis: 50% mortality in oliguric/diuretic phases

C. Intrarenal ARF: due to primary damage to kidney cells

1. Toxic antibiotics

2. Ingestion of poisons

D. Postrenal ARF: due to obstruction to flow of urine out of kidney. Back pressure causes necrosis of nephrons.

1. BPH

2. Stones

# ALTERATIONS IN NUTRITION AND METABOLISM

I. Disorders of Nutrition

A. Alterations in the processes of ingesting, digesting, and absorbing nutrients and eliminating waste.

B. Ingestion

1. Anorexia

2. Pica

3. Nausea and vomiting

4. Esophageal atresia

tracheoesophageal fistula

5. Esophageal stenosis

6. Cleft lip/palate

7. Anorexia nervosa

8. Pyloric stenosis

projectile vomiting

B. Maldigestion: Digestion is initiated in stomach but most occurs in the small intestine. Maldigestion usually results from enzyme deficiencies.

1. Lactase deficiency: "milk intolerance"

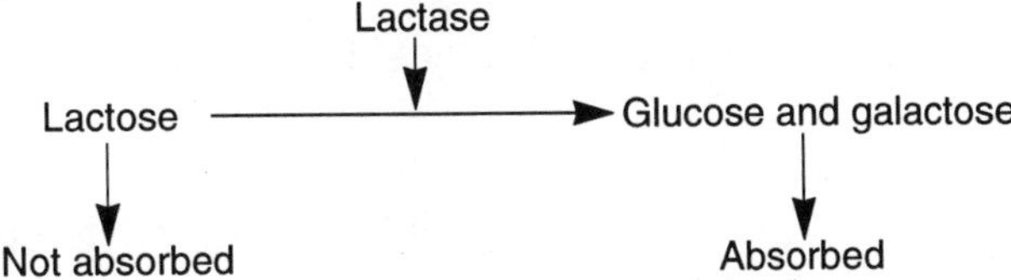


build up of lactose in bowel and bacteria break it down, causing bloating, gas, cramps, diarrhea.

2. Pancreatitis: Pancreatic enzymes are not secreted into bowel

3. Cystic fibrosis: Autosomal recessive gene defect. Abnormally thick secretions.

pancreatic ducts blocked and eventually destroyed

C. Malabsorption: Signs and symptoms of maldigestion and malabsorption are similar: (1) malnutrition, (2) abnormal intestinal contents → (3) diarrhea. Maldigestion can be a cause of malabsorption.

1. Intestinal parasites

2. Gastrectomy: removal of all or part of stomach; usually for ulcers or cancer

loss of stomach as reservoir for food

dumping syndrome

loss of intrinsic factor

3. Celiac disease (Sprue): inflammatory response in small intestine due to ingestion of gluten-containing foods (wheat, corn, oats, rye, barley)

inflammation → sloughing of intestinal villi

mechanism ?

4. Cholecystitis/cholelithiasis: gall bladder disorders resulting in lack of bile salts secreted into small intestine

malabsorption of fats (steatorrhea)

fat intolerance

5. Regional enteritis, "Crohn's disease": inflammation, scarring, and thickening of the bowel wall.

general malabsorption

D. Elimination: Disorders are generally either an obstruction of elimination or diarrhea.

1. Diarrhea: Major problem is fluid and electrolyte disorder as well as discomfort.

a. causes

osmotic changes

secretory changes

mucosal damage

altered motility

b. Crohn's disease

etiology: unknown, runs in families; stress-related

patho: inflammation, swelling, thickening of bowel wall. Involves all layers of the bowel wall. Bowel becomes scarred, stiff, nonfunctional for absorption. Lesions are skip lesions.

S/S: characterized by remissions and exacerbations

malabsorption
bloody diarrhea

complication: Fistula formation between loops of bowel

treatment: no cure—palliative

diet: ↑cal, low fat, low fiber

steroids

stress management

bowel resection

c. ulcerative colitis: many similarities to Crohn's disease

etiology: unknown—familial; triggered by emotional upset; stress related.

patho: inflammation and sloughing of mucosal layer only of the colon; lesions continuous with the rectum.

S/S: bloody diarrhea

complication: after 10 years, an increased potential for malignant changes in colon

treatment: palliative

diet: ↑calcium, ↓fiber

steroids

stress management

surgery colostomy

d. compare and contrast Crohn's and ulcerative colitis

| | Crohn's | UC |
|---|---|---|
| Lesion type | | |
| Location | | |
| Diarrhea | | |
| Malignant potential | | |
| Fistula formation | | |

2. Constipation and bowel obstruction

a. mechanical obstruction: Hyperactive peristalsis upstream from obstruction often causes crampy pain, N&V. Eventually increased pressure in bowel leads to absence of bowel activity. Major complications are necrosis of bowel and peritonitis. Treatment is usually surgery.

intussusception "telescoping"

volvulus "twisting"

adhesions

strangulated hernia

tumors

impaction

b. functional bowel obstruction: No peristaltic movement, but no mechanical obstruction. No bowel sounds are present; less cramping and pain. Treatment is bowel decompression and time.

bowel manipulation (surgery)

narcotic anesthesia

peritonitis

II. Inflammatory Disorders of GI System: very common problems

A. Esophagitis: often secondary to hiatal hernia. Gastric acid irritates esophageal mucosa.

1. Treatment

small meals
do not lie down after eating
antacids
surgery

B. Gastritis: inflammation of stomach

1. Acute gastritis: Transient inflammation of stomach lining. Commonly associated with ETOH and aspirin ingestion.

2. Chronic gastritis: Progressive atrophy of stomach lining. May lead to:

a. pernicious anemia
b. ↓ HCl production
c. gastric ulcer

C. Peptic ulcer disease (PUD): Ulcerations of the GI tract due to acid-pepsin activity. Common locations are esophagus, stomach, duodenum.

1. Etiology

a. ↑ Pepsin secretion, "Cushings"

b. ↓ Mucosal barrier, "Curlings"

c. "Stress" ulcers common development in pts with severe trauma or physiologic stress.

2. S/S: pain, often relieved by food/antacids

3. Complications

a. bleeding
b. perforation

4. Treatment

a. diet (avoid ETOH)
b. antacids
c. $H_2$ antagonists
d. vagotomy
e. surgical removal of ulcerated area

D. Appendicitis: inflammation of appendix. The appendix is a blind pouch that is often obstructed (by stool) and becomes inflamed.

1. Signs and symptoms

   right lower quadrant pain
   low grade fever
   rebound tenderness

2. Treatment: surgical removal of appendix

3. Complication: rupture and peritonitis. Peritonitis is infection/ inflammation of peritoneal cavity.

   a. manifestations

      fever
      paralytic ileus
      board-like abdomen
      shock/sepsis

   b. treatment

      antibiotics
      F & E replacement
      often leave wound open to drain

E. Diverticulosis/diverticulitis: Diverticulosis is a herniation of the mucosal layer through the muscle layer of the colon. If pouches become inflamed, it is diverticulitis.

1. Etiology: due to increased intraluminal pressure

   a. ↓ bulk in diet
   b. ↓ volume of stool
   c. irregular bowel habits

2. Signs and symptoms: asymptomatic unless inflamed (diverticulitis)

   a. abdominal pain, cramping, bloating, gas
   b. blood in stool
   c. systemic signs of inflammation

3. Complication: potential for perforation

4. Treatment

   a. prevention: dietary fiber

b. treatment of diverticulitis

rest the bowel

stool softeners

bed rest

low fiber diet

F. Pancreatitis: inflammation of pancreas

1. Etiology: Normally pancreatic digestive enzymes are inactive while in the pancreas. They are somehow activated in the pancreas, causing autodigestion and necrosis. The cause is unclear.

   a. alcohol?

   b. gallstones with reflux of bile?

2. Acute pancreatitis: severe, sudden onset

   a. severe abdominal pain

   b. huge fluid loss into abdomen
      shock

   c. ↑ serum amylase and lipase (diagnostic)

   d. hyperglycemia

   e. may be life threatening

3. Treatment of acute pancreatitis

   fluid replacement

   pain relief

   antibiotics (peritonitis)

   decrease pancreatic activity

      NPO

      gastric suction

      parenteral nutrition

4. Chronic pancreatitis: Progressive destruction of pancreatic tissue. Associated with chronic alcoholism and chronic biliary obstruction.

   a. less dramatic signs and symptoms

   b. progressive loss of exocrine and endocrine function

G. Cholecystitis: inflammation of gallbladder

1. Etiology: cholelithiasis (gallstones) which block the drainage of bile

   a. ↑ pressure in gallbladder

   b. ↑ concentration of bile, irritation

   c. Reason gall stones form is not clear. They occur more often with obesity, pregnancy, and oral contraceptive use. May be altered cholesterol metabolism.

2. Signs and symptoms: stones may be asymptomatic

   a. pain: colicky flank pain

   b. fat intolerance

   c. steatorrhea

3. Treatment: cholecystectomy

III. Disorders of the Liver and Nutrient Metabolism

A. Functions of the liver

1. Metabolism of nutrients, storage of vitamins. Production of many serum proteins and enzymes.

2. Detoxification of drugs, hormones, alcohol, steroids

3. Formation and excretion of bile: conjugation of bilirubin

4. Synthesis of urea

B. General signs and symptoms of liver dysfunction

1. Malnutrition due to inadequate nutrient metabolism

   a. Inborn errors of metabolism, e.g., galactosemia and phenylketonuria (PKU). Person lacks an essential liver enzyme necessary to break down these nutrients.

b. Hypoalbuminemia and generalized edema. Liver synthesizes inadequate amounts of proteins into the blood.

c. Inadequate production of immune globulins, which also require protein. Leads to susceptibility to infection.

d. Inadequate production of protein clotting factors leads to bleeding tendencies.

2. Accumulations of toxins and hormones due to inadequate detoxification.

a. People with liver disease usually must receive lower doses of drugs.

b. Accumulation of hormones such as steroids (estrogen) may lead to feminization of males.

3. Inadequate conjugation and excretion of bilirubin will cause it to accumulate in tissues where it is toxic (jaundice). Jaundice may be caused by

a. liver disease

b. increased RBC destruction (hemolysis)

c. obstruction in biliary system

4. If liver is unable to convert nitrogenous waste (ammonia) to urea which can be excreted by kidney, there will be increased blood ammonia. Ammonia is toxic to cells, especially nerve cells.

C. Liver inflammation: hepatitis

1. Etiology

a. viral: hepatitis A, hepatitis B, hepatitis C

b. toxic: alcohol, drugs

c. biliary obstruction

2. Acute viral hepatitis: general signs and symptoms include

fatigue
flu-like symptoms
anorexia
hepatomegaly
jaundice
elevated liver enzymes (SGOT, SGPT)

3. Comparison of hepatitis A and B

| | Hepatitis A | Hepatitis B |
|---|---|---|
| Common route of transmission | Fecal/oral | Blood and body fluids |
| Other names | “Infectious” | “Serum” |
| Risk group | Institutionalized poor sanitation | IV drug abusers and health-care workers |
| Incubation | About 30 days<br>No carriers | About 90 days<br>Carriers (5–10%) |
| Symptoms | Less severe | More severe |
| Treatment | Rest and fluids | Rest and fluids |

4. Acute alcoholic hepatitis: Similar signs and symptoms as viral hepatitis. May follow acute ingestion of large amounts of alcohol.

D. Liver cirrhosis: Liver is irreversibly destroyed with accumulation of fibrous scar tissue. Loss of liver function, hepatocellular failure, and liver becomes an obstruction to blood flow from the gut; portal hypertension.

1. Etiology

a. Most commonly due to chronic alcohol use. Alcohol is toxic to liver cells. Liver cells use alcohol as fuel source and do not metabolize fats and other substances. “Fatty liver” has accumulations of fat in cells; cells eventually die.

b. Biliary cirrhosis is due to obstruction in biliary drainage, which leads to building pressure, irritation of the liver.

c. Postnecrotic cirrhosis is a complication of viral or toxic hepatitis in which there is massive liver necrosis.

d. Cardiac cirrhosis is due to severe right heart failure which causes prolonged venous liver congestion and eventual liver necrosis and fibrosis.

2. Signs and symptoms: due to hepatocellular failure and to portal hypertension. (Recall normal function and determine what would happen if nonfunctional.)

a. hepatocellular failure

| Hepatocyte Function | Hepatocyte Dysfunction |
|---|---|
| Excrete bilirubin | Jaundice |
| Protein synthesis | Hypoalbuminemia and generalized edema |
| | ↓ Clotting factors/bleeding tendencies |
| | ↓ Immunoglobulins |
| Metabolize steroid hormones | Gynecomastia<br>Testicular atrophy<br>Palmar erythema<br>Spider nevi |
| Synthesis of urea and excretion of ammonia | Hepatic encephalopathy |

b. hepatic encephalopathy is a mental deterioration associated with increased blood ammonia levels. It may be triggered by an increase in blood proteins (diet, GI bleed).

(i) stages:

confusion, personality change

asterixis "flapping tremor"

combative

coma

(ii) treatment: decrease protein intake; remove blood from GI tract

c. portal hypertension: The portal vein drains blood from the gut to the liver. A cirrhotic liver obstructs blood flow through the liver and pressure builds up in the portal system.

(i) ascites: fluid in the abdominal cavity due to leakage of fluid from liver (hypoalbuminemia also contributes to development of ascites)

(ii) pressure reflected back through the venous system of GI tract

splenomegaly

hemorrhoids

esophageal varices: often severe bleeding risk

(iii) treatment

balloon tamponade of bleeding varices

portacaval shunt

E. Liver cancer: May also have signs and symptoms similar to cirrhosis. Liver cancer is almost always metastatic. The survival rate is less than 5%.

F. Liver failure: This term is usually used if a person has hepatocellular failure and loss of liver function, but does not necessarily have a fibrotic, cirrhotic liver. They may not have signs/symptoms of portal hypertension.

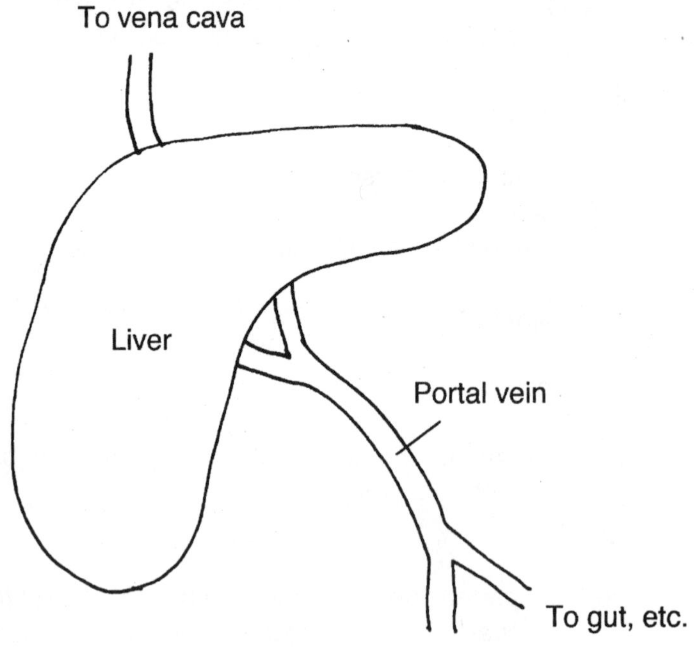

# ALTERATIONS IN ENDOCRINE FUNCTION

I. Functions of Classic Endocrine System

A. A communication network that uses hormones to send information about the state of the organism from cell to cell, organ to organ

B. Involved in many functions that require interaction among several systems

1. Response to stress or injury

2. Growth and development

3. Reproduction

4. Fluid and electrolyte balance

C. Numerous hormonal peptides have endocrine-like functions but are not part of the classic endocrine system. These are called diffuse or putative hormones. Examples are endorphins, prostaglandins, vasoactive intestinal peptides, etc.

II. Pituitary Hormones and Feedback Regulation

A. Pituitary hormones

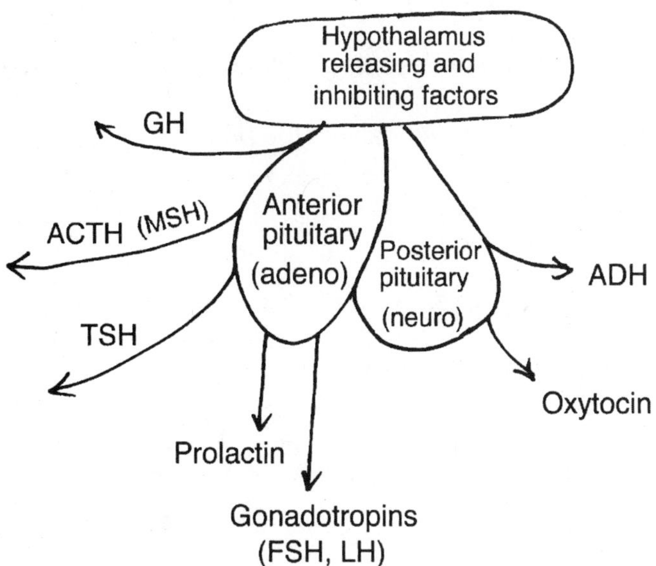


B. Negative feedback regulation

1. Hypothalamus is very involved in hormone regulation via several releasing factors and inhibiting factors that act on the pituitary.

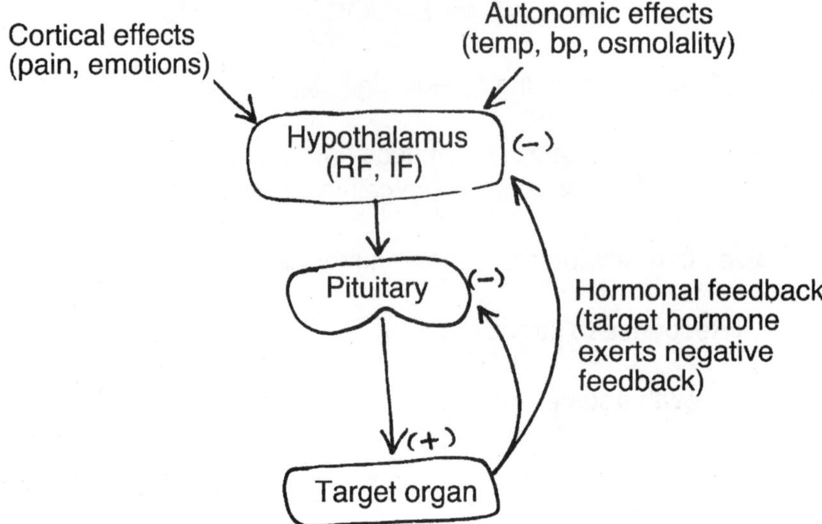


2. Other hormone systems that are not under pituitary control also use negative feedback:

   a. aldosterone ⟶ blood volume

   b. parathyroid hormone ⟶ blood calcium

   c. insulin ⟶ blood glucose

C. Primary versus secondary endocrine disorders

1. Primary: defect is within the target gland (thyroid, adrenal)

2. Secondary: defect originates with the pituitary

III. Two Disorders of Endocrine System

| | Hypersecretion | Hyposecretion |
|---|---|---|
| Etiology | Idiopathic<br>Secreting tumors | Autoimmune destruction<br>Nonsecreting tumors<br>Ischemia/infarction<br>Surgical removal<br>Receptor defects |
| Treatment | Surgical removal of all or part of gland<br>Drugs to destroy gland | Hormone replacement |

IV. Disorders of Growth and Development

A. Growth hormone

| Normal Function | Excess | Deficit |
|---|---|---|
| Growth of body cells. Glucose metabolism (↑ in GH ↑ blood glucose) | Giantism (child)<br>Acromegaly (adult)<br>↑ bone bulk<br>Course facial features<br>Large hands/feet<br>Widely spaced teeth<br>Hyperglycemia<br>↑ Serum GH | Dwarfism (child)<br>No S/S (adult) |

B. Diagnosis: Xray, glucose, and GH assay. A pituitary tumor is often responsible for excess GH. Other pituitary hormones are often affected. May have S/S of increased ICP if due to tumor.

C. Treatment: Trans sphenoidal hypophysectomy (removal of pituitary). The treatment usually results in panhypopituitarism and then requires life-long replacement of hormones affected. The surgery often leads to short-term diabetes insipidus due to swelling of posterior pituitary.

V. Disorders of Stress Response

A. Adrenocortical hormones: glucocorticoids (ACTH)

| Normal Function | Excess | Deficit |
|---|---|---|
| Gluconeogenesis<br>Maintenance of bp<br>Response to stress<br>Some mineral corticoid activity<br>↑ $Na^+$ ↓ $K^+$ inhibit immune response | Cushings<br><br>Muscle wasting<br>Fat redistribution<br>Moon face<br>Buffalo hump<br>Truncal obesity<br>Easy bruising<br>Hyperglycemia<br>↑ Infection risk<br>↓ $K^+$<br>Osteoporosis<br>Mood changes | Addisons or adrenal insufficiency<br>Hypoglycemia<br>↑ $K^+$<br>↓ bp<br>↓ Blood volume<br>Primary: blotchy dark skin pigmentation |

B. Diagnosis: Blood and urine assay of cortisol and metabolites. ACTH assay. ACTH assay is important to determine if problem is primary or secondary. An injection of ACTH may be given to see if it affects cortisol levels.

C. Treatment: Cushings may be caused by excess steroid administration, and a decrease in dosage is indicated. A secreting tumor (either pituitary or adrenal) is usually surgically removed. Steroid replacement is given for adrenocortical insufficiency. Periods of stress (i.e., surgery) require an increase in dosage.

D. Addison's crisis: may be precipitated by stress

E. Adrenogenital syndrome: a form of adrenocortical insufficiency that results in the production of large amounts of androgens

1. Etiology: a gene defect that results in absence of one or more enzymes necessary for making cortisol in the adrenal cortex (primary) Autosomal recessive.

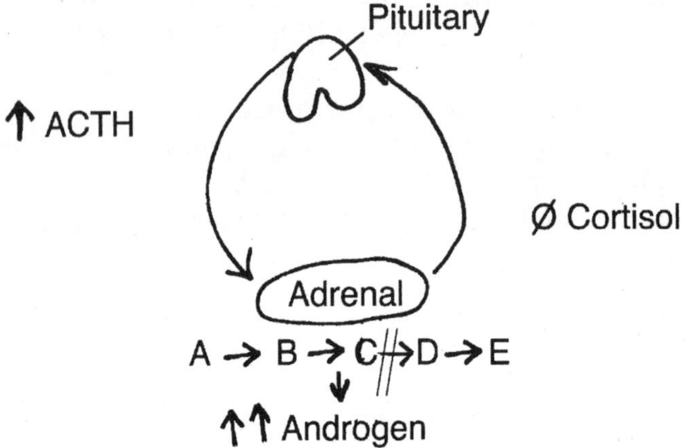


2. Patho: Lack of cortisol causes the pituitary to secrete large amounts of ACTH which stimulates the adrenal gland. This results in adrenal hyperplasia and formation of large amounts of cortisol precursors (A & B). These are also precursors for androgens.

3. Signs and symptoms: In addition to adrenal insufficiency, there is masculinization.

4. Treatment: Cortisol

F. Catecholamines: dopamine, epinephrine, norepinephrine; from adrenal medulla

| Normal Function | Excess | Deficit |
|---|---|---|
| "Fight or flight" <br> ↑ bp <br> ↑ hr <br> ↑ blood glucose | Pheochromocytoma <br> Benign tumor <br> Hypertension <br> Tachycardia <br> Palpitations <br> Hyperglycemia <br> Headache <br> Nausea <br> Blurred vision | No problem: SNS compensates |

1. Diagnosis: Signs and symptoms tend to come and go as spurts of catecholamines are released by the tumor. This makes diagnosis harder. Measure plasma and urine catecholamines. 24-hr urine for VMA (vanillylmandelic acid. X-ray—,may see tumor.

2. Treatment: Prior to surgery, may need sympathetic blocking drugs. After adrenalectomy may need sympathomimetics for a time. Major complication is stroke. Adrenalectomy usually cures the hypertension.

VI. Disorders of Fluid and Electrolyte Balance

A. Aldosterone (adrenal cortex)

| Normal Function | Excess | Deficit |
|---|---|---|
| ↑ Blood volume <br> ↑ $Na^+$ reabsorption <br> ↑ $K^+$ excretion | Aldosteronism <br> Hypertension <br> Edema <br> Weight gain <br> ↓$K^+$ | Usually occurs with primary adrenal insufficiency (see Addisons) |

1. Etiology: Aldosterone secretion is regulated by the Renin-Angiotensin-Aldosterone system. Too much aldosterone secretion occurs when renal perfusion is inadequate such as in heart failure.

2. Treatment: Treat underlying cause. Angiotensin-converting enzyme inhibitors (Captopril)

B. Parathyroid hormone

| Normal Function | Excess | Deficit |
|---|---|---|
| To ↑ serum calcium levels<br>1. bone resorption<br>2. gut absorption<br>3. renal absorption | Hyperparathyroidism<br>↑Serum calcium<br>Bone resorption<br>↓Neuromuscular activity<br>constipation<br>weakness<br>CNS depression | Hypoparathyroidism<br>↓Serum calcium<br>↑Neuromuscular activity<br>tetany,spasm<br>convulsion<br>+ Chvostek's<br>+ Trousseau's |

1. Etiology: The parathyroid glands (four to six pairs) are imbedded in the thyroid gland. Benign tumor is most common cause of hyperparathyroidism. Thyroidectomy (with removal of parathyroids) is common cause of hypoparathyroidism.

2. Treatment: Parathyroidectomy for hyperparathyroidism. High calcium intake and vitamin D supplements for hypoparathyroidism.

VII. Disorders of Hormonal Control of Metabolism

A. Thyroid hormones: $T_3$ triiodothyronine, $T_4$ thyroxine (TSH)

| Normal Function | Excess | Deficit |
|---|---|---|
| ↑Energy production<br>Thermogenesis<br>Growth and development | Hyperthyroidism<br>Thyrotoxicosis<br>Toxic goiter<br>Graves disease<br>±Goiter<br>↑BMR<br>↑HR, ↑BP<br>Palpitations<br>Heat intolerance<br>Weight loss<br>Nervousness<br>Tremors<br>Diarrhea<br>Exophthalmos | Hypothyroidism<br>Cretinism (child)<br>Myxedema (adult)<br><br>±Goiter<br>↓BMR<br>Slow mentation<br>Weight gain<br>Cold intolerance<br>Constipation<br>Nonpitting edema<br>Child: mental and physical retardation |
| | Thyroid storm | Myedema coma |

1. Diagnosis of thyroid disorders

    a. radioactive iodine uptake

    b. $T_3$ and $T_4$ levels

    c. TSH levels (differentiate between primary and secondary)

2. Treatment

    a. hyperthyroid

        thyroidectomy (partial or total)
        radioactive iodine therapy
        antithyroid drugs (propylthiouracil) block thyroxine synthesis
        diet: high calorie, high carb, high protein
        exophthalmos does not reverse

    b. hypothyroid

        thyroid hormone replacement
        careful adjustment of drug dosages (e.g., narcotics) due to ↓metabolism
        diet: low calorie, weight loss diet, restrict goitrogens? (cabbage, peanuts, brussel sprouts, peaches,etc.), iodized salt.

B. Insulin (from pancreas)

| Normal Function | Excess | Deficit |
|---|---|---|
| Increase uptake of blood glucose into cells and lower blood glucose levels | Hypoglycemia<br>Hunger<br>Weakness<br>Tremor<br>Sweaty<br>Cold<br>Clammy<br>Coma<br>↓Blood glucose | Diabetes mellitus<br>Hyperglycemia<br>Elevated blood glucose<br>Polydipsia<br>Polyphagia<br>Polyuria<br>Dehydration |

1. Insulin excess: Usually due to exogenous insulin administration or secreting pancreatic tumor (rare). Functional hypoglycemia: exaggerated response to sugar. Insulin secretion overshoots and causes hypoglycemia. Exact cause unknown. It tends to occur in tense, anxious individuals.

2. Treatment for insulin excess:

    a. emergency: give quick-acting sugar source

    b. functional: avoid sweets/simple sugars

    c. tumor: surgical removal

3. Insulin deficit: Major sign is elevated blood sugar and slow or absent insulin response to sugar load. Often diagnosed by glucose tolerance test.

VIII. Diabetes Mellitus

A. Incidence: Affects more than 12 million in the U.S. One in five people born today will go on to develop DM; 600,000 new cases diagnosed each year. Until 1921 when insulin was discovered, there was no treatment, and still today there is no cure.

B. Causes: A wide variety of factors are associated with the development of diabetes, but exact cause is unknown.

1. Genetic predisposition

2. Diet: excessive carbohydrate and sugar intake

3. Obesity

4. Pregnancy (gestational diabetes)

5. Autoimmune destruction of beta cells

6. Lack of insulin receptors on cells

C. Two major classifications of DM

| | Insulin-dependent DM (IDDM) | Non-Insulin-dependent DM (NIDDM) |
|---|---|---|
| Other names | | |
| | Juvenile onset | Adult onset |
| | Type I | Type II |
| | Brittle | |
| Onset | | |
| | Any age | Usually after 40 years of age<br>9/10 obese |
| Pathophysiology | | |
| | No insulin production (beta cells nonfunctional) | Produce insulin, but not enough or tissues are resistant to insulin |
| Major complication | | |
| | Diabetic ketoacidosis (cell starvation) | Less ketosis prone, problem is hyperosmolar (hyperglycemia) |

D. Basic problem in both types of DM is the same: blood sugar is not transported into cells. This leads to two major problems: (1) cell starvation and (2) hyperglycemia.

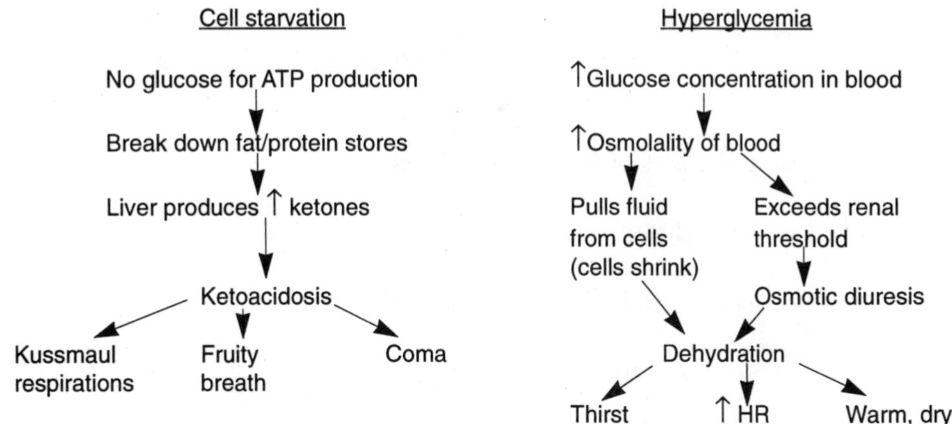


E. Hormonal control of blood sugar and the Somogyi phenomenon

1. Many hormones affect blood sugar levels. All but insulin serve to increase blood sugar. A drop in blood sugar will stimulate the secretion of these hormones.

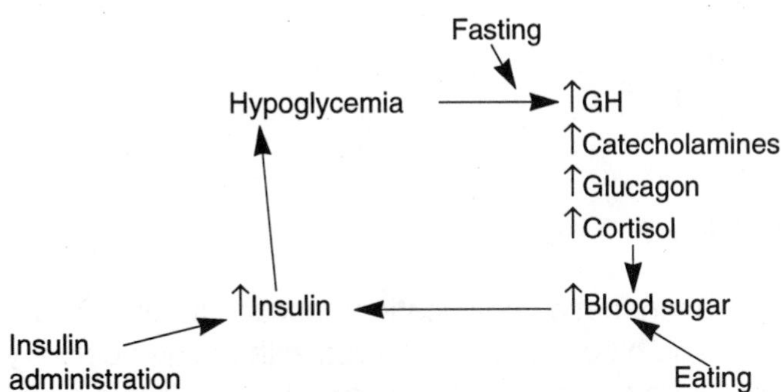


2. Administration of too much insulin in the diabetic causes transient hypoglycemia, which stimulates release of GH, cortisol, etc., leading to hyperglycemia. This circular chain of events is called Somogyi phenomenon.

F. Treatment of diabetes

1. Diet: low in simple carbohydrates and sweets. Often a weight loss diet for the NIDDM, but not for the IDMM, who is often underweight.

2. Exercise: increases uptake of glucose by muscle cells and decreases insulin requirements.

3. Hypoglycemic drugs

   a. oral: stimulate beta cells to secrete insulin. May increase cellular receptors; only used for NIDDM.

   b. insulin: must be given parenterally. Used for both NIDDM and IDDM.

G. Complications of diabetes mellitus

1. Short term

   a. diabetic coma (hyperglycemia)

   b. insulin shock (hypoglycemia)

   important to be able to differentiate S/S of each

| Diabetic coma | Insulin shock |
| --- | --- |
| S/S due to hyperosmolality and/or ketoacidosis: | S/S due to sympathetic response to low blood sugar |
| Dehydration | Cool/clammy |
| Warm/dry | Tremors/weakness |
| ↑ Respirations | Headache |
| Fruity breath | |
| ↓ | ↓ |
| Coma | Coma |

   When in doubt, give sugar.

2. Long term: The reason these complications occur with diabetes is unclear. Possibly high blood sugar interferes with oxygen delivery to tissues. (The RBCs have a higher affinity for $O_2$.) Diabetes cuts life expectancy by one-third. The long-term problems occur 15–20 years after diagnosis.

   a. retinopathy/blindness

   b. nephropathy

   c. neuropathy

   d. arterial insufficiency

   e. myocardial infarction

   f. CVA

   g. increased susceptibility to infection

# ALTERATIONS IN NEUROLOGIC FUNCTION

I. Increased Intracranial Pressure (ICP)

A. Normal ICP is 0–15 mm Hg.

1. Head contains: brain tissue, CSF, blood supply

2. An increase in any of these increases pressure in noncompliant skull.

B. Causes of increased ICP: many possible: brain infection, rupture of blood vessels, hydrocephalus, fluid and electrolyte imbalance, and most common—head trauma

1. Primary injury: due to direct blow to head

2. Secondary injury: due to subsequent brain swelling (related to hypoxia, intracranial bleeding, ischemia, inflammation)

C. Mechanisms of secondary injury

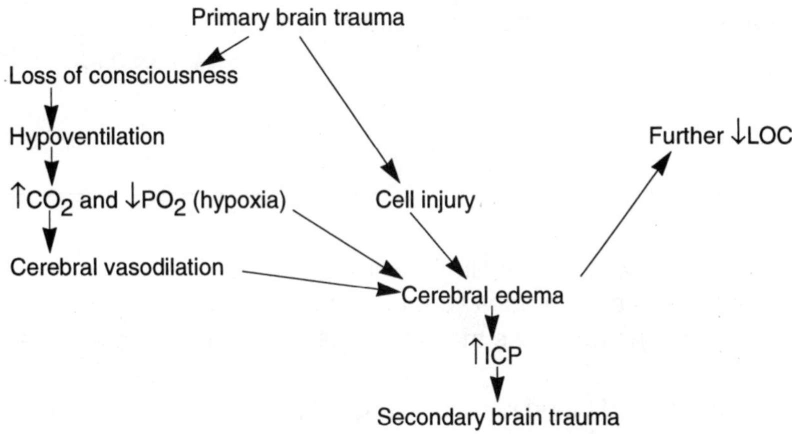


D. Compensation for increased ICP due to brain swelling

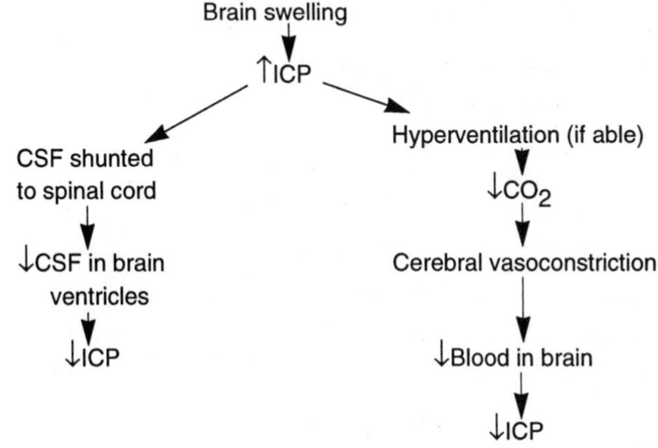

E. Progression of signs and symptoms with increasing ICP

| ↑ICP | Brain area affected | Signs and symptoms |
|---|---|---|
| Mild to moderate | Cortical | headache, ↓LOC<br>projectile vomiting<br>localized pain/follow commands<br>decorticate posturing |
| Moderate to severe | Midbrain | pupil changes<br>hyperventilation<br>decerebrate posturing<br>seizures |
| Severe | Pons | loss of resp control<br>apnea/sigh |
| Severe | Medulla | resp arrest<br>flaccidity<br>ischemic response |
| Severe | Brain herniation | brain death<br>no spontaneous resp for 3 min<br>unresponsive<br>fixed pupils<br>flat EEG |

F. Ischemic response: "Cushing's reflex"
When ICP reaches a point where the brain tissue is not getting blood supply, ischemic response tries to reestablish blood supply to brain.

1. Increased blood pressure, especially systolic
2. Wide pulse pressure
3. Decreased heart rate
4. Loss of respiration

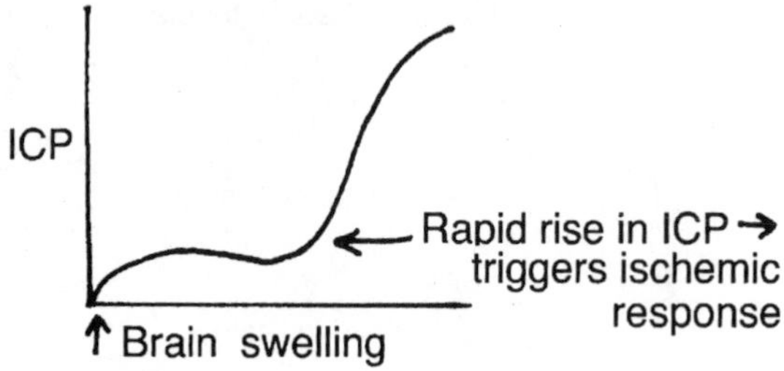

G. Diabetes insipidus

H. General therapy for increased ICP

1. Elevate head of bed

2. Diuretics (mannitol, furosemide)

3. Dilantin/phenobarb (seizures and decrease metabolic rate)

4. Hyperventilation (respirator)

5. Decompression → burr holes

→ventriculostomy

6. Steroids

I. Prognosis for brain injury: extremely difficult to predict; swelling peaks at 48–72 hours after injury

II. Classification of Head Trauma

A. Concussion: transient

B. Contusion: S/S depend on area contused (temporal, frontal, etc.)

C. Brainstem contusion

D. Hemorrhage: high mortality rate

1. Epidural: arterial bleeding (middle meningeal)

2. Subdural: venous bleeding

a. acute
b. subacute/chronic

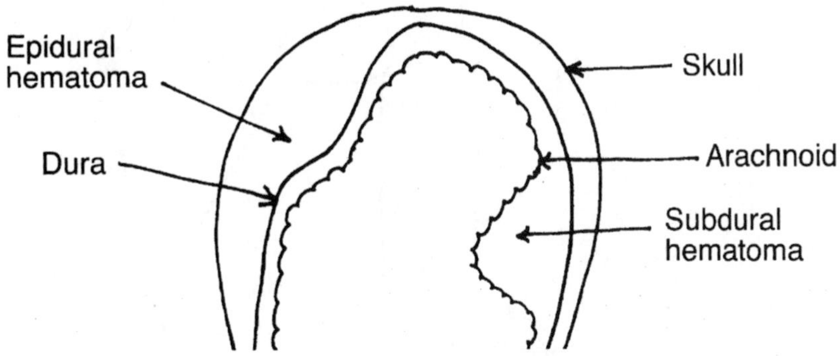

III. Cerebral Vascular Accident (CVA): Stroke

A. Etiology of stroke

1. Rupture of blood vessel (aneurysm)—rare

2. Embolism—25%

3. Thrombotic—most common; related to atherosclerotic vessels in brain

   Narrowed vessel—thrombus formation; disrupts blood supply to portion of brain

B. Stages of thrombotic stroke

1. Transient ischemic attacks (TIA): no residual damage

2. Stroke in evolution: most critical time

3. Completed stroke: stable neurologic status for 24 hrs

C. Signs and symptoms of stroke: depends greatly on location of brain lesion

1. Contralateral hemiplagia

2. Eye ptosis

3. Loss of bladder/bowel control

4. Inappropriate emotional outbursts

5. Aphasia

   expressive (Broca's)
   receptive (Wernicke's)

6. Homonymous hemianopsia (contralateral field blindness)

7. Neglect

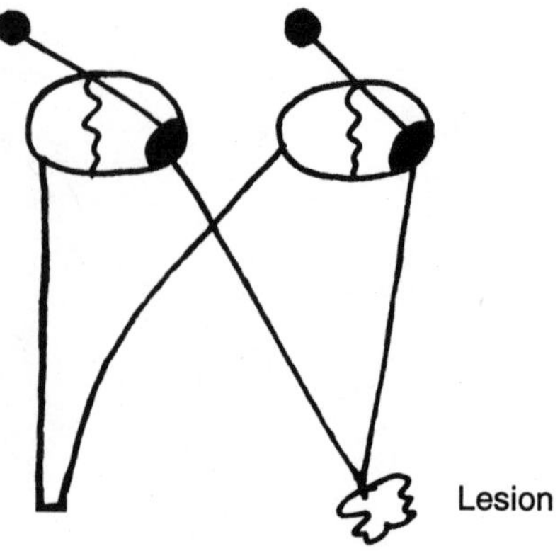

D. Therapy for stroke

1. Prevention

2. Surgery: carotid endarterectomy

3. Anticoagulation

4. Treat high blood pressure

5, Rehabilitation

IV. Other Brain Disorders

A. Aneurysm: aneurysm precautions

B. Hydrocephalus: accumulation of CSF in brain

C. Brain infections: encephalitis, meningitis

1. Nuchal rigidity

V. Organic Brain Syndrome (OBS)

A. Definition: deterioration of mental function due to deterioration of brain tissue—atrophy, e.g., Alzheimers

B. Signs and symptoms (JAMCO)

J—Judgment

A—Affect

M—Memory

C—Confusion

O—Orientation

VI. Seizures

A. Definition: spontaneous, uncontrolled neuronal discharge from cortical brain cells

B. Epilepsy: recurrent seizure

C. Classification of seizures

| Partial (one hemisphere, local) | Generalized (both hemispheres) |
|---|---|
| Simple (no ↓ LOC)<br>Complex (↓ LOC)<br>Secondarily generalized | Absence<br>Tonic-clonic |

D. Care and Treatment

1. Observation, documentation, protection

2. Drug therapy

VI. Neuromuscular Disorders

A. Upper motor neruon disorders (cortex, basal ganglia)

1. Stroke or head injury

2. Cerebral palsy, nonprogressive brain cell damage; 70% mental retardation

   causes: hypoxia at birth, head trauma, encephalitis, etc.

3. Huntington's chorea: rapidly progressing; autosomal dominant; onset at 40-50 years

   cortical and basal ganglia atrophy

   chorea—involuntary rapid, jerky movements

   also severe mental deterioration

4. Parkinson's disease: slowly progressive; degeneration of basal ganglia with deficiency of the neurotransmittor dopamine

   a. three cardinal signs and symptoms

      tremor
      rigidity
      akinesia

b. associated signs and symptoms

masklike facies
shuffling, propulsive gait
monotonous speech
drooling
intelligence and lifespan not necessarily affected

c. Treatment

Levodopa/carbodopa

anticholinergics

B. Brainstem and spinal cord disorders

1. Multiple sclerosis: chronic, progressive

a. etiology: unknown—viral? autoimmune?

b. pathology: demyelination of white matter in cord/brain. Myelin normally insulates and speeds conduction.

c. S/S: remissions and exacerbations, weakness, paresthesias, double vision, loss of bowel/bladder control

d. treatment: symptomatic, steroids

2. Poliomyelitis: not progressive (post-polio syndrome?)

a. etiology: polio virus

b. pathology: destroys anterior horn cells (motor) in cord

c. S/S: generally flaccid paralysis

d. treatment: symptomatic (prevention)

3. Spinal cord injury: function of nerves below the injury is usually lost.

complete: no sensory/motor function

incomplete: may regain some function

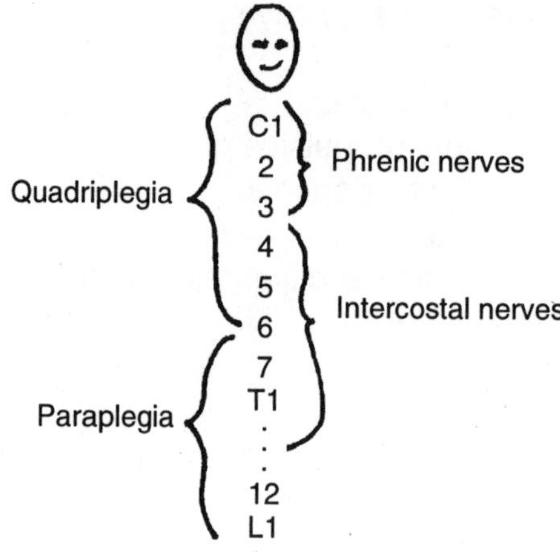


a. spinal shock

2 weeks to 2 months after injury

spinal cord is in "shock"—no reflex activity

no bladder or bowel tone
decreased vascular tone
loss of temperature control
flaccid paralysis with no reflexes

after shock subsides—reflexes return

motor control and sensation do not return

b. autonomic dysreflexia (or hyperreflexia)

exaggerated autonomic response to a stimulus occurs in SCI above T6

S/S: hypertension, decreased heart rate, headache, flushing/sweating above SCI area, unable to dilate below SCI

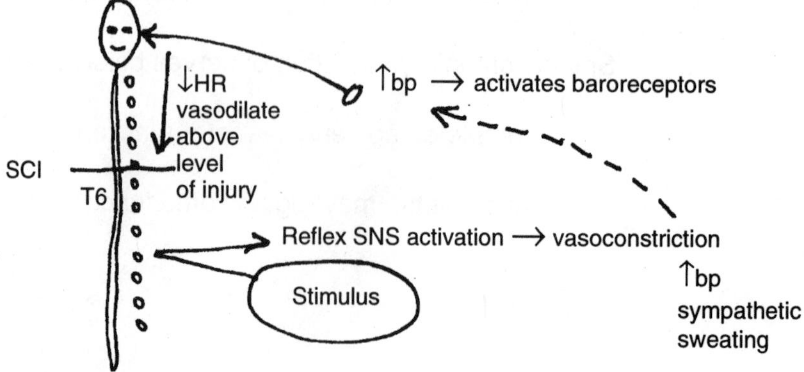


treatment: remove stimulus

C. Cranial and peripheral nerve disorders (LMN)

1. Bells palsy: 7th cranial nerve (facial nerve)

loss of motor function: paralysis

etiology: usually unknown; often spontaneous recovery

S/S: similar facial appearance to stroke;
ipsilateral droop of face, eyelid, mouth

2. Guillian-Barré: acute inflammation of peripheral and cranial nerves.

etiology: unknown: viral? autoimmune?

S/S: bilateral weakness/paralysis that progressively ascends the body, feet to head; sensation remains intact

treatment: supportive care: mechanical ventilation, avoid complications of immobility, paralysis spontaneously subsides in weeks to years.

D. Neuromuscular junction disorders

1. Myasthenia gravis: "grave weakness"

etiology: thought to be from autoimmune destruction of muscle receptor sites for acetylcholine

S/S: weakness increases with use of muscles, bilateral ptosis, double vision, respiratory distress

treatment: drugs—steroids, anticholinesterase

E. Muscle disorders

1. Muscular dystrophy: progressive atrophy of muscle cells—replaced by fat and scar tissue.

etiology: thought to be genetic defects; runs in families; several different types of MD

S/S: weakness, bulky muscles

treatment: symptomatic

# ALTERATIONS IN SENSATION

I. Pain

A. Physiology of pain

1. Pain has both physical and psychologic components.

2. Transmission of pain signals

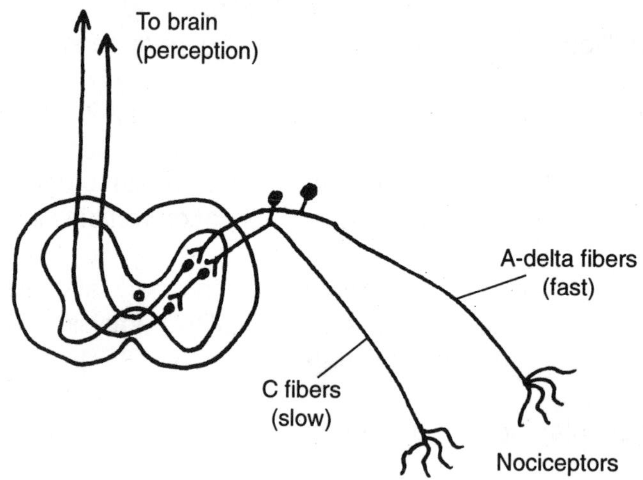


3. Gate control theory

4. Endogenous endorphins/enkephalins

B. Neuralgia: severe, brief, recurrent attacks of pain along the distribution of a spinal or cranial nerve

1. Trigeminal neuralgia: "tic douloureax" trigeminal nerve (CN5) is affected.

etiology: unknown—nerve compression?

S/S: severe pain triggered by minor stimulation

treatment: anticonvulsants Dilantin, Tegretol; craniotomy for nerve decompression

II. Alteration in the Special Senses

A. Hearing loss

1. Conductive deafness: sound not transmitted through external or middle ear

otosclerosis

2. Sensorineural deafness: degeneration or destruction of structures of the inner ear

   loud noises, drugs (ototoxic)

   presbycusis—"old age"

3. Central deafness: damage to auditory nerve or brain centers for perception

4. Ménière's disease: increased pressure and dilation of the labyrinth of the inner ear

   due to: increased production of endolymph and/or decreased absorption of endolymph

   S/S: severe vertigo, tinnitus, unilateral sensorineural hearing loss

   treatment: bed rest, sodium restriction

B. Eye

1. Disorders of refraction

   a. hyperopia

   b. myopia

   c. astigmatism

   d. presbyopia

2. Cataract: increased opacity of the lens; 3rd leading cause of blindness

   etiology: trauma, heat, toxins, infections, UV light, congenital, advancing age

   S/S: decreasing visual acuity, night glare

   treatment: remove lens → lens transplant or contacts

3. Retinal holes, tears, detachment

   etiology: trauma, degeneration

   S/S: fluid may leak under retina and cause separation from underlying pigment layer; not painful, loss of portion of visual field "curtain," floaters, blindness if not treated treatment: bed rest (on back), scleral buckling, laser

4. Glaucoma: increased intraocular pressure, may cause optic nerve degeneration and blindness, normal IOP 10–20 mm Hg

   a. closed angle glaucoma: forward displacement of iris causes narrowed opening through canal of Schlemm

      S/S: acute attacks with pupil dilation, eye pain, halos, headache, N&V

      treatment: avoid precipitating factors, miotic drugs

   b. open angle glaucoma: normal size anterior chamber, but drainage network in canal of Schlemm does not drain well

      S/S: usually painless, loss of vision

      treatment: carbonic anhydrase, miotics, diagnose by tonometry

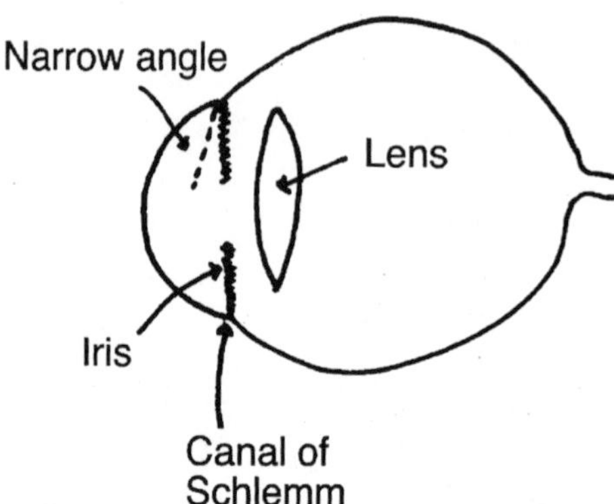

# ALTERATIONS IN SKELETAL FUNCTION

I. Bone Injuries and Fractures

A. Types

1. Longitudinal
2. Dislocation
3. Compound (open)
4. Comminuted
5. Greenstick
6. Spiral
7. Compression

B. Complications

1. Fat emboli
2. Compartment syndrome

II. Arthritis

A. Definition: joint inflammation/degeneration with loss of joint mobility

B. Rheumatoid arthritis: systemic connective tissue disease. Joints are progressively destroyed by chronic inflammation.

1. Onset: young adulthood
2. Etiology: unknown, possibly autoimmune
3. S/S: remission and exacerbations, pain, swelling, stiffness, calcification, deformities
4. Treatment: ASA, steroids, non-steroidal anti-inflammatory drugs (indocin), gold compounds, surgical joint replacement

B. Osteoarthritis: arthritis of aging. Joint degeneration due to long-term wear and tear

1. Incidence: very prevalent in older people

2. Pathology: local joint disorder, erosion of cartilage

3. S/S: stiffness, pain, grating, crepitus

4. Treatment: ASA, physical therapy, joint replacement

# SECTION FIVE

## *Transparency Masters*

# *Transparency Masters*

| Transparency Number | Textbook Figure Number | Description |
|---|---|---|
| 1. | 1-18 | Etiologic Classification of Disease |
| 2. | 2-2 | Structure of Cell Membrane |
| 3. | 2-16 | Mitochondrial Electron Transport Chain |
| 4. | 2-17 | Schematic of ATP Synthetase |
| 5. | 2-20 | Membrane Channels and Carriers |
| 6. | 2-23 | The Sodium-Potassium Ion Pump |
| 7. | 2-24 | Membrane Calcium Ion Pumps |
| 8. | 2-27 | Effect of Potassium Concentration on Resting Membrane Potential |
| 9. | 2-29 | Ion Conductance During Action Potential |
| 10. | 2-31 | Action Potential in Ventricular Myocardium |
| 11. | 2-33 | Receptor Mechanisms |
| 12. | 3-4 | Cellular Responses to Injury |
| 13. | 5-1 | Chromosome Nondisjunction |
| 14. | 5-9 | Autosomal Dominant Inheritance Patterns |
| 15. | 5-11 | Autosomal Recessive Inheritance Patterns |
| 16. | 5-13 | Periods of Fetal Vulnerability |
| 17. | 6-4 | Mechanisms of Oncogene Activation |
| 18. | 6-6 | Mechanisms of Altered Growth Control |
| 19. | 7-1 | Sympathetic Alarm Reaction |
| 20. | 7-7 | Organs of the Immune System |
| 21. | 7-12 | Potential Stress Reactions |
| 22. | 8-4 | Factors Affecting Infectious Processes |
| 23. | 9-1 | Hematopoietic Cells |
| 24. | 9-11 | Typical Immunoglobulin Structure |
| 25. | 10-10 | HIV Structure |
| 26. | 10-11 | Sequence of HIV Infection |
| 27. | 13-1 | The Clotting Cascade |
| 28. | 14-13 | Factors Affecting Transcapillary Filtration |
| 29. | 16-12 | Sarcomere Structure |
| 30. | 16-15 | Proteins of the Thin Filament |
| 31. | 16-18 | The Role of Calcium Ion in Crossbridge Formation |
| 32. | 16-19 | Mechanisms of Calcium Ion Removal from the Sarcoplasm |
| 33. | 16-22 | Conduction System of the Heart |
| 34. | 17-2 | Subendocardial (A) and Transmural (B) Infarct |
| 35. | 17-6 | Mitral Stenosis |
| 36. | 17-7 | Mitral Regurgitation |
| 37. | 17-10 | Aortic Stenosis |
| 38. | 17-15 | Fetal Circulation |
| 39. | 18-1 | Compensatory Mechanisms in Heart Failure |
| 40. | 18-4 | Pathophysiology of Left Heart Failure |
| 41. | 18-5 | Manifestations of Left Heart Failure |
| 42. | 18-6 | Pathophysiology of Right Heart Failure |
| 43. | 18-7 | Manifestations of Right Heart Failure |
| 44. | 19-5 | Pulmonary Alveoli |
| 45. | 19-8 | Lobes and Segments of the Lungs |

*(continued)*

| Transparency Number | Textbook Figure Number | Description |
|---|---|---|
| 46 | 19-12 | Functional Zones of the Lungs |
| 47 | 20-10 | Pathophysiology of Emphysema |
| 48 | 21-1 | Mechanism of Tension Pneumothorax |
| 49 | 26-6 | Microanatomy of Glomerular Membrane |
| 50 | 26-11 | Functional Anatomy of the Nephron |
| 51 | 27-8 | Nephrotic Syndrome |
| 52 | 40-1 | Major Pituitary Hormones, Target Tissues and Feedback Mechanisms |
| 53 | 40-4 | Mechanism of ADH Action on Renal Tubule Cells |
| 54 | 40-13 | Negative Feedback in Primary Adrenocortical Insufficiency |
| 55 | 41-4 | Metabolic Effects of IDDM |
| 56 | 41-5 | Metabolic Effects of NIDDM |
| 57 | 42-1 | Anatomy of a Neuron |
| 58 | 42-9 | Spinal Nerves |
| 59 | 42-13a | Functional Areas of Cerebral Cortex |
| 60 | 46-3 | Transverse Section of Spinal Cord Showing Pain Pathways |
| 61 | 46-4 | Mechanism of Pain Transmission and Inhibition |
| 62 | 50-1 | Types of Bone Fractures |
| 63 | 50-5 | Open and Closed Fractures |
| 64 | 51-2 | Affected Joints in Rheumatoid and Osteoarthritis |
| 65 | 52-13 | Accessory Structures of the Skin |
| 66 | 53-1a | Primary Skin Lesions |
| 67 | 53-1b | Secondary Skin Lesions |
| 68 | 53-3 | Fingernail Abnormalities |
| 69 | 54-9 | Mechanisms of Endotoxin Activity |
| 70 | 56-1 | Nutritional Assessment and Intervention |
| 71 | 56-2 | Catabolic Response to Starvation |
| 72 | 56-3 | Immediate Catabolic Response to Stress |
| 73 | 56-5 | Malnutrition and CHF |
| 74 | 56-6 | Malnutrition and COPD |

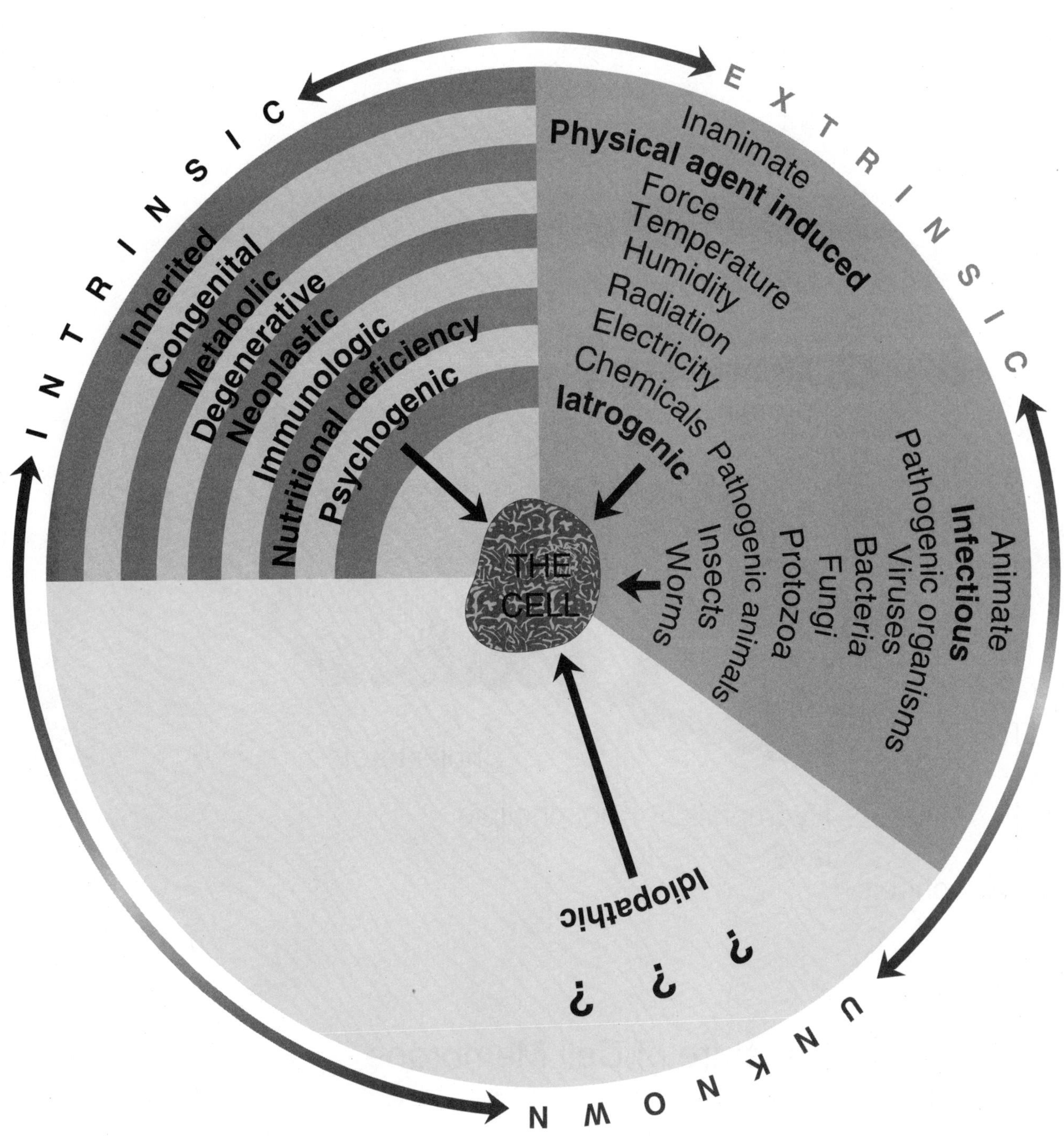


Etiologic Classification of Disease

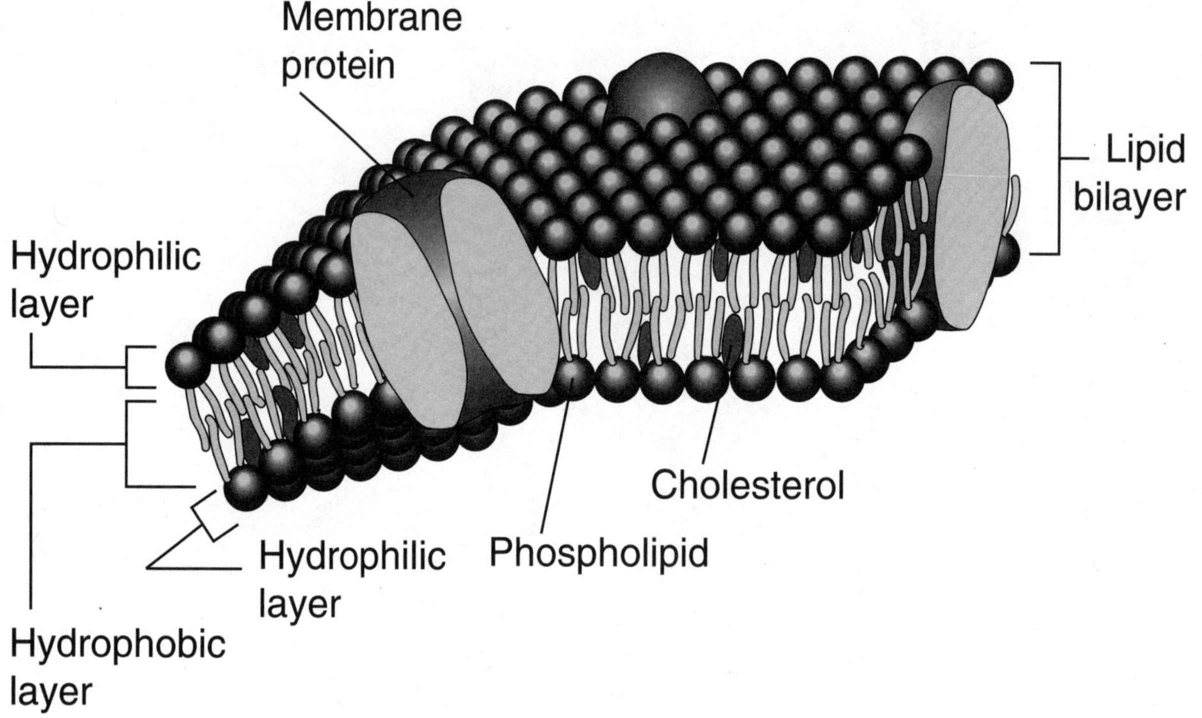


Structure of Cell Membrane

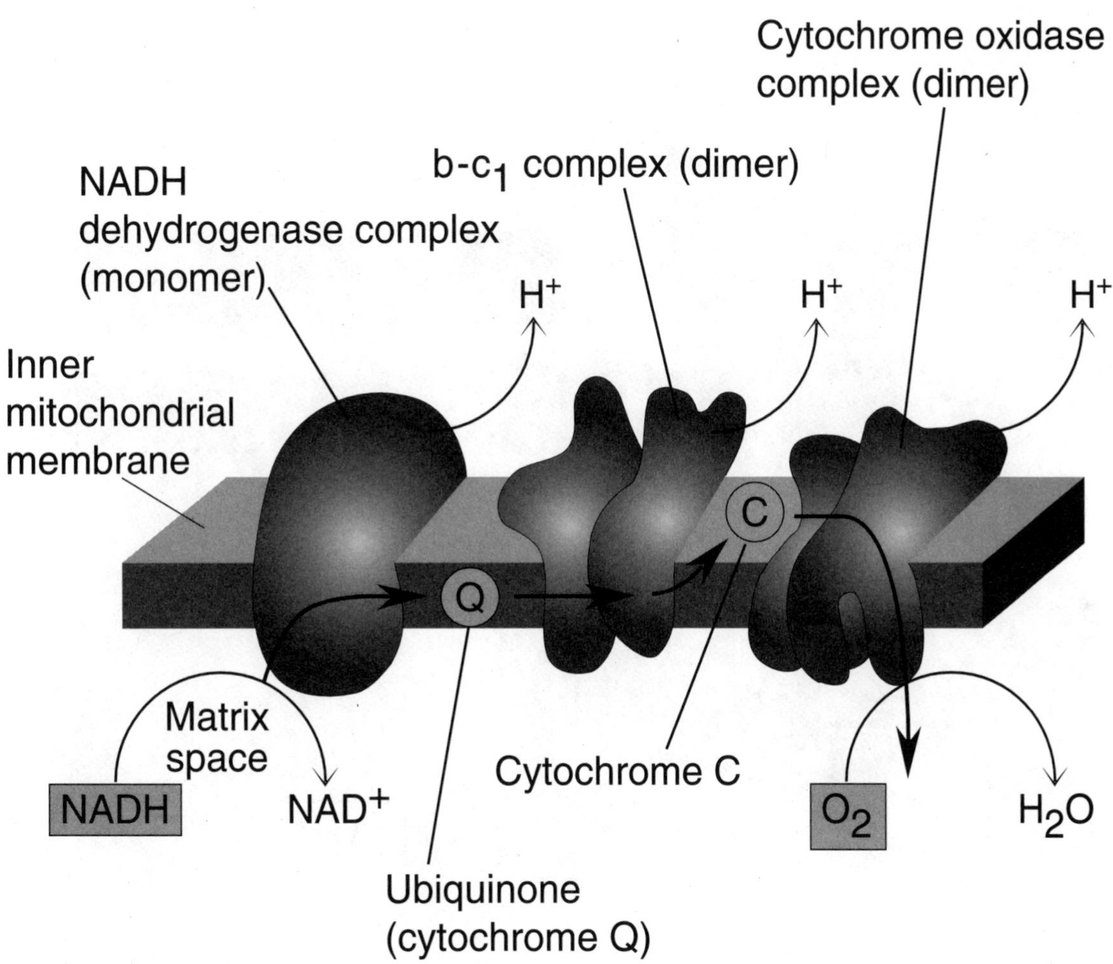


Mitochondrial Electron Transport Chain

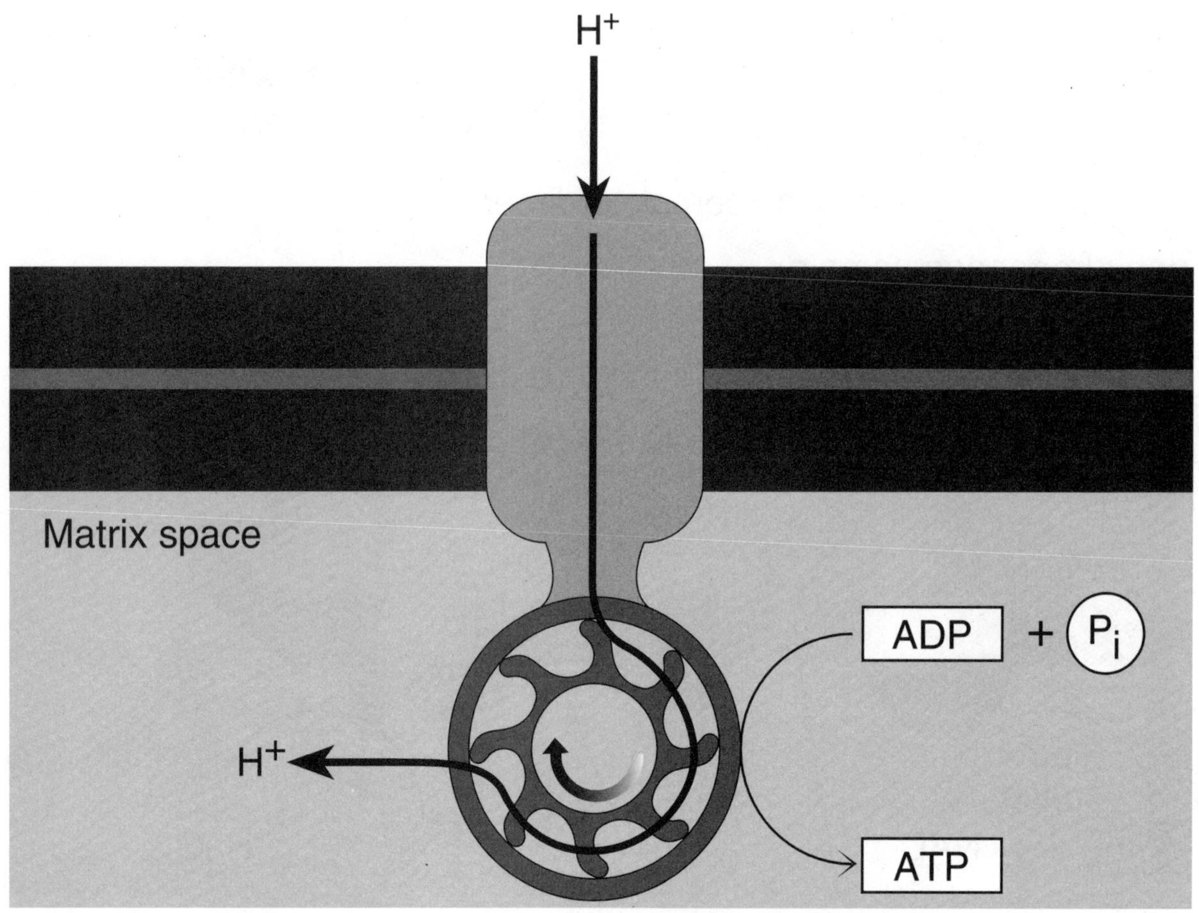


# Schematic of ATP Synthetase

Adapted with permission from Alberts B, et al (eds): *Molecular Biology of the Cell*, 2nd ed. New York, Garland Press, 1989, p 357.

W. B. Saunders Company

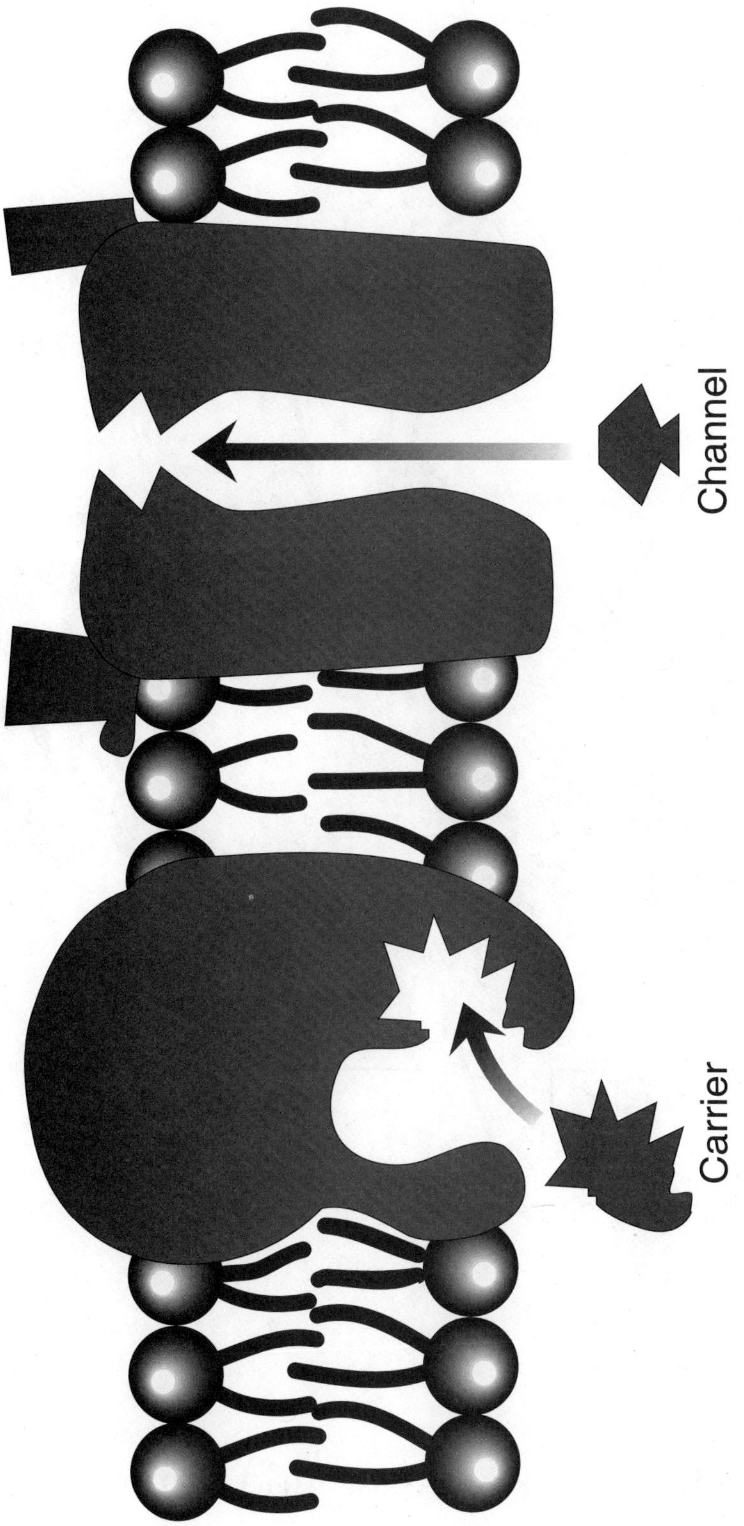

Channel

Carrier

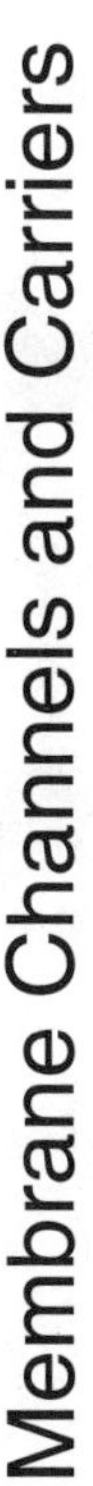

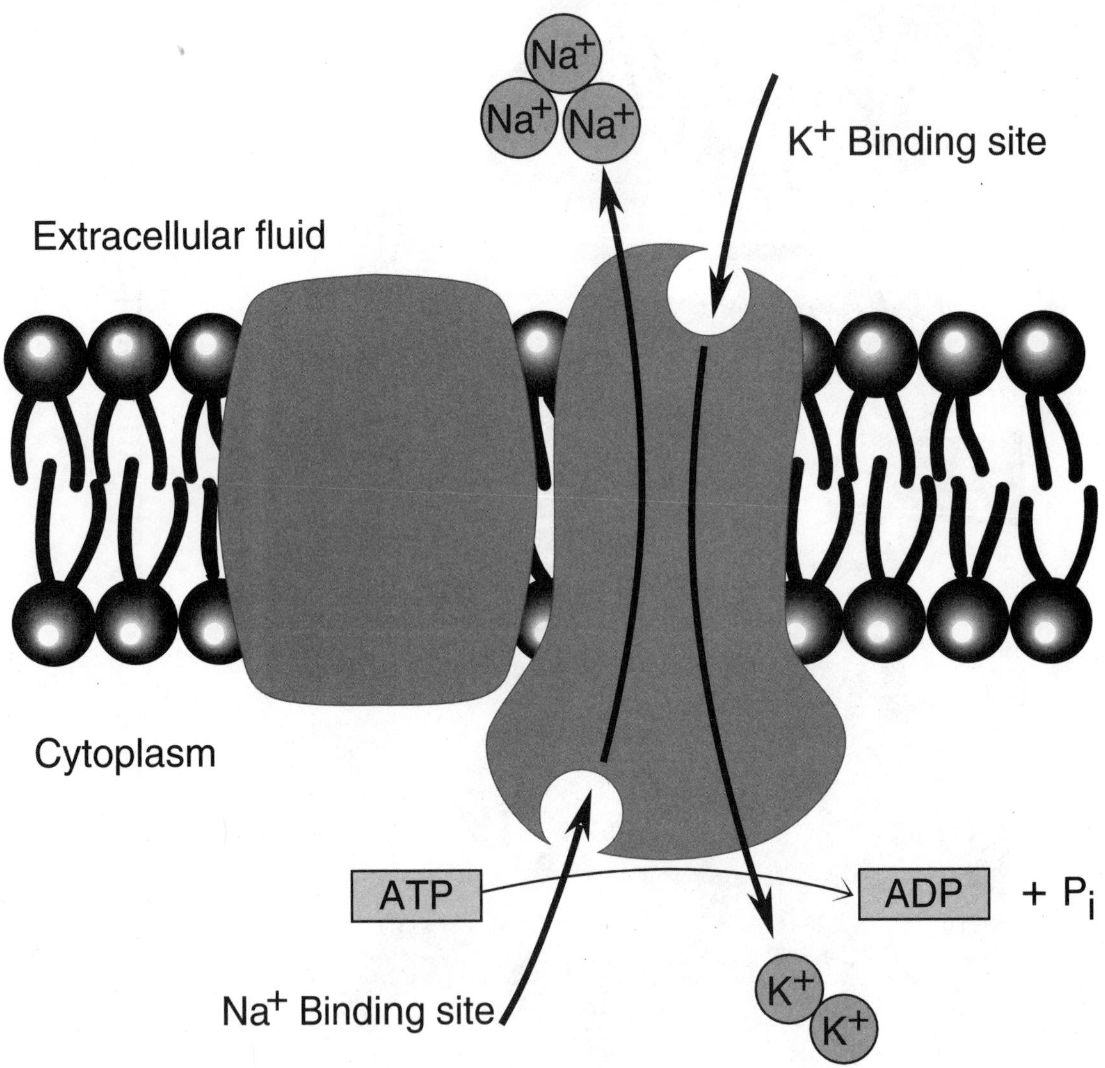


The Sodium-Potassium Ion Pump

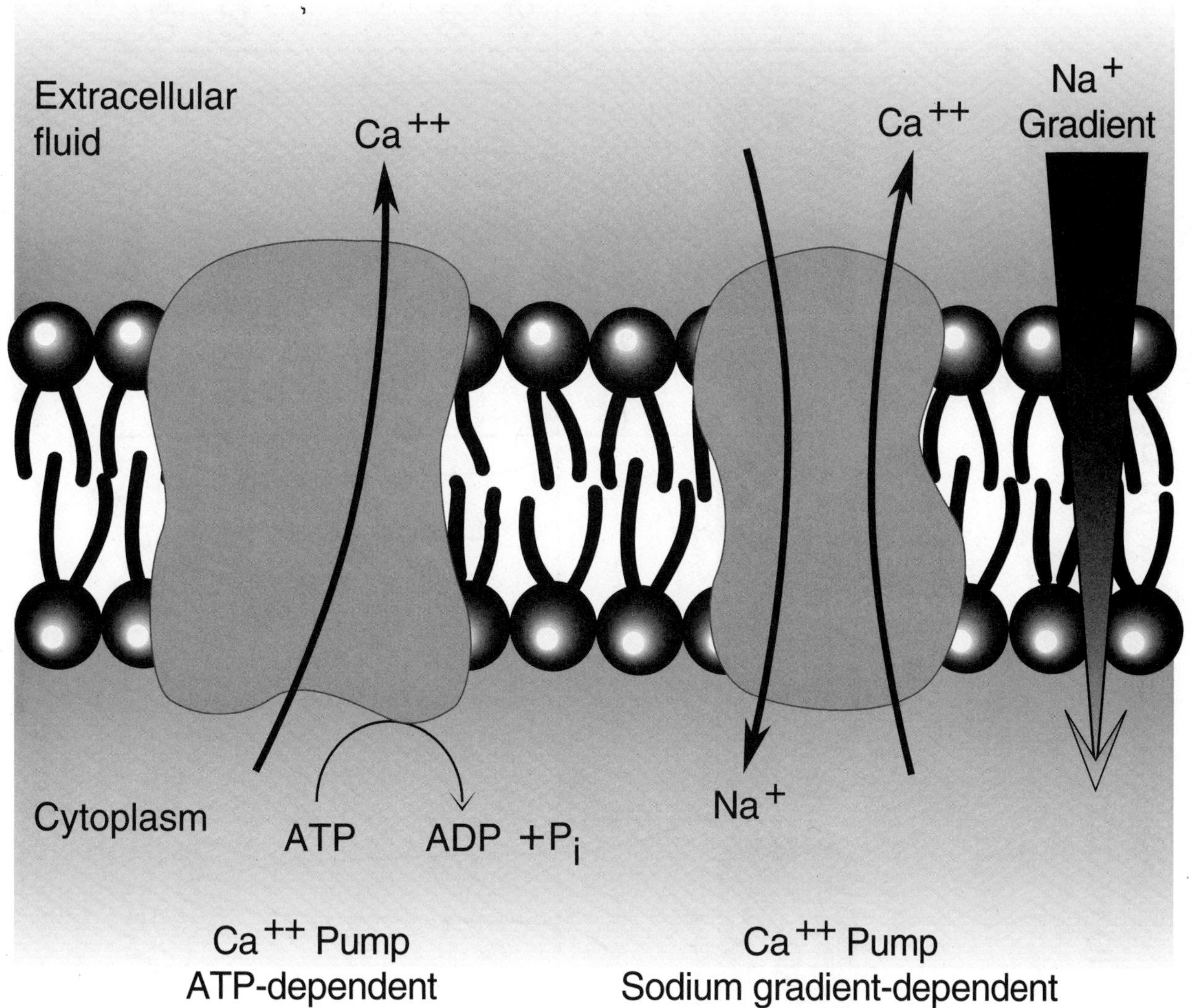


Membrane Calcium Ion Pumps

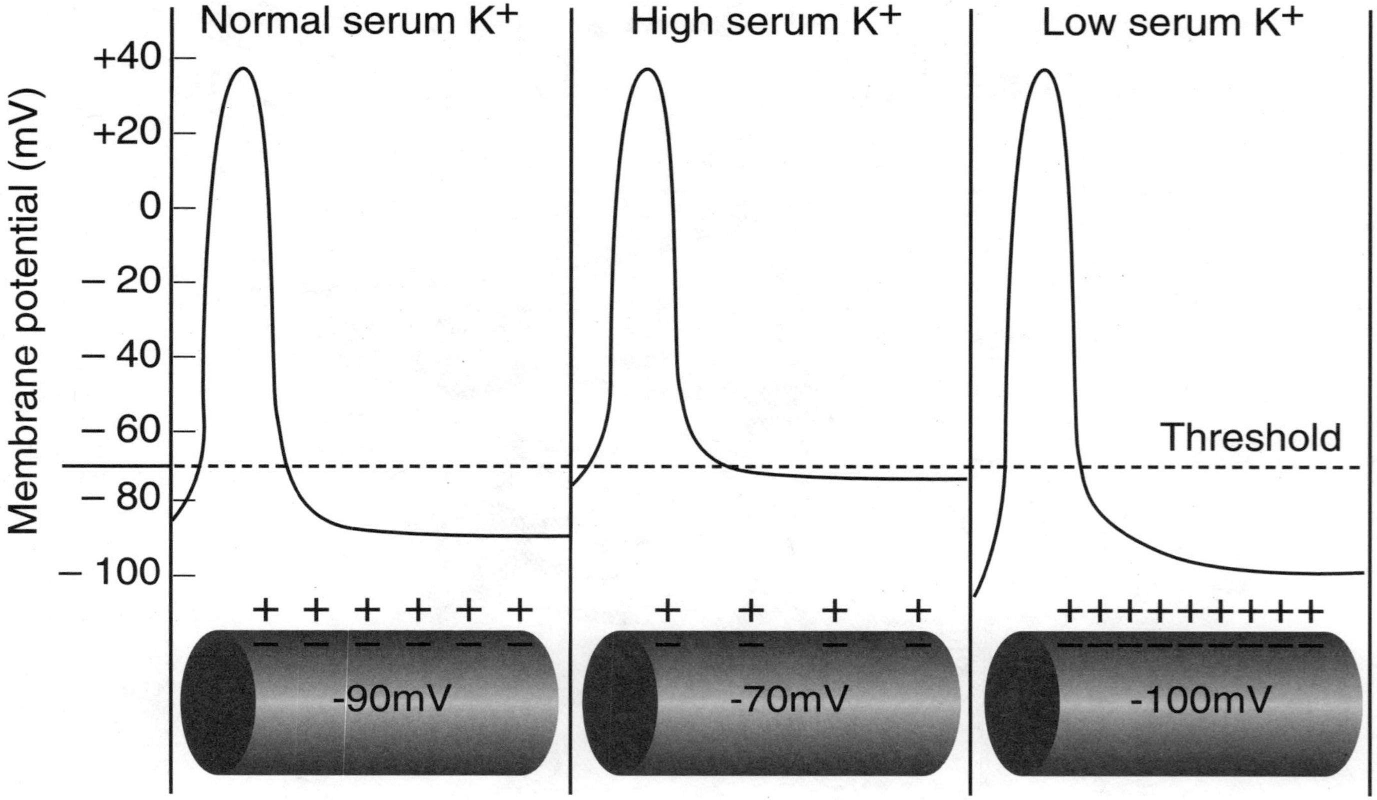

# Effect of Potassium Concentration on Resting Membrane Potential

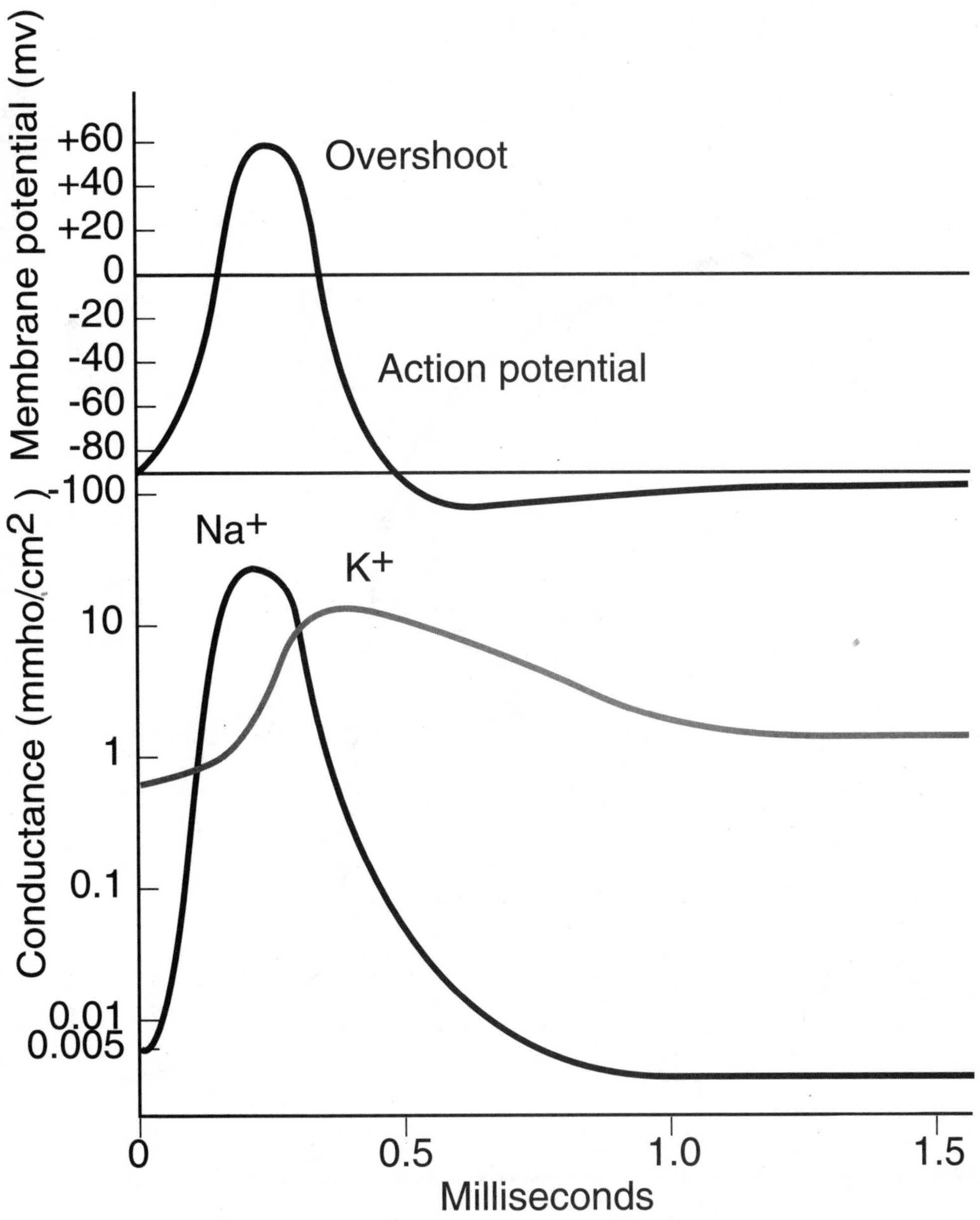


Ion Conductance During Action Potential

Transparency #10

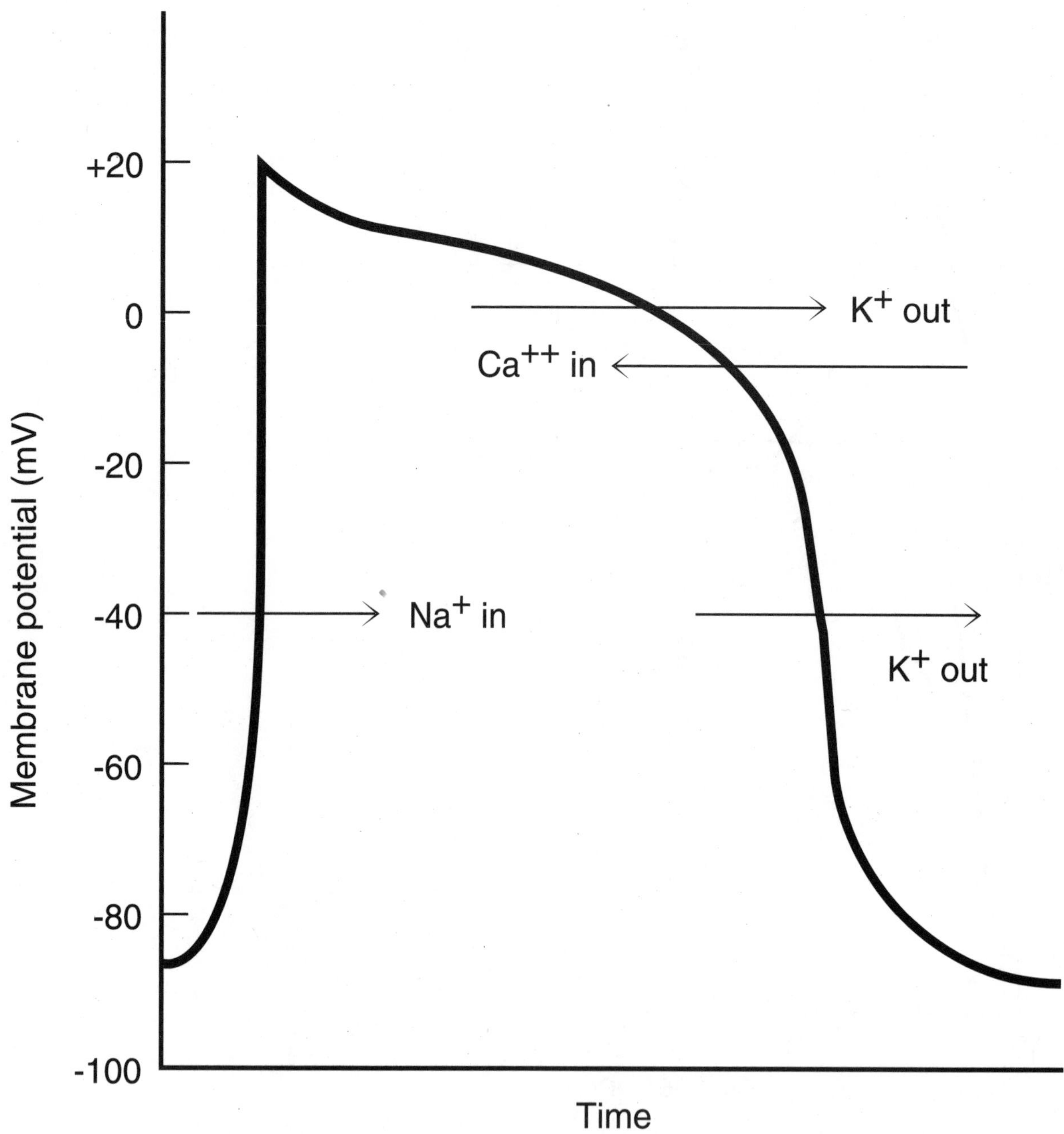


Action Potential in Ventricular Myocardium

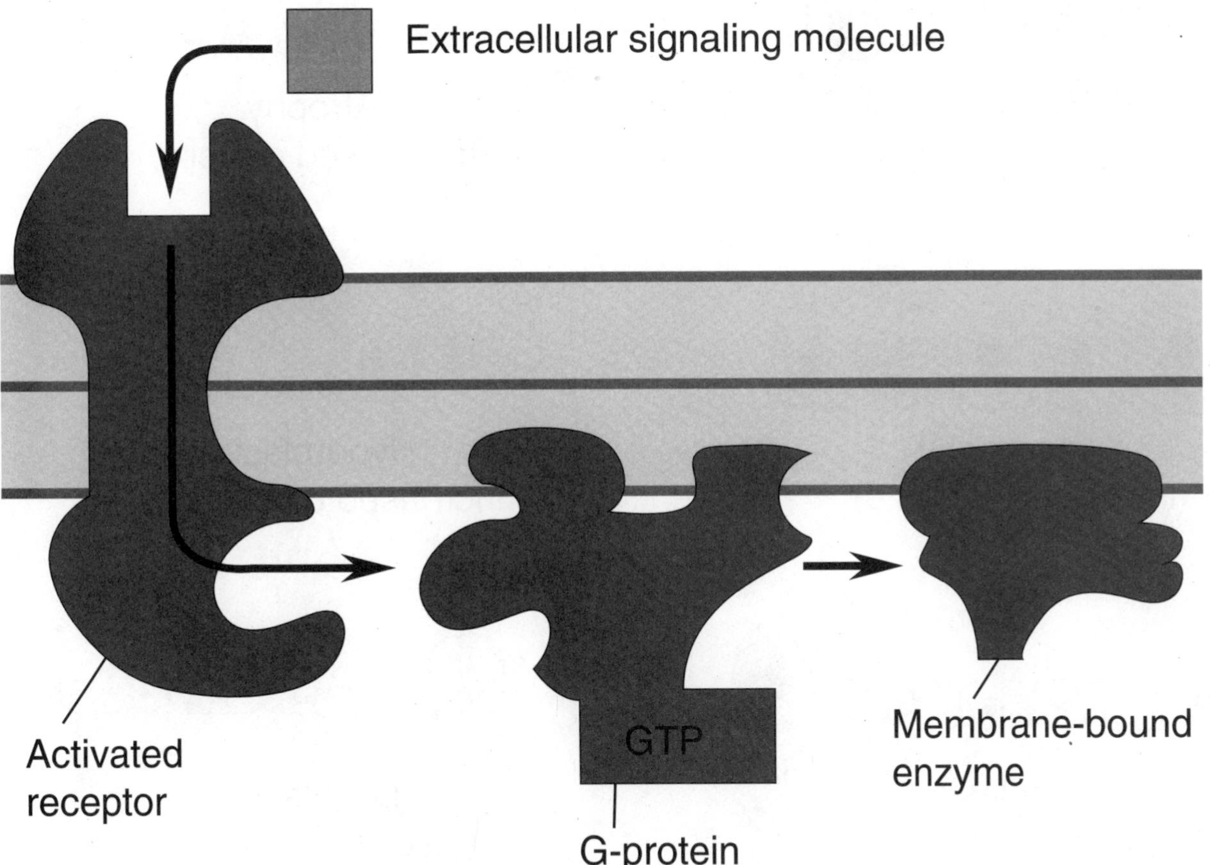


Receptor Mechanisms

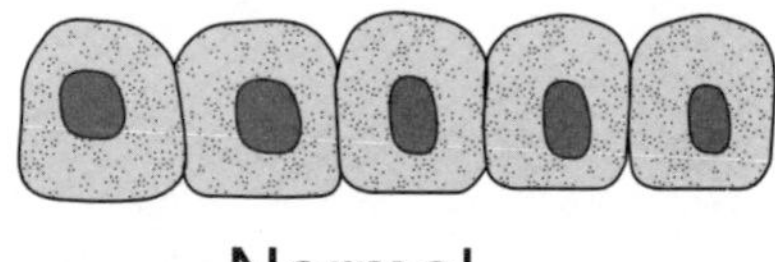

Normal

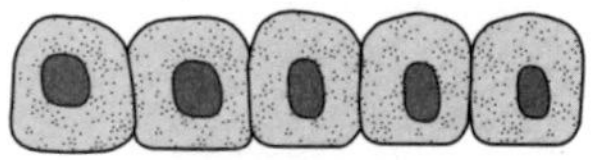

Atrophy
(decreased cell size)

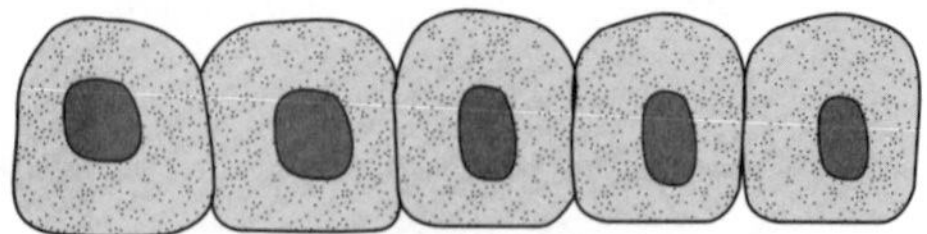

Hypertrophy
(increased cell size)

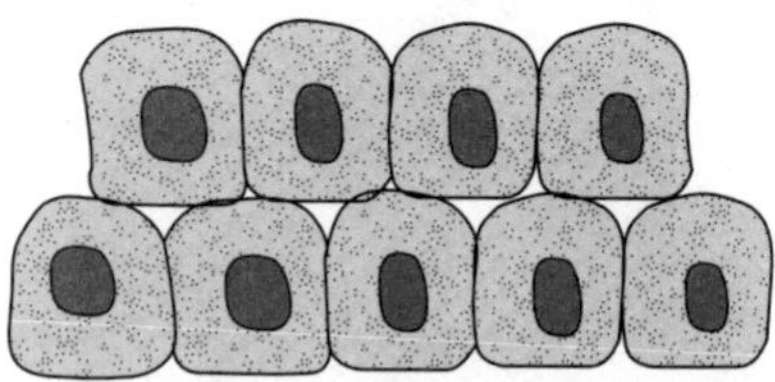

Hyperplasia
(increased cell number)

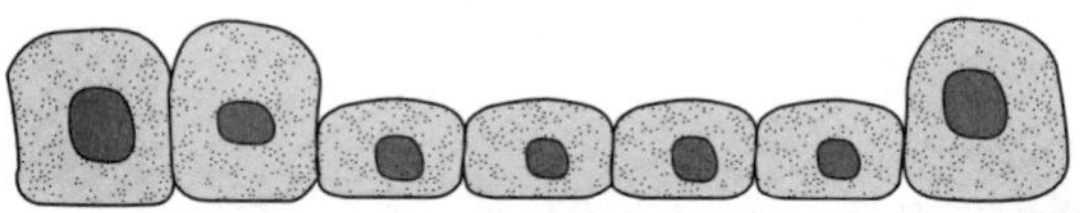

Metaplasia
(conversion of one cell type to another)

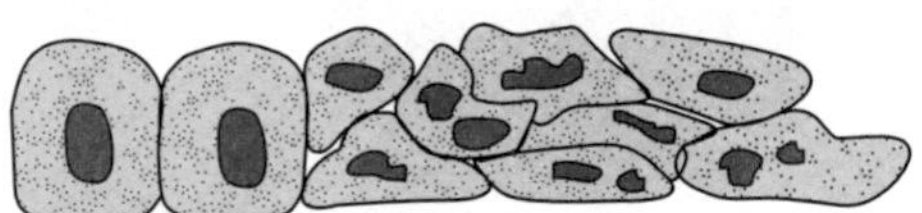

Dysplasia
(disorderly growth)

# Cellular Responses to Injury

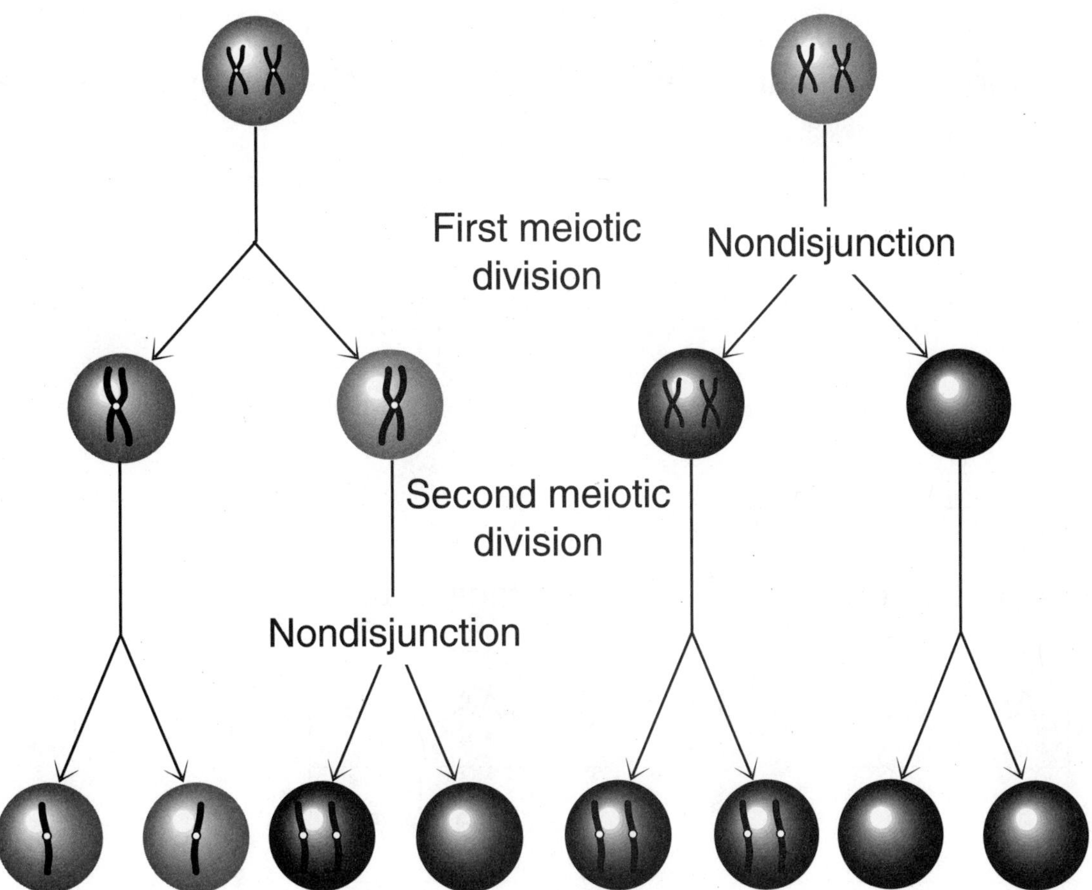


Chromosome Nondisjunction

## A PEDIGREE CHART

### One affected parent (Aa)

One normal parent (aa)

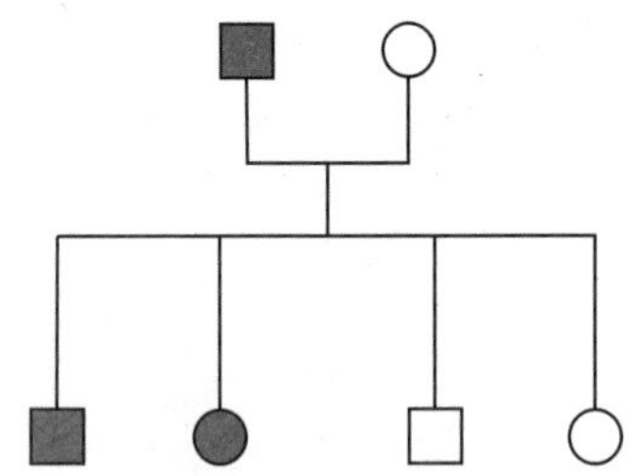

### Two affected parents (both Aa)

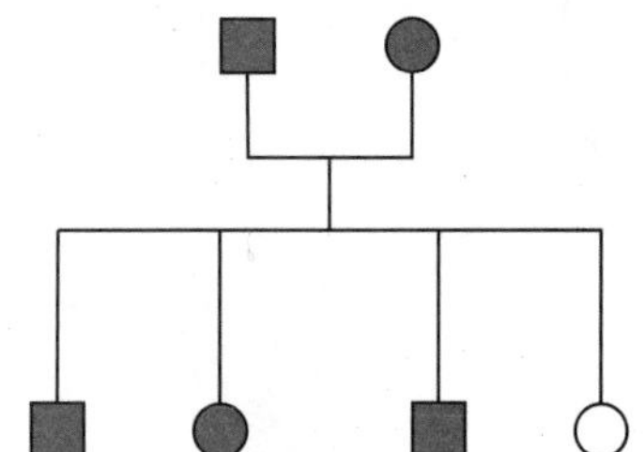

## B PUNNETT SQUARE

| Normal parent \ Affected parent | A | a |
|---|---|---|
| a | Aa | aa |
| a | Aa | aa |

| Affected parent \ Affected parent | A | a |
|---|---|---|
| A | AA | Aa |
| a | Aa | aa |

# Autosomal Dominant Inheritance Patterns

## A PEDIGREE CHART

One heterozygous carrier parent (Aa)
One affected parent (aa)

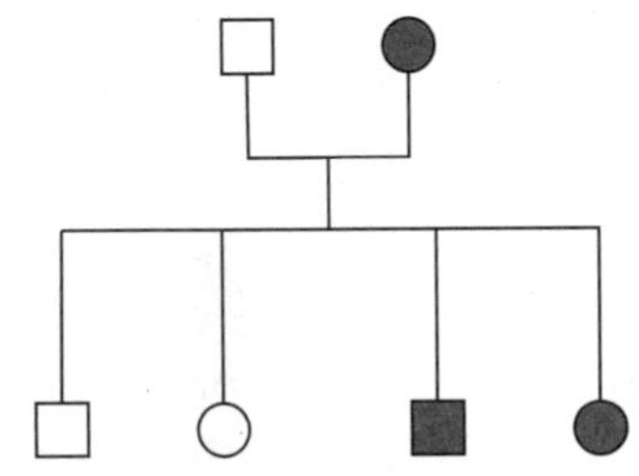

Two heterozygous carrier parents (both Aa)

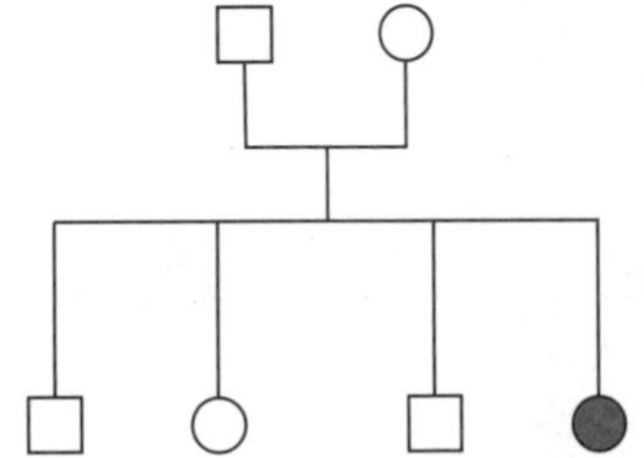

## B PUNNETT SQUARE

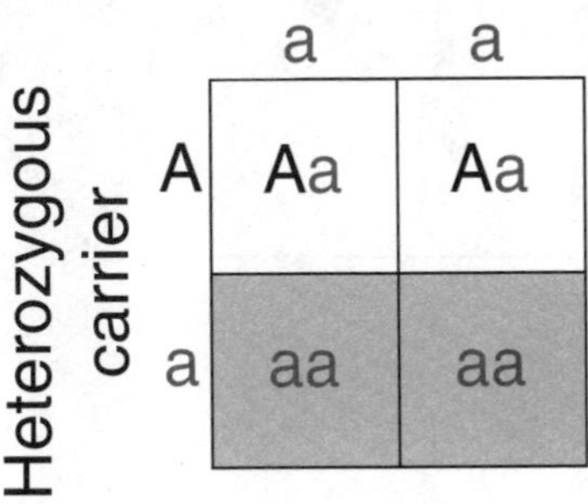


Heterozygous carrier

| Heterozygous carrier | A | a |
|---|---|---|
| A | AA | Aa |
| a | Aa | aa |

# Autosomal Recessive Inheritance Patterns

Transparency #16

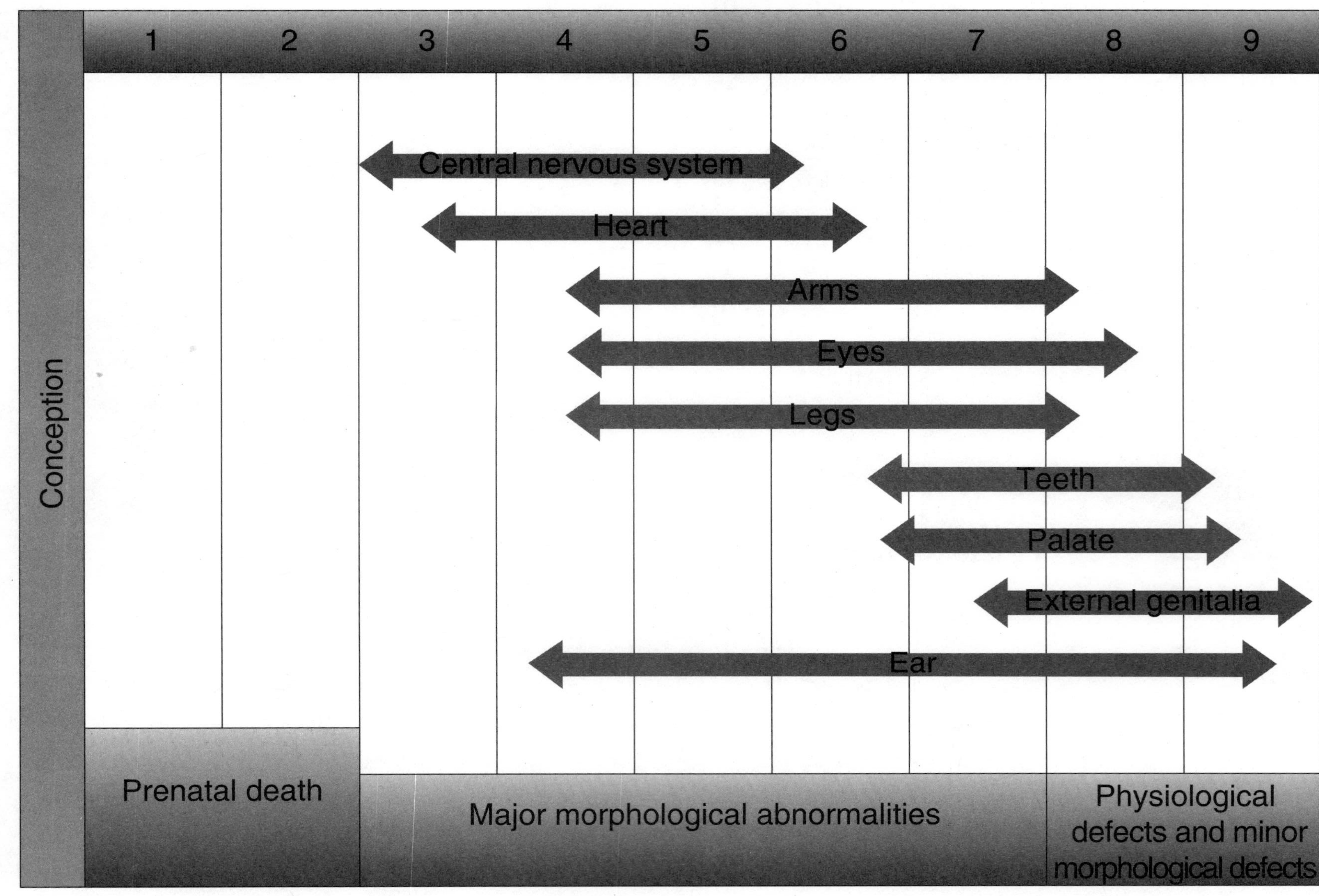


# Periods of Fetal Vulnerability

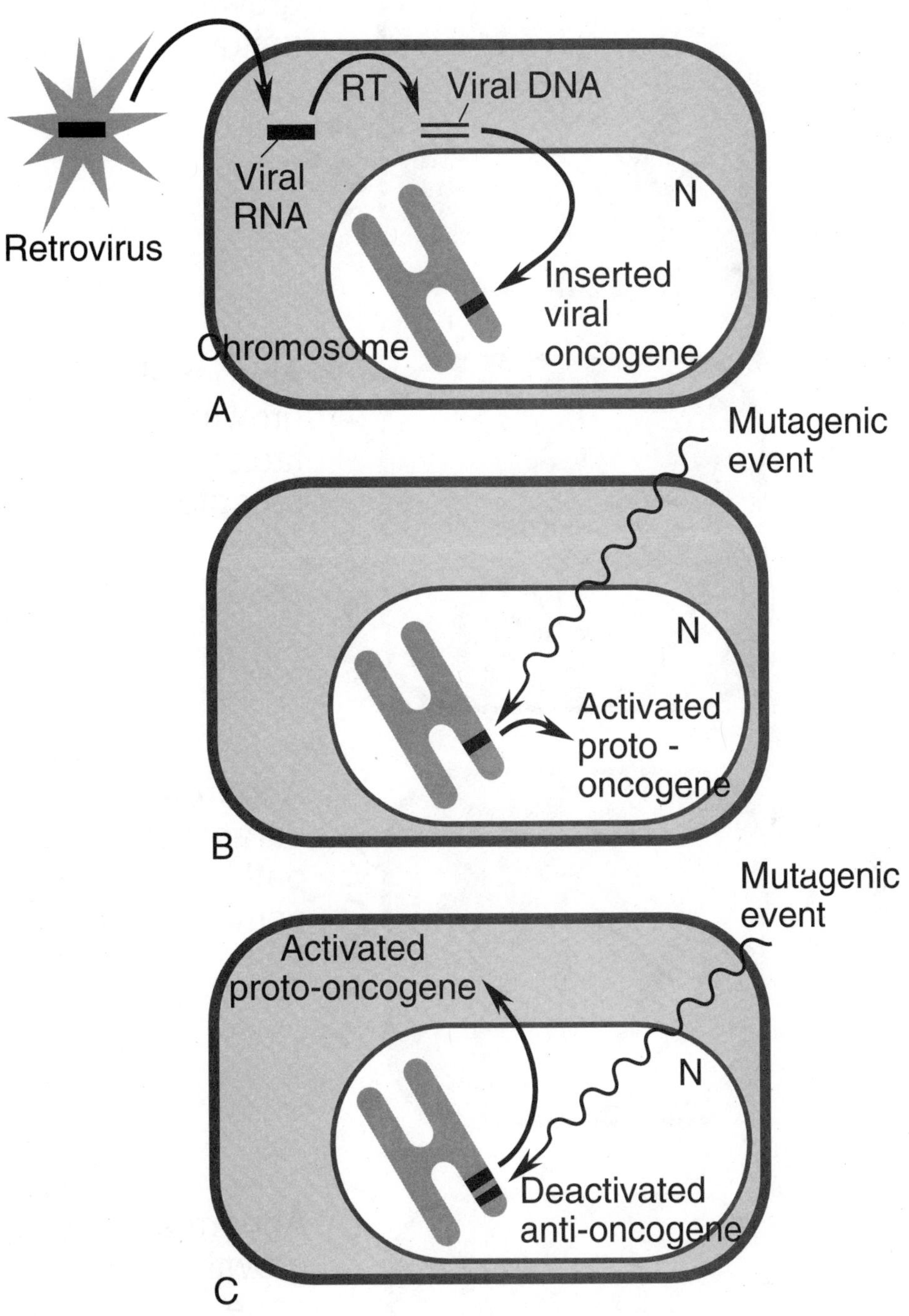


Mechanisms of Oncogene Activation

Transparency #18

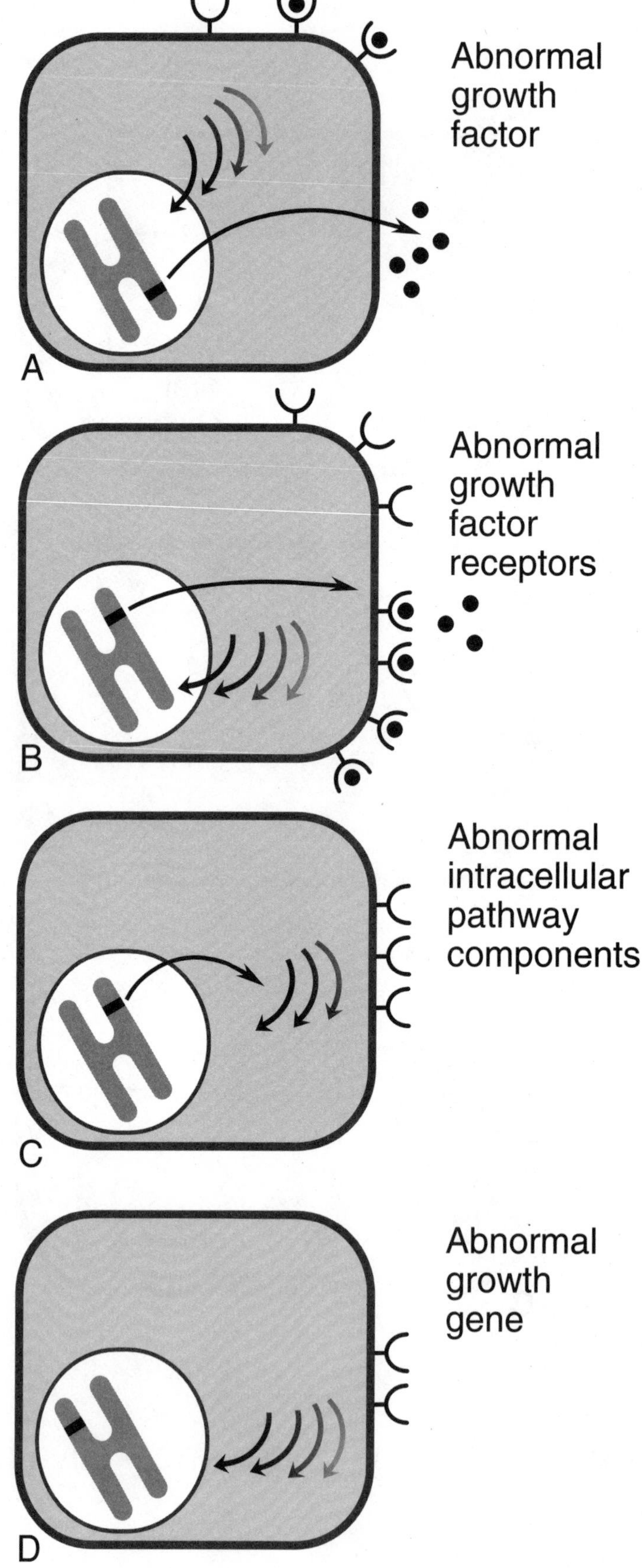


Mechanisms of Altered Growth Control

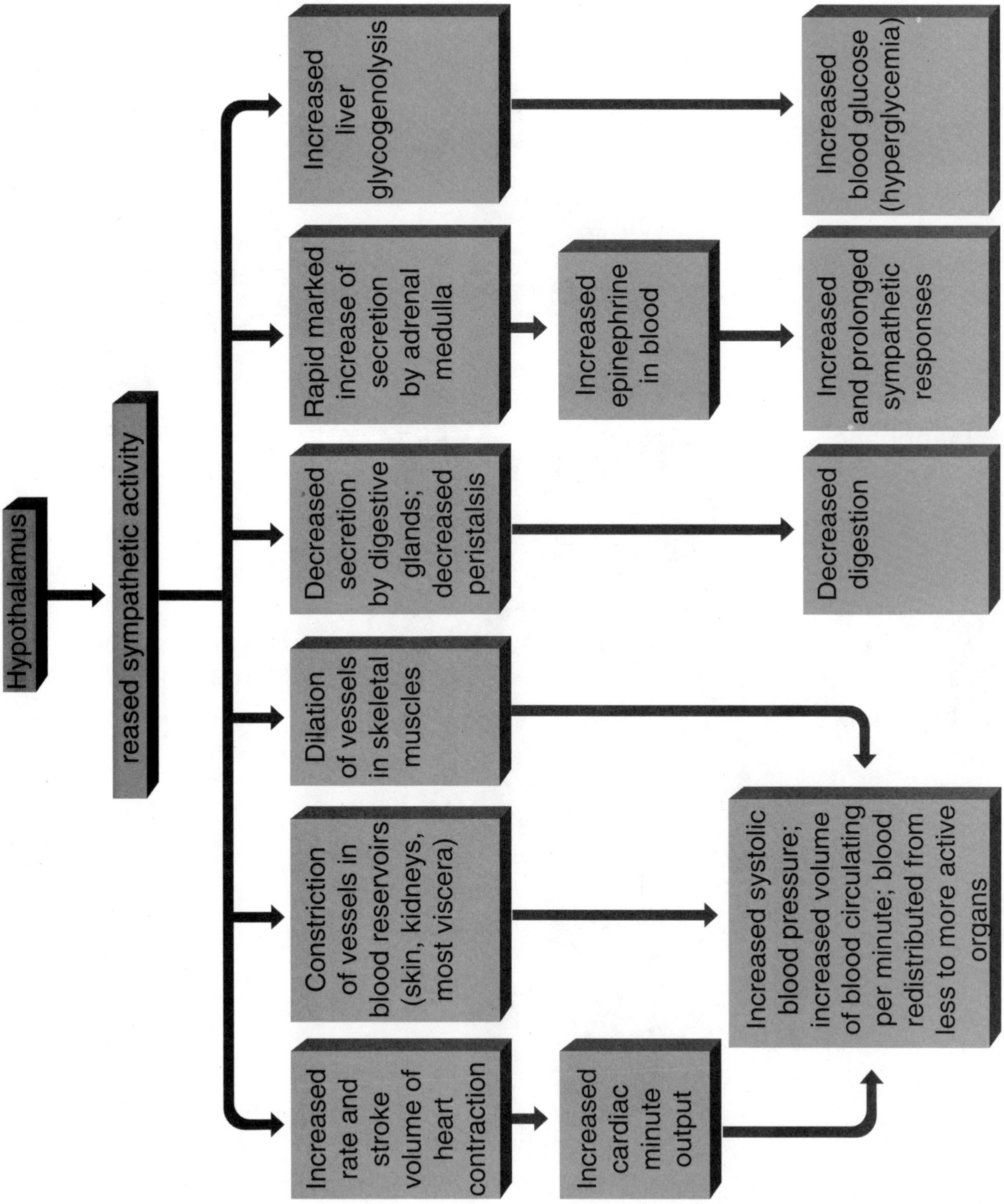

# Sympathetic Alarm Reaction

Hypothalamus

reased sympathetic activity

Increased rate and stroke volume of heart contraction

Increased cardiac minute output

Constriction of vessels in blood reservoirs (skin, kidneys, most viscera)

Dilation of vessels in skeletal muscles

Increased systolic blood pressure; increased volume of blood circulating per minute; blood redistributed from less to more active organs

Decreased secretion by digestive glands; decreased peristalsis

Decreased digestion

Rapid marked increase of secretion by adrenal medulla

Increased epinephrine in blood

Increased and prolonged sympathetic responses

Increased liver glycogenolysis

Increased blood glucose (hyperglycemia)

Adapted with permission from Thibodeau GA, Patton KT: *Anatomy and Physiology*, 2nd ed. St Louis, Mosby-Year Book, 1993, p 570.

W. B. Saunders Company

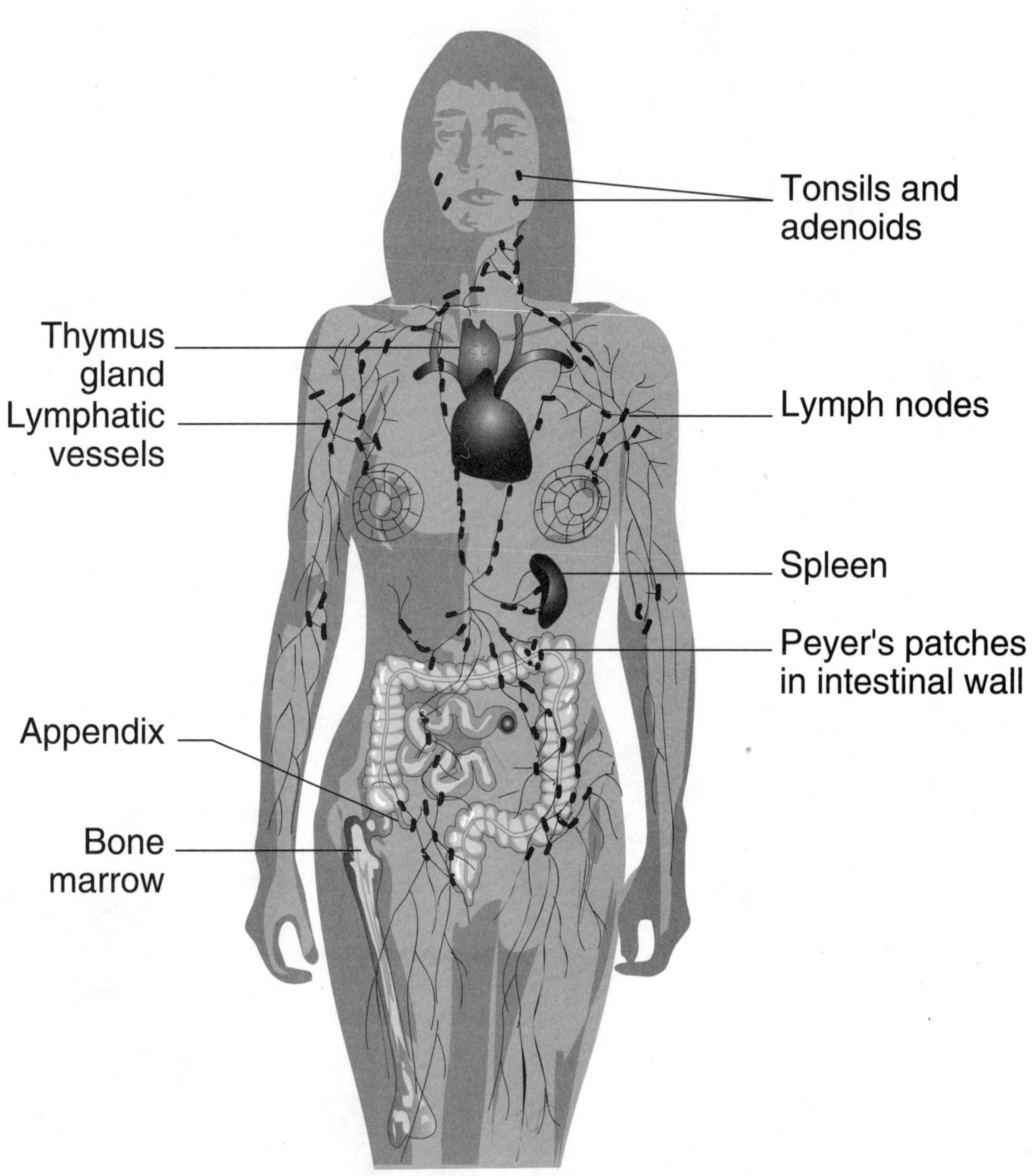


Organs of the Immune System

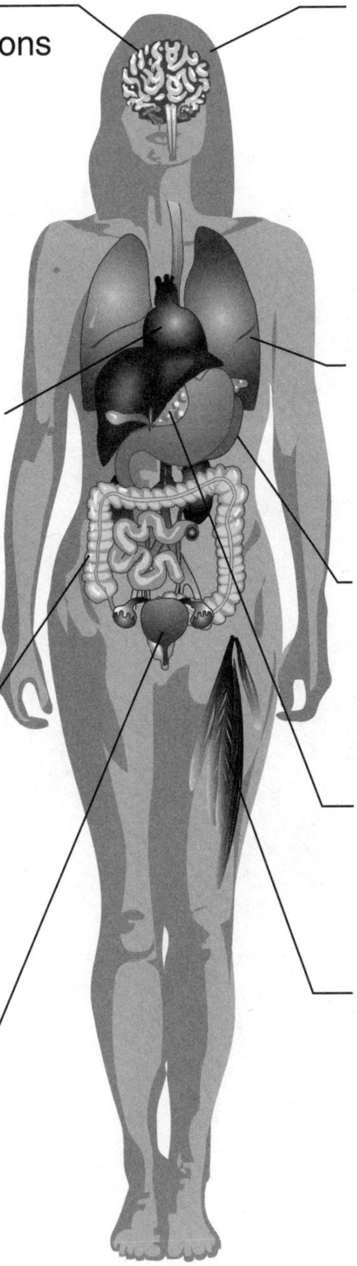

NERVOUS SYSTEM

Neuropsychological Manifestations

- Nervous tic
- Fatigue
- Loss of motivation
- Anxiety
- Overeating
- Depression
- Insomnia

INTEGUMENTARY SYSTEM

- Eczema
- Psoriasis
- Neurodermatitis
- Acne
- Hair loss

RESPIRATORY SYSTEM

- Increased respiration
- Asthma
- Hay fever

CARDIOVASCULAR SYSTEM

- Disturbances of heart rate and rhythm
- Hypertension
- Stroke
- Coronary artery disease

IMMUNE SYSTEM

- Immunodeficiency
- Immunosuppression
- Autoimmune disease

GASTROINTESTINAL SYSTEM

- Gastritis
- Irritable bowel syndrome
- Diarrhea
- Nausea and vomiting
- Ulcerative colitis

ENDOCRINE SYSTEM

- Hyperglycemia
- Diabetes mellitus

MUSCULOSKELETAL SYSTEM

- Tension headache
- Muscle contraction backache
- Rheumatoid arthritis
- Inflammatory diseases of connective tissue

GENITOURINARY SYSTEM

- Diuresis
- Irritable bladder
- Impotence
- Frigidity
- Menstrual irregularity

# Potential Stress Reactions

Transparency #22

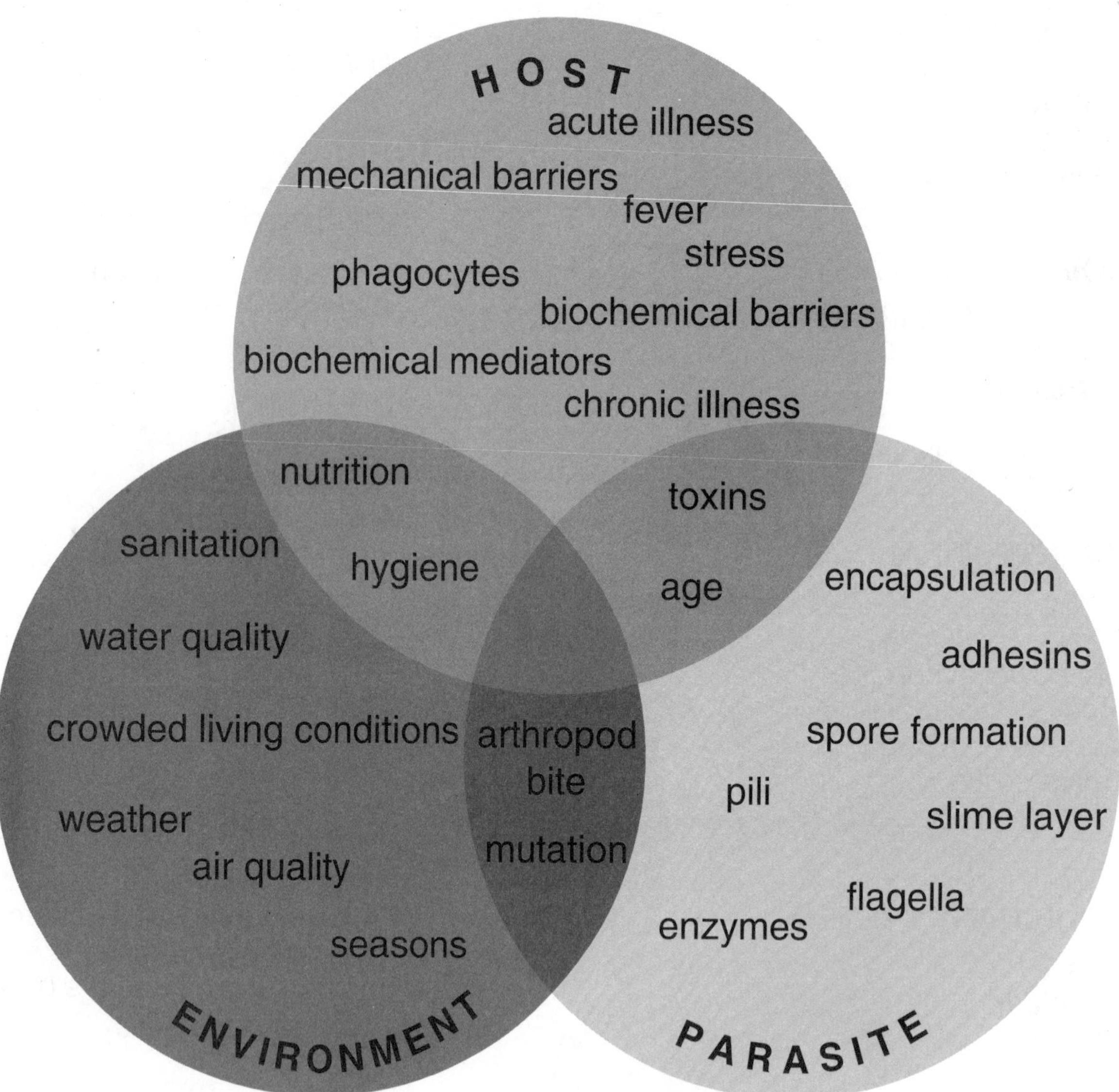


Factors Affecting Infectious Processes

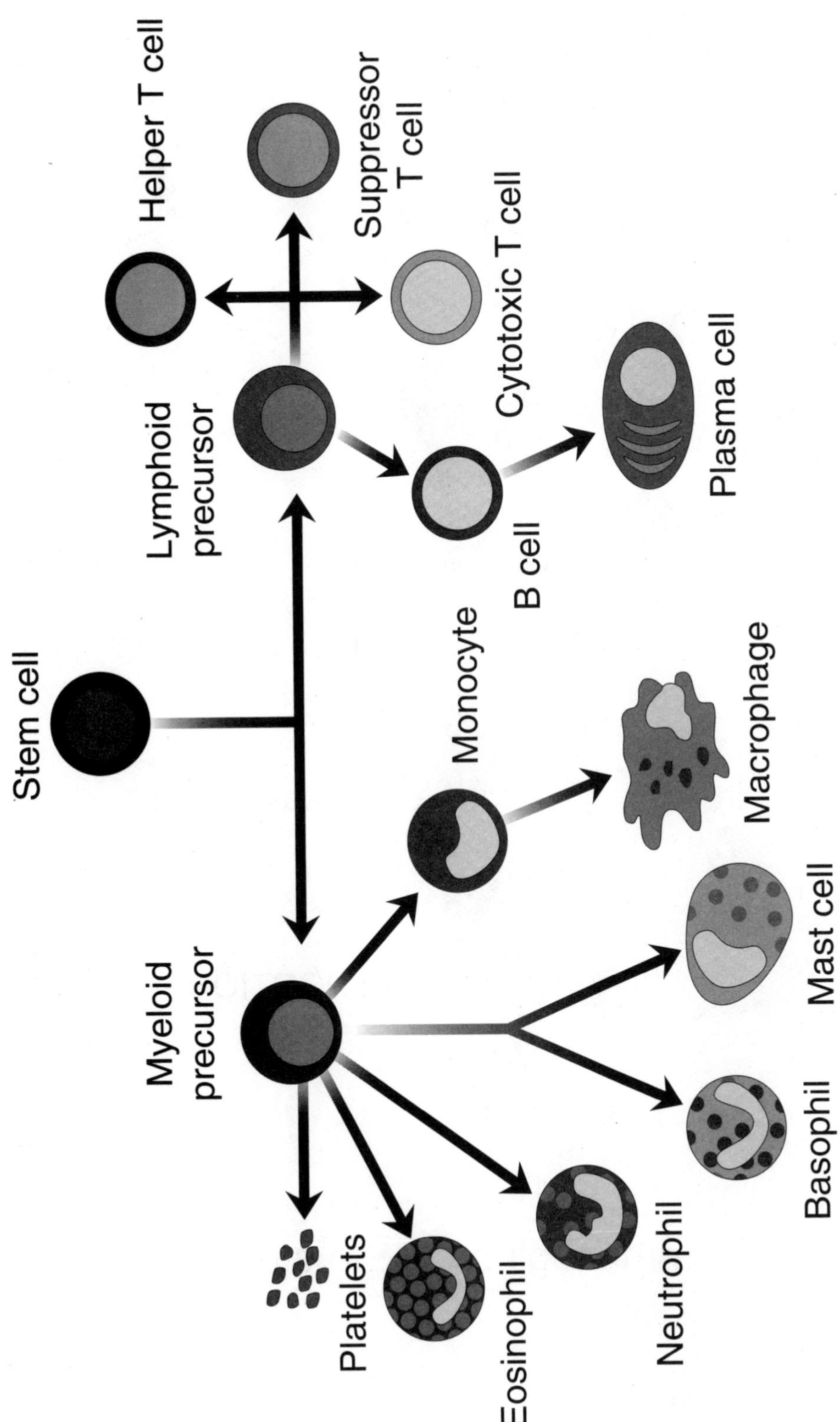


Redrawn from Schindler LW: *Understanding the Immune System.* NIH Publication No. 92-529. U.S. Department of Health and Human Services, 1991, p.5.

W. B. Saunders Company

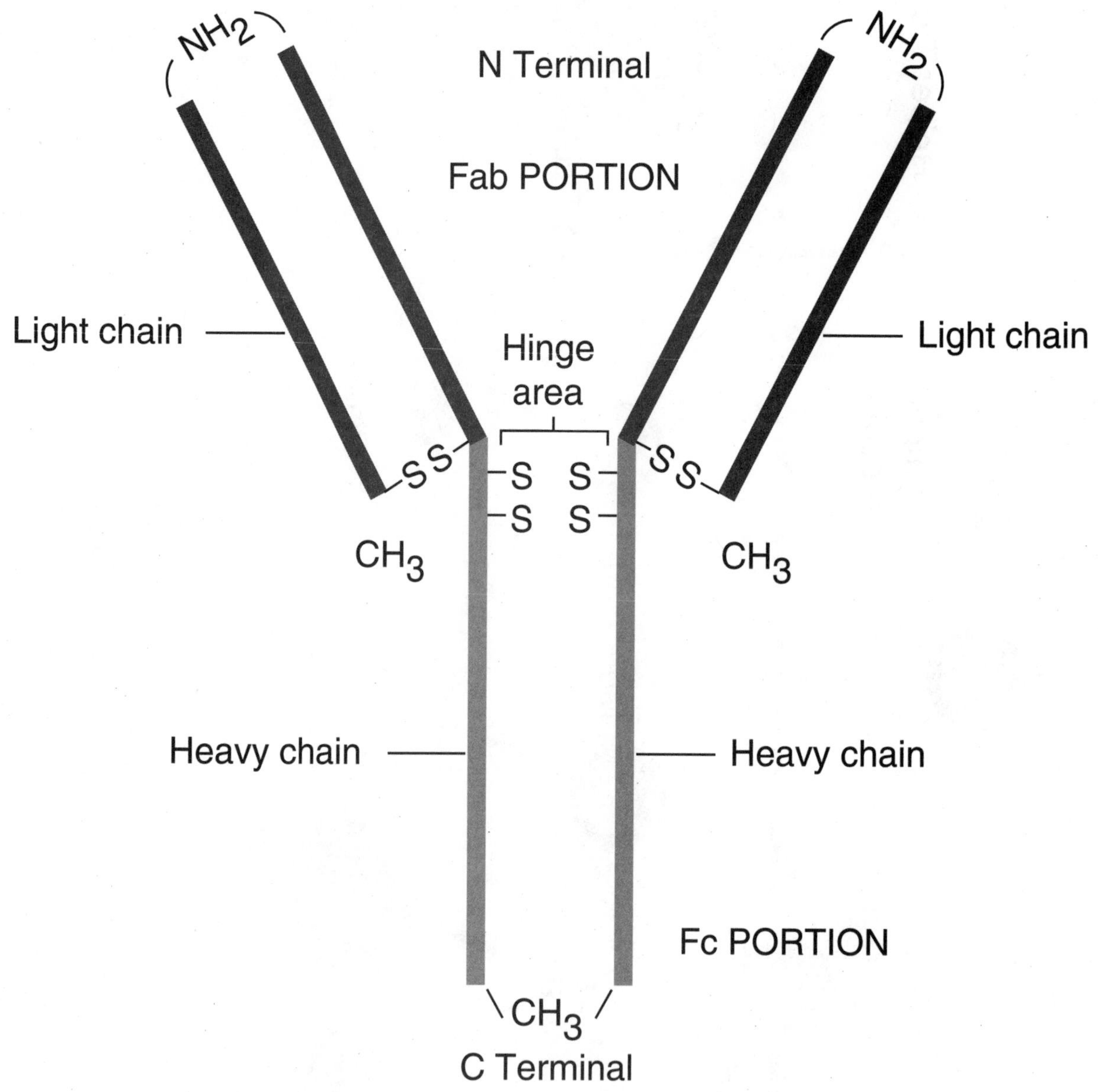


Typical Immunoglobulin Structure

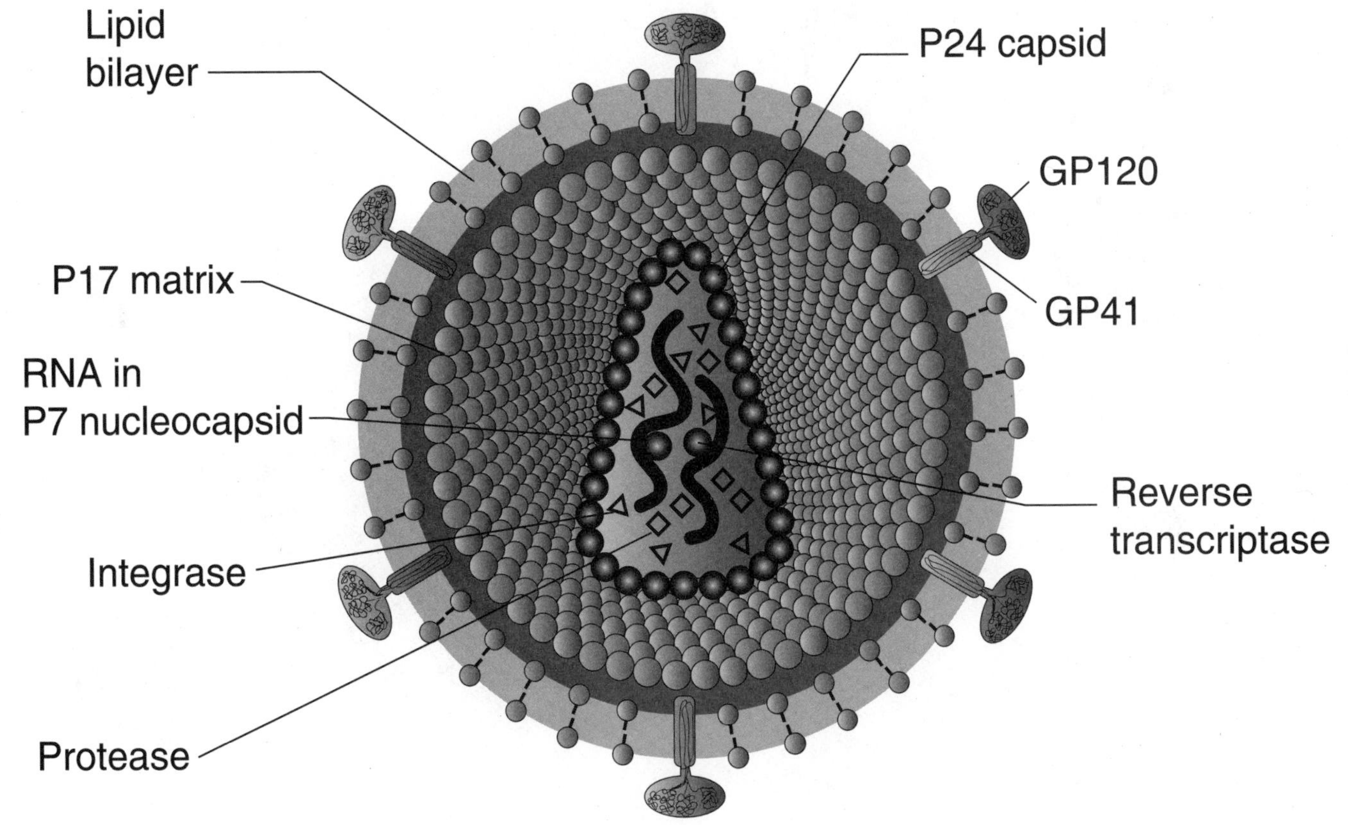


HIV Structure

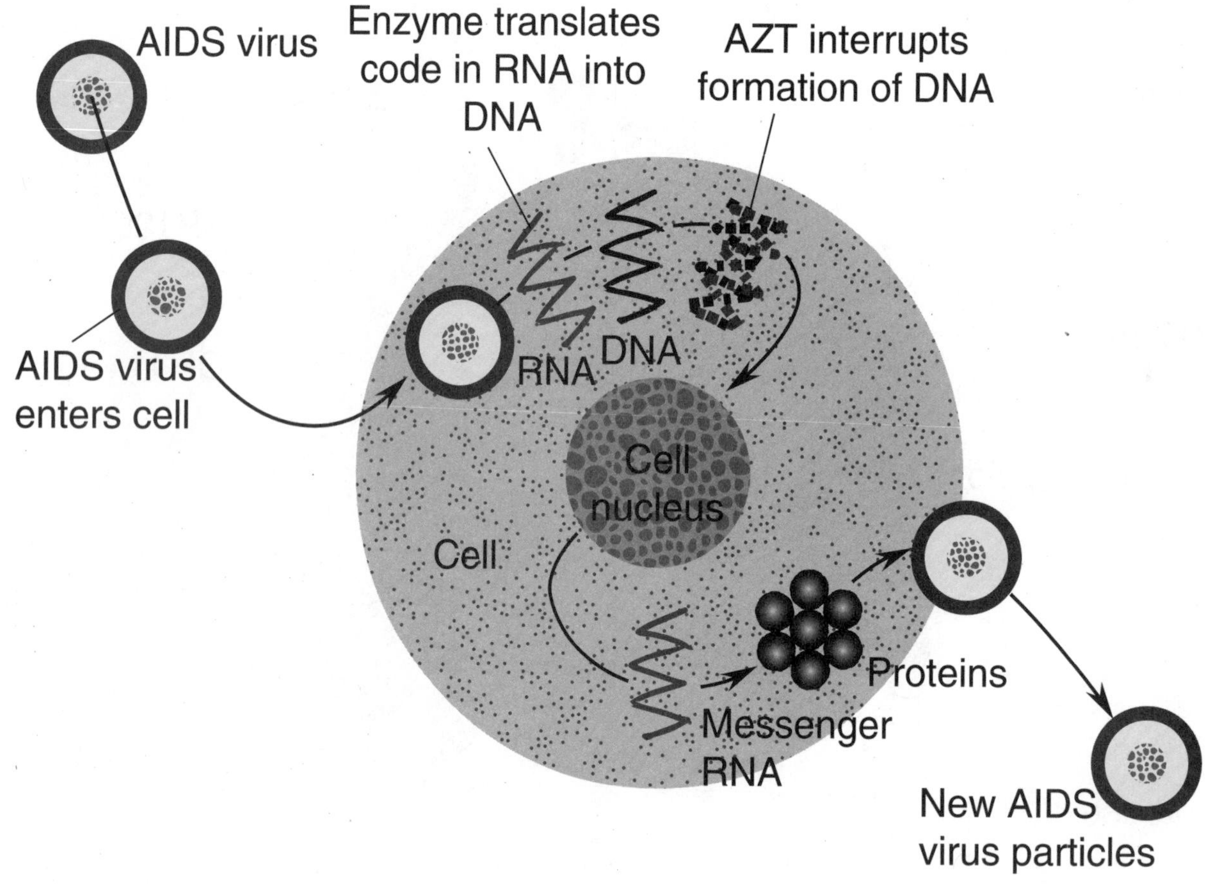


## Sequence of HIV Infection

Redrawn with permission from Schecter J: The frustrating fight against AIDS, *Technol Rev* 1987;90:65.

W. B. Saunders Company

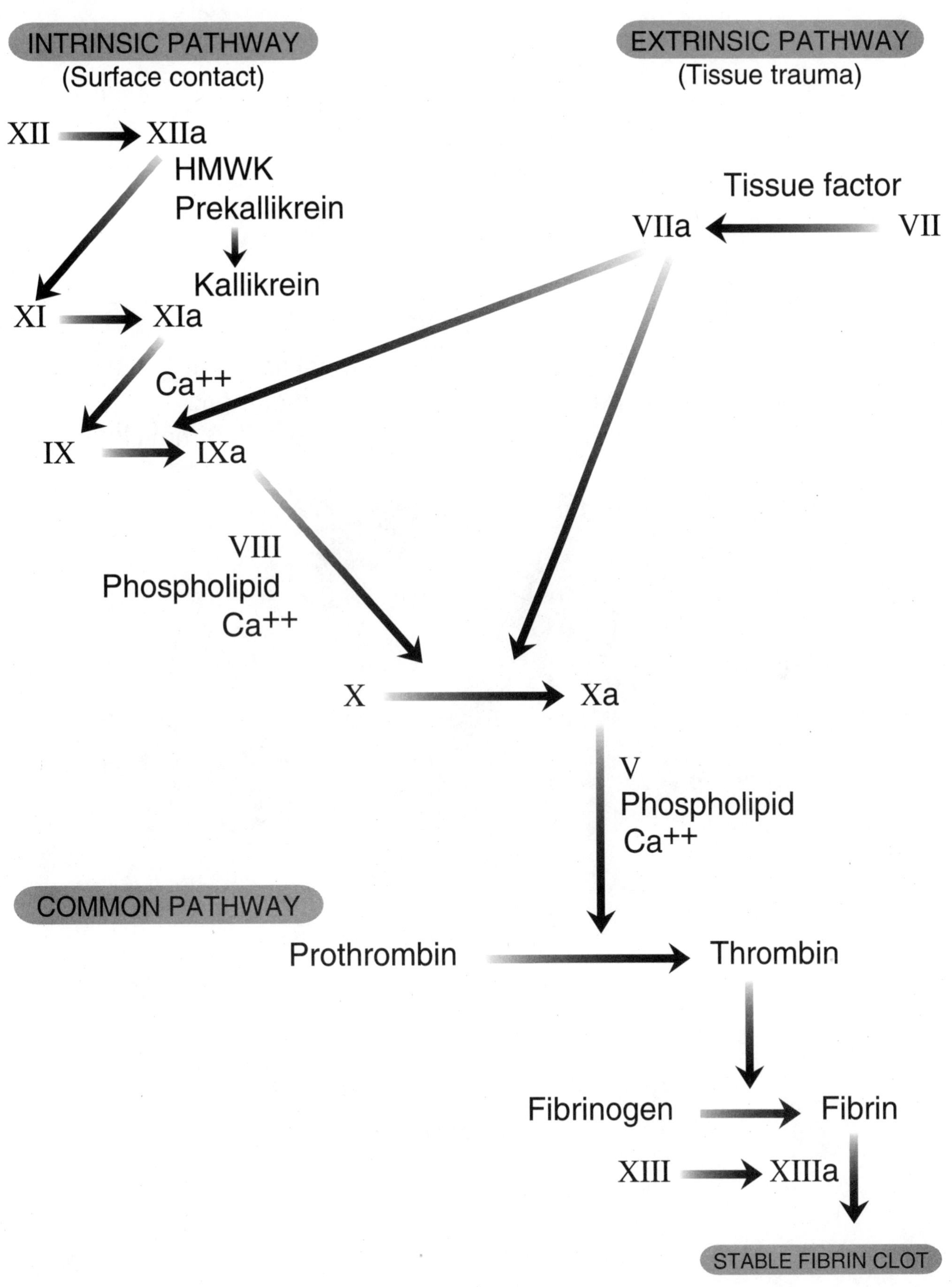


The Clotting Cascade

Transparency #28

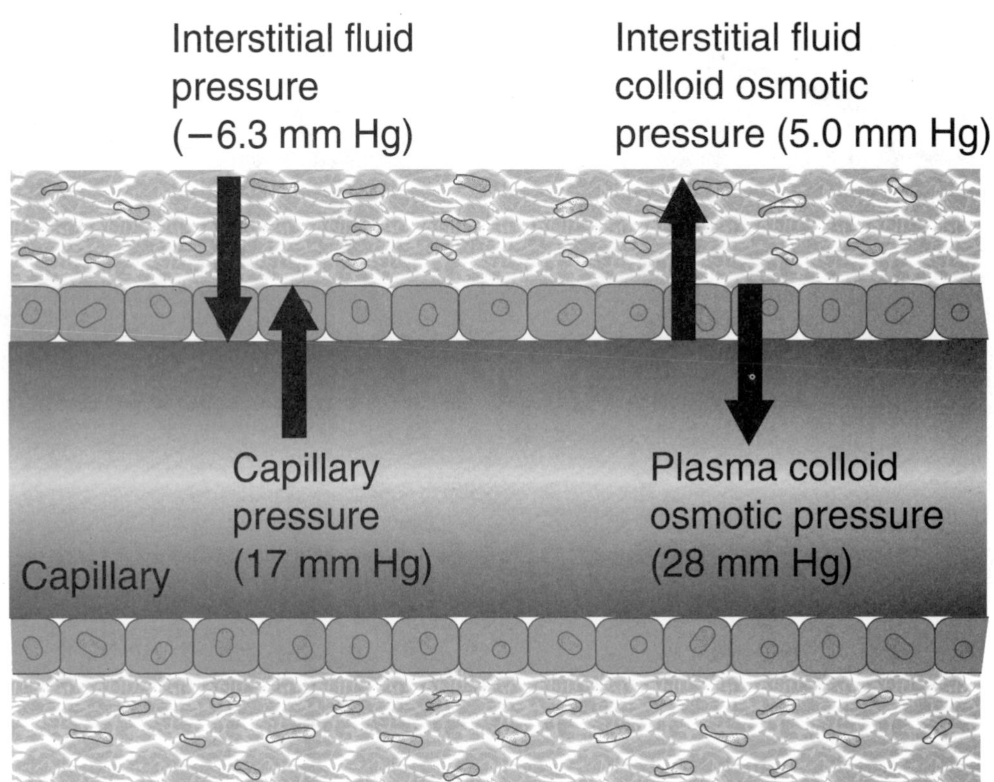


# Factors Affecting Transcapillary Filtration

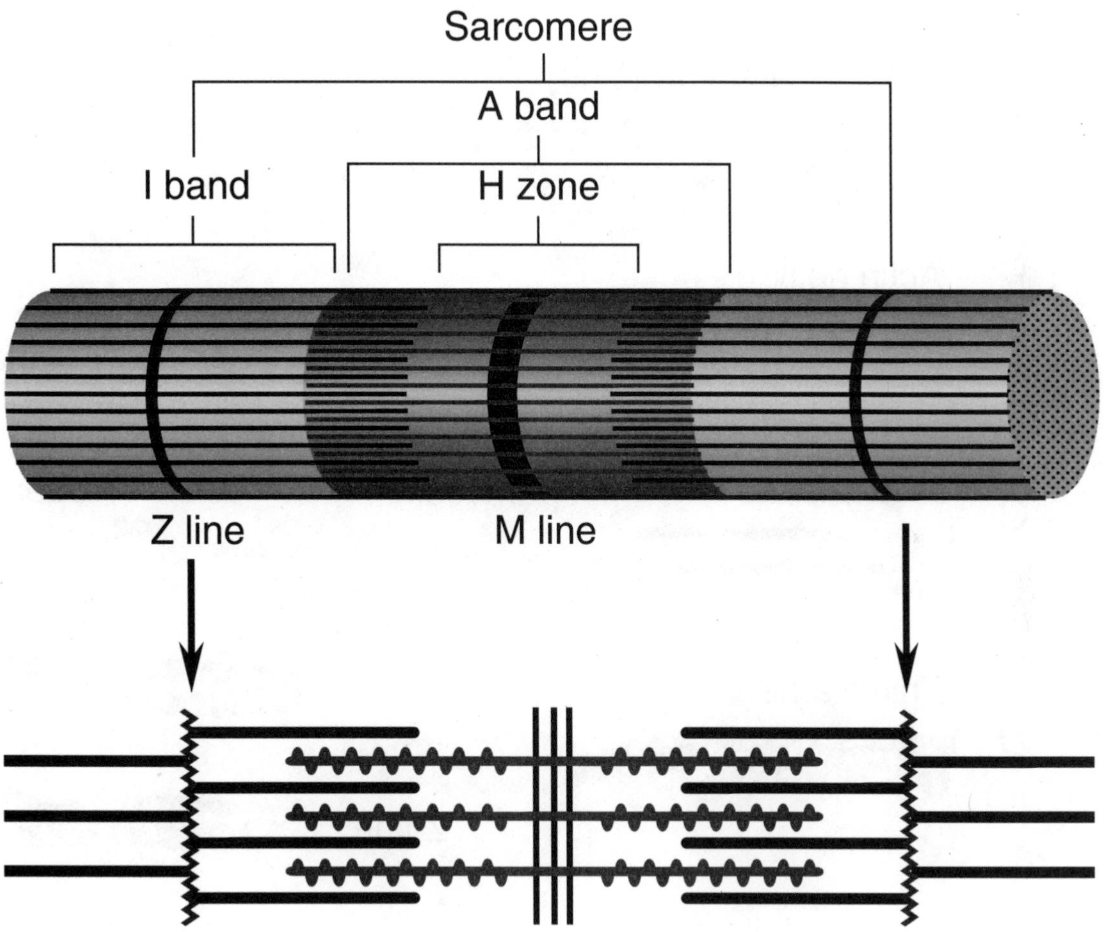


Sarcomere Structure

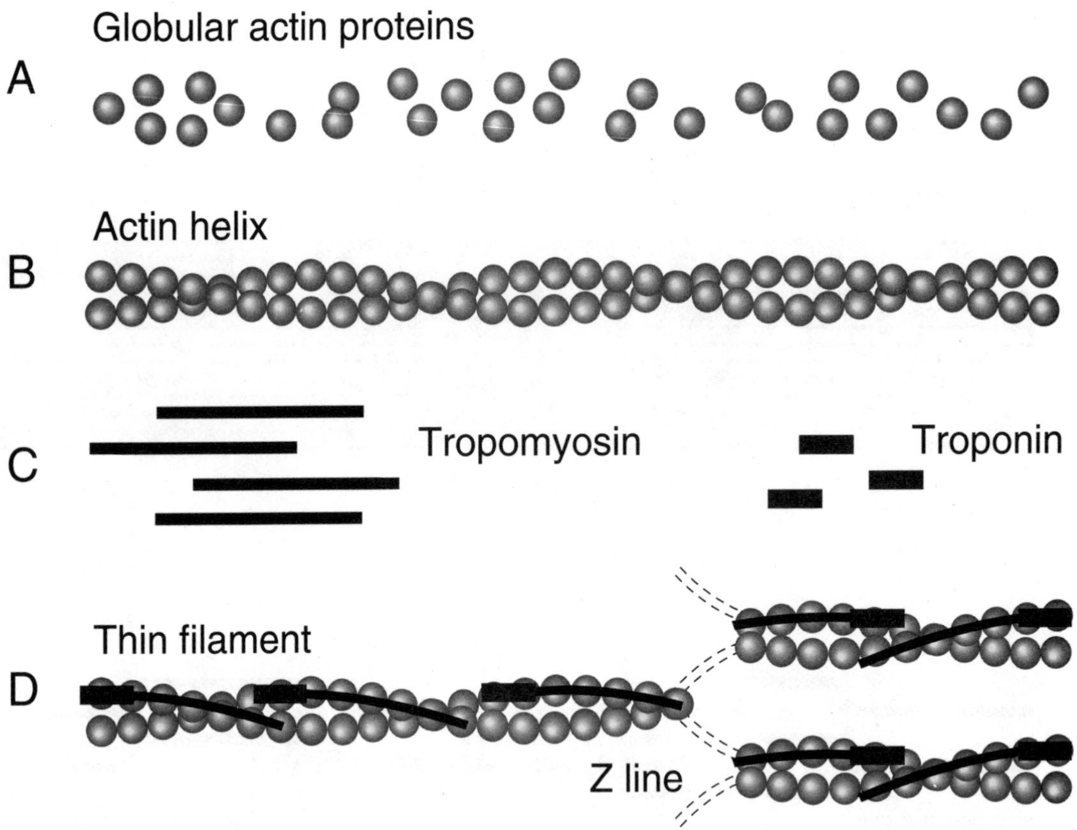


Proteins of the Thin Filament

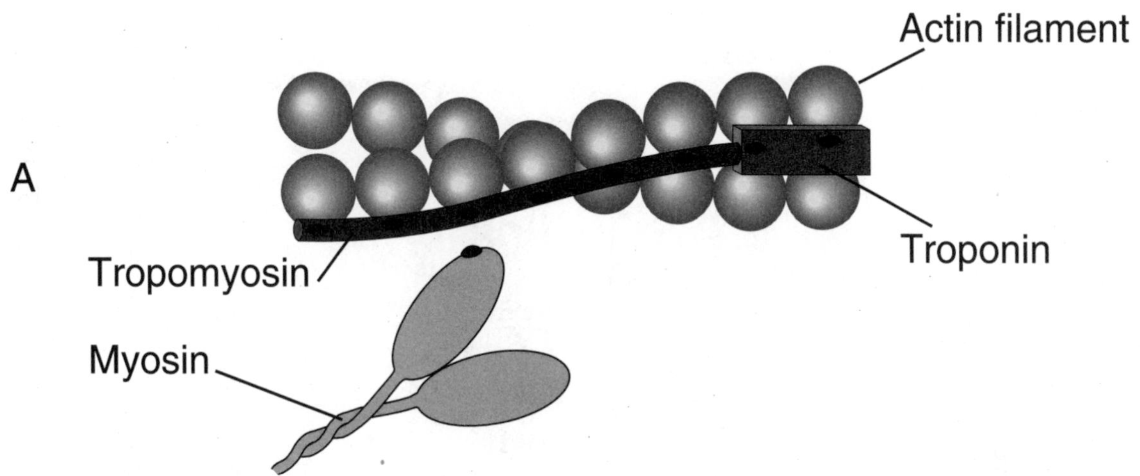


CROSSBRIDGE BINDING SITE BLOCKED BY TROPOMYOSIN

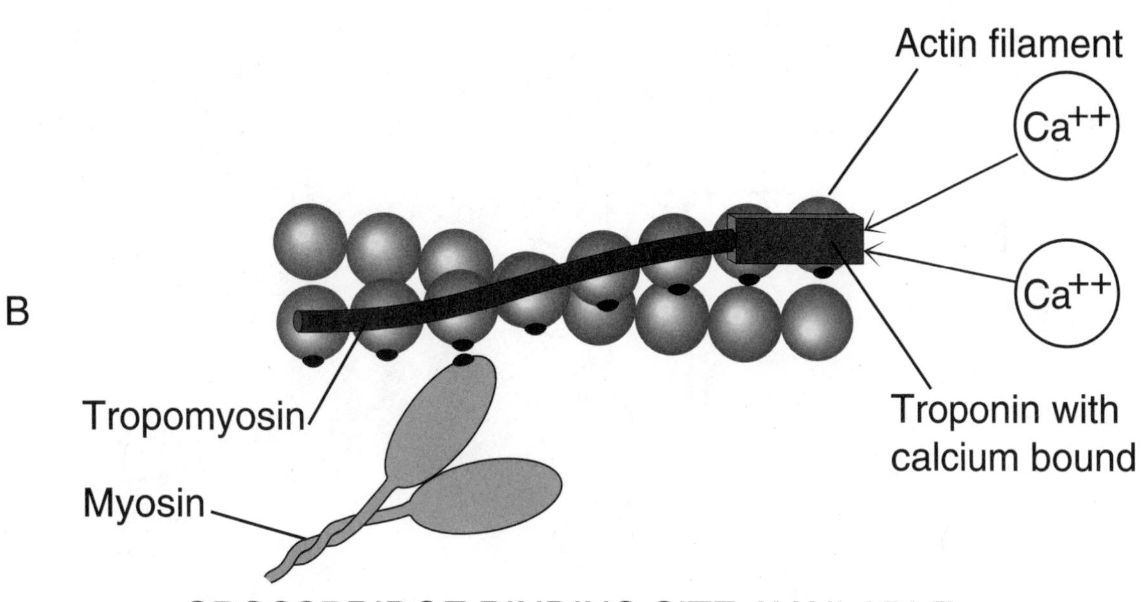


CROSSBRIDGE BINDING SITE AVAILABLE

# The Role of Calcium Ion in Crossbridge Formation

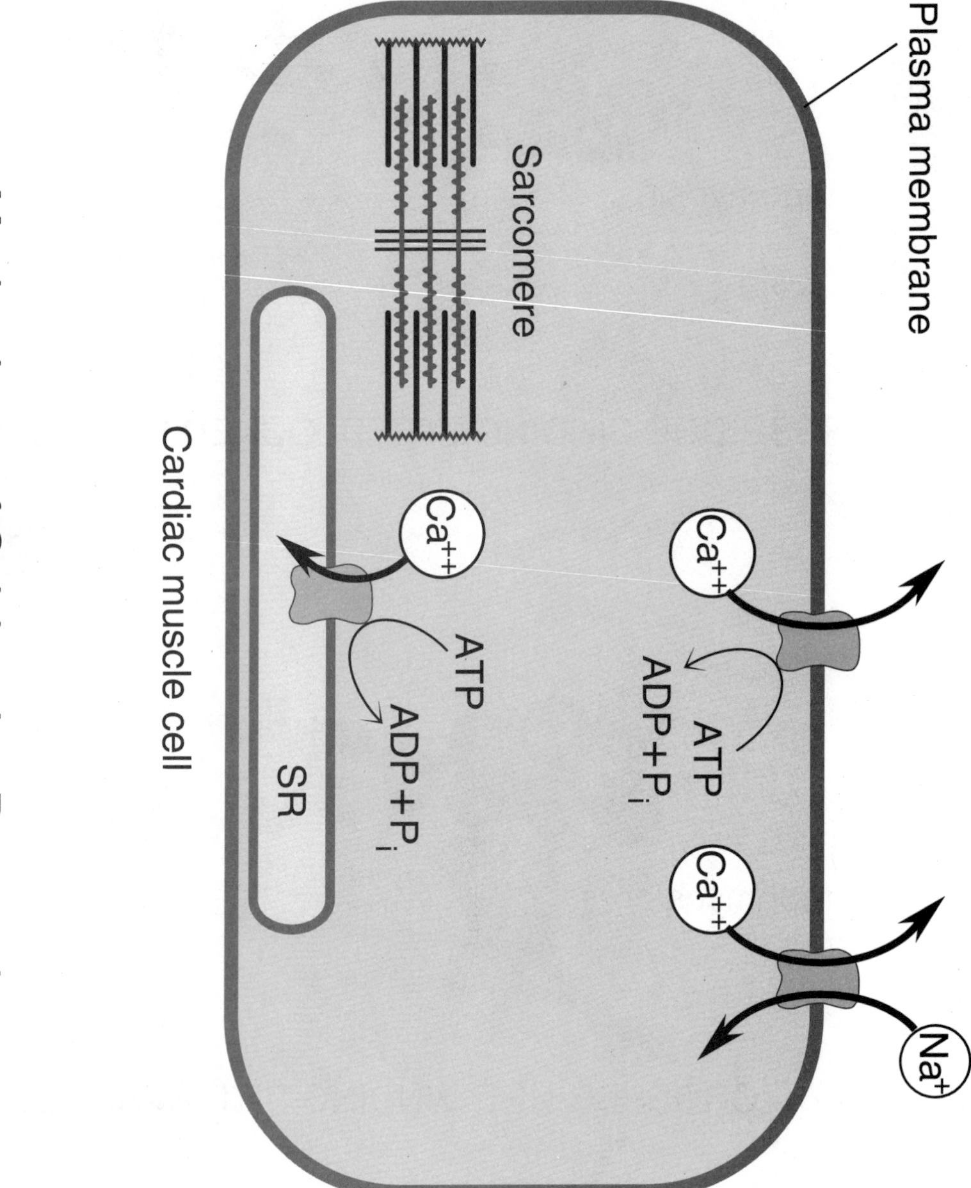


# Mechanisms of Calcium Ion Removal from the Sarcoplasm

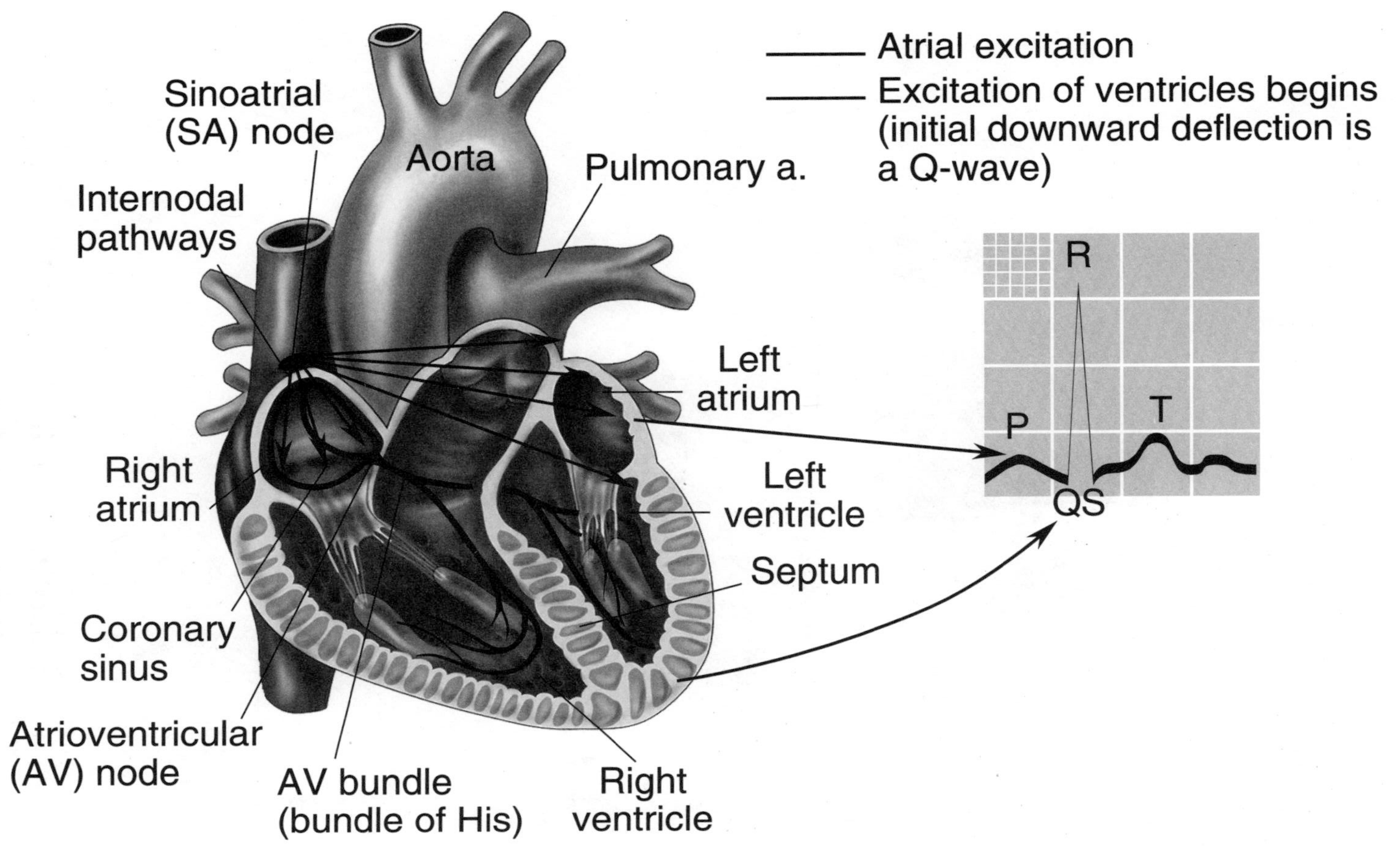


Conduction System of the Heart

Transparency #34

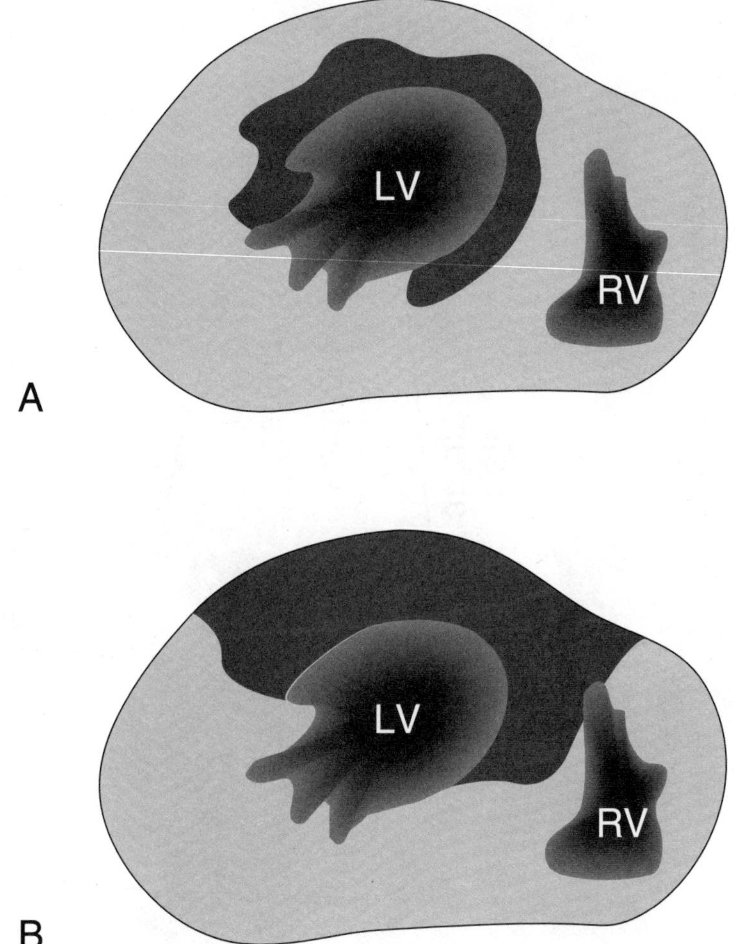


Subendocardial (A) and
Transmural (B) Infarct

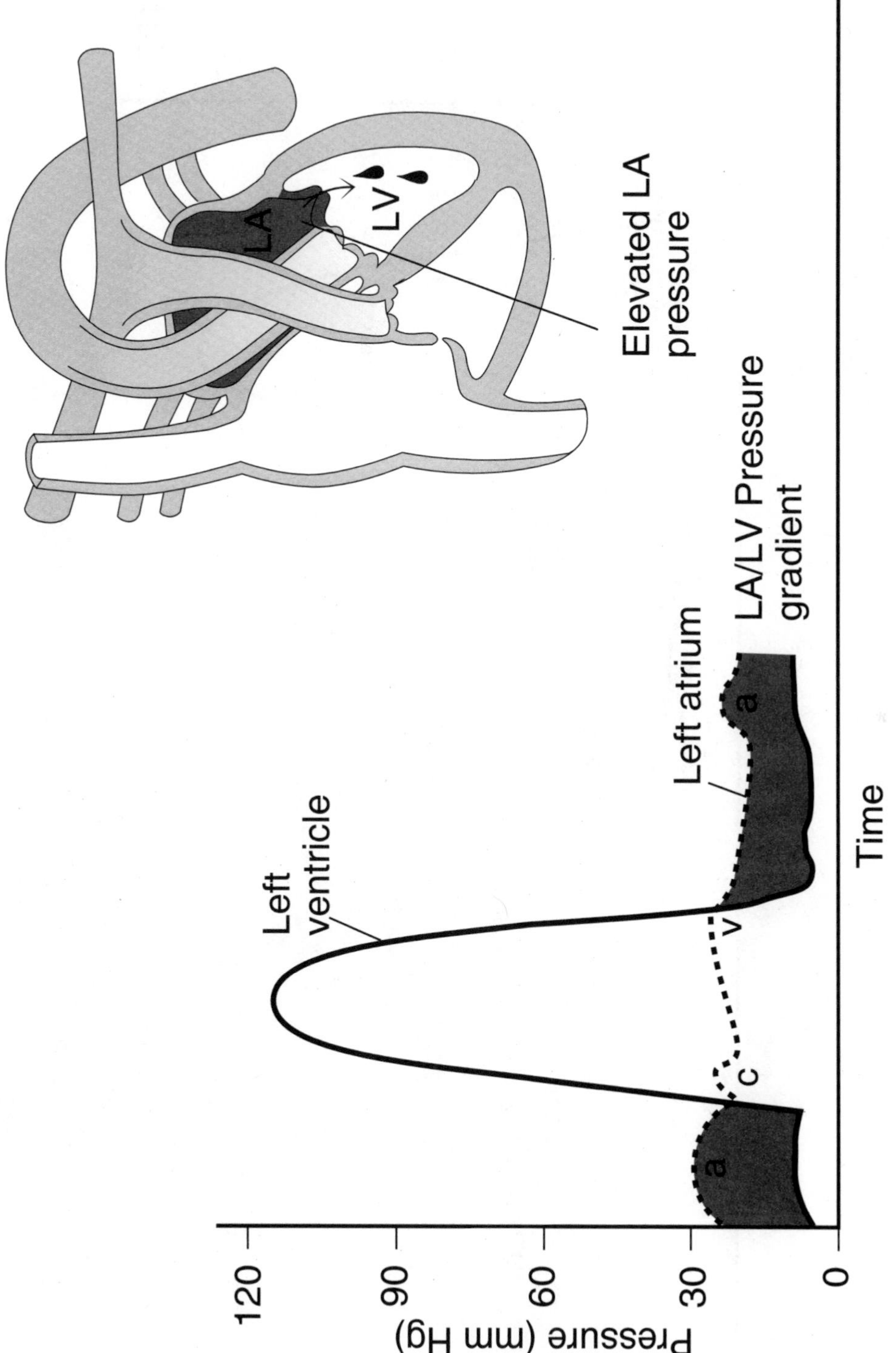


Mitral Stenosis

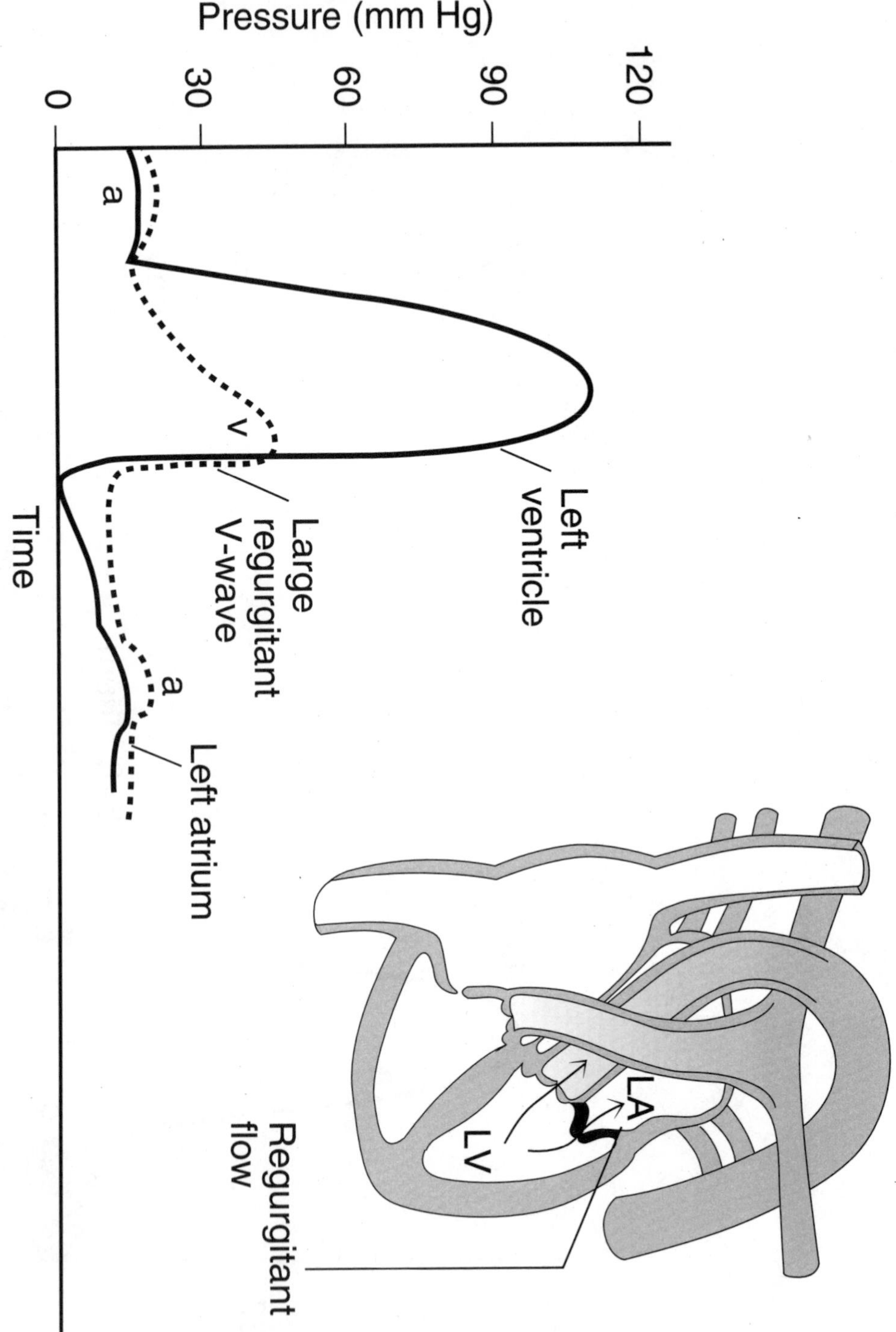


Mitral Regurgitation

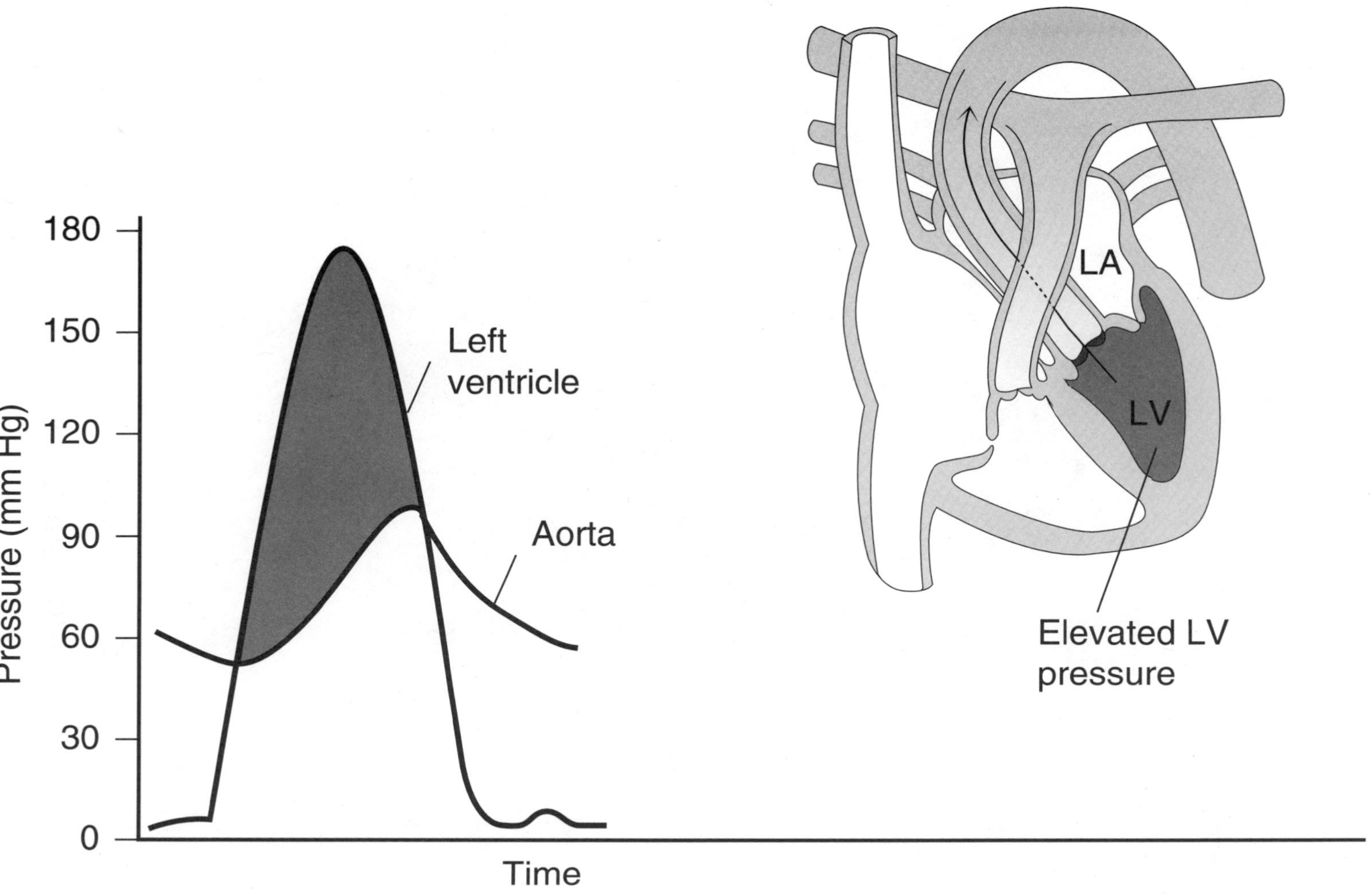


Aortic Stenosis

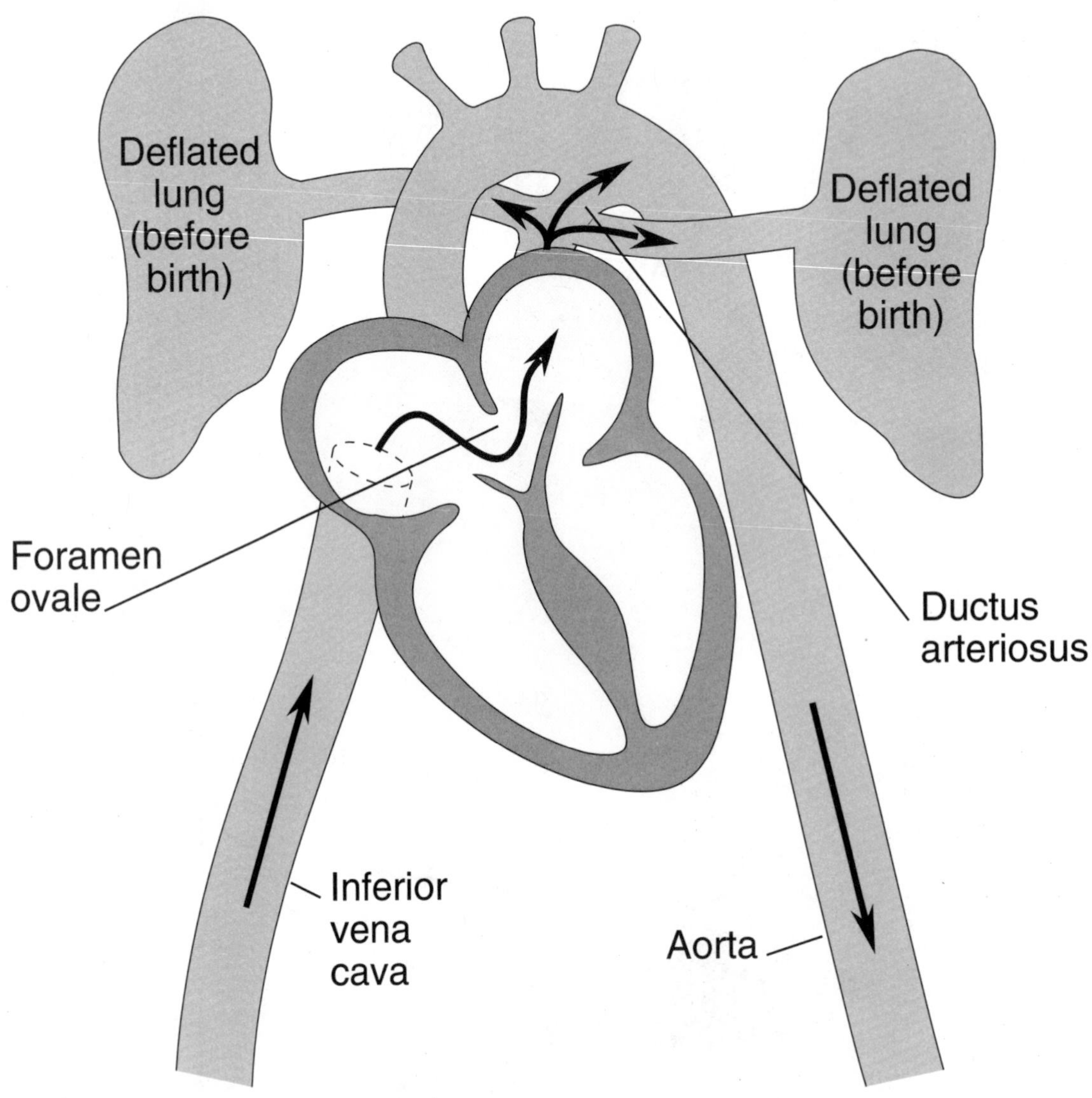


Fetal Circulation

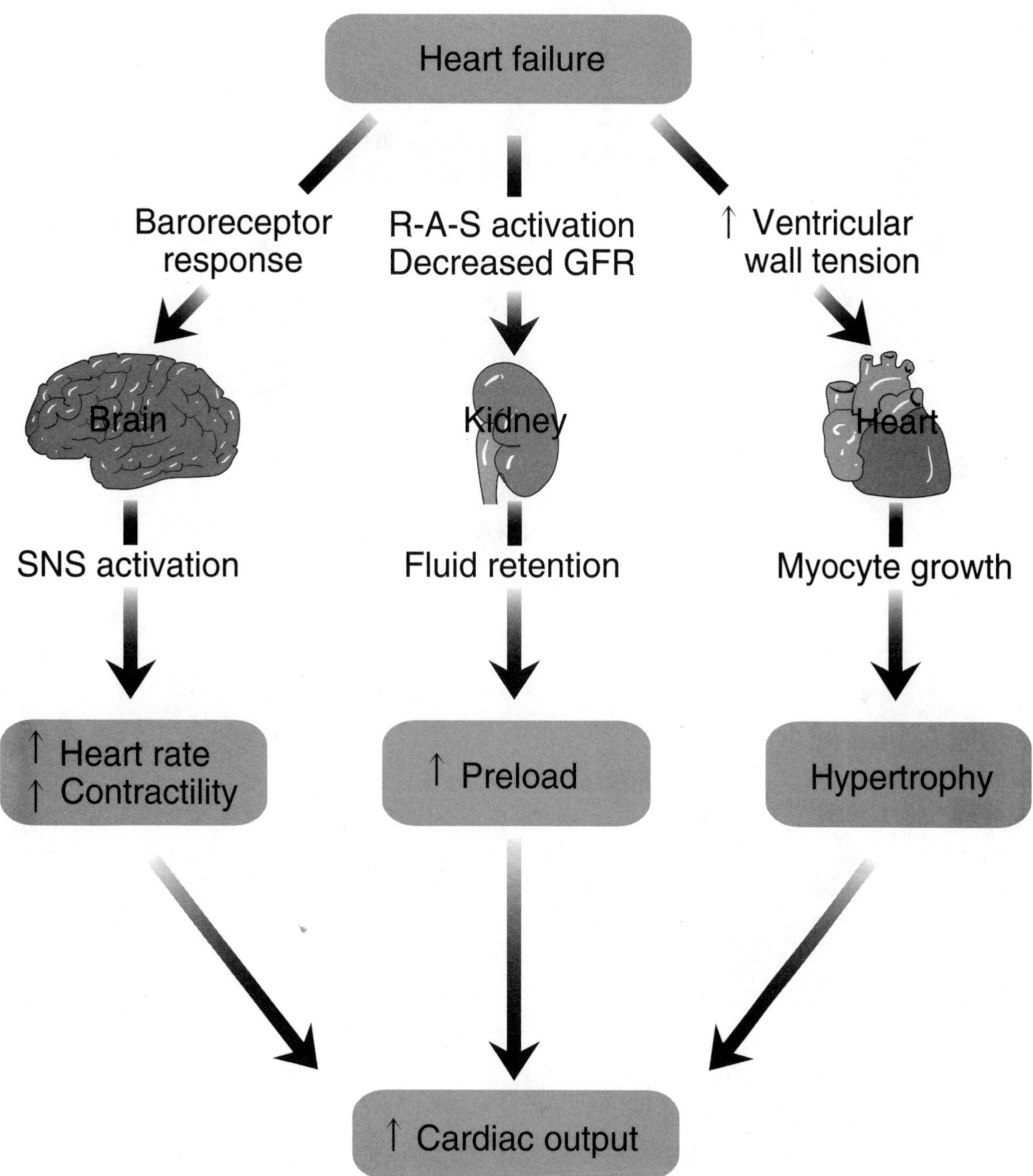


Compensatory Mechanisms in Heart Failure

Transparency #40

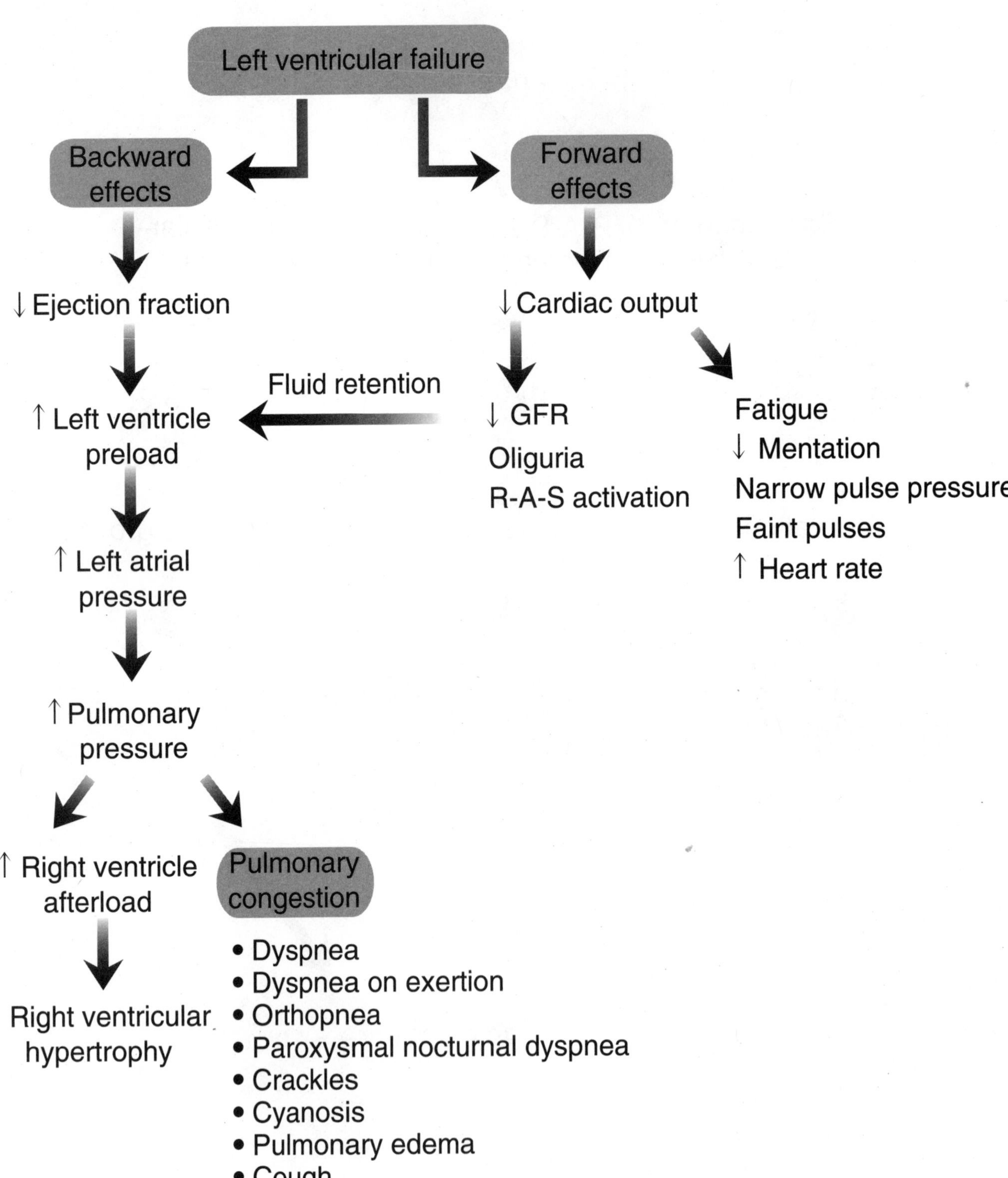


## Pathophysiology of Left Heart Failure

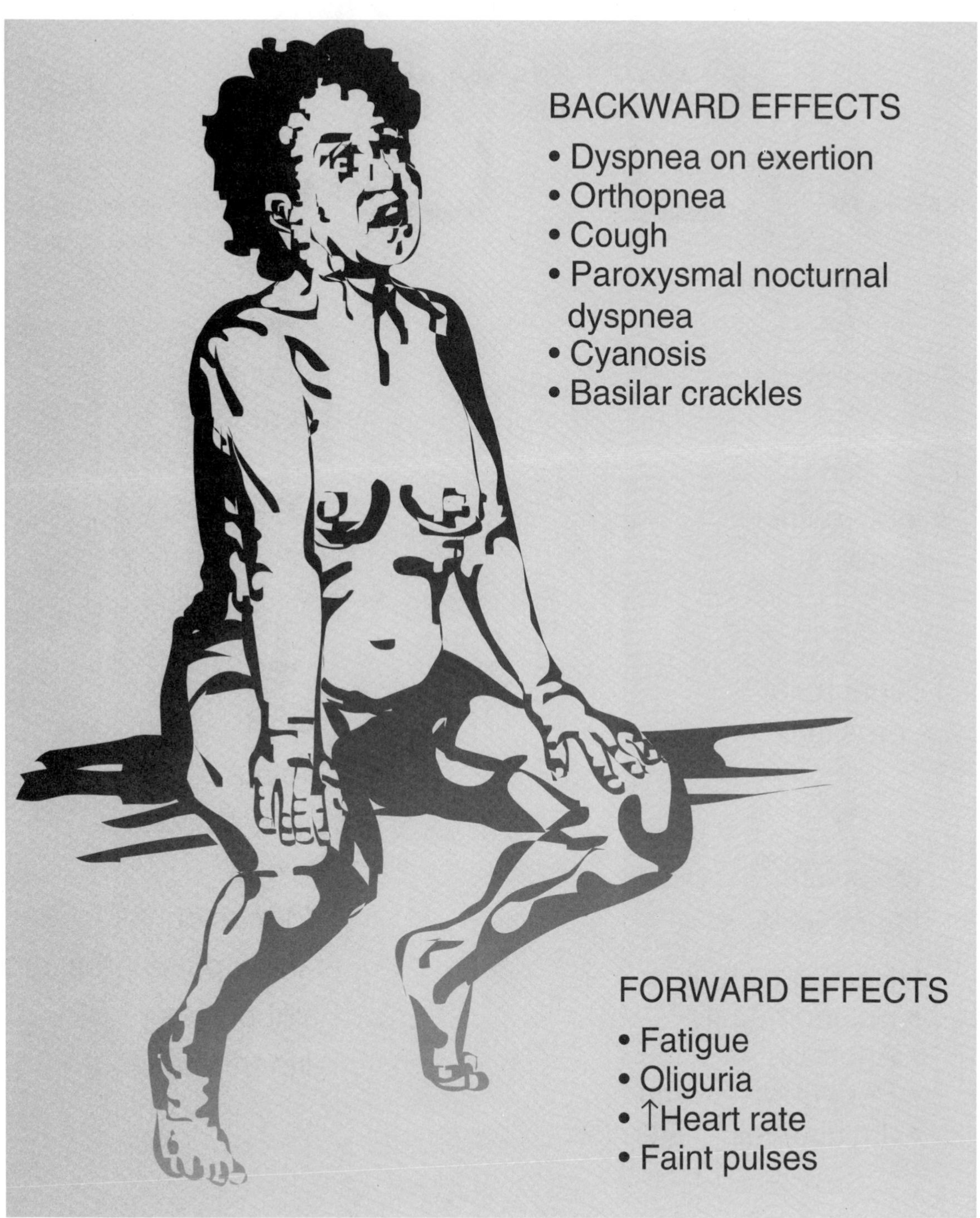


Manifestations of Left Heart Failure

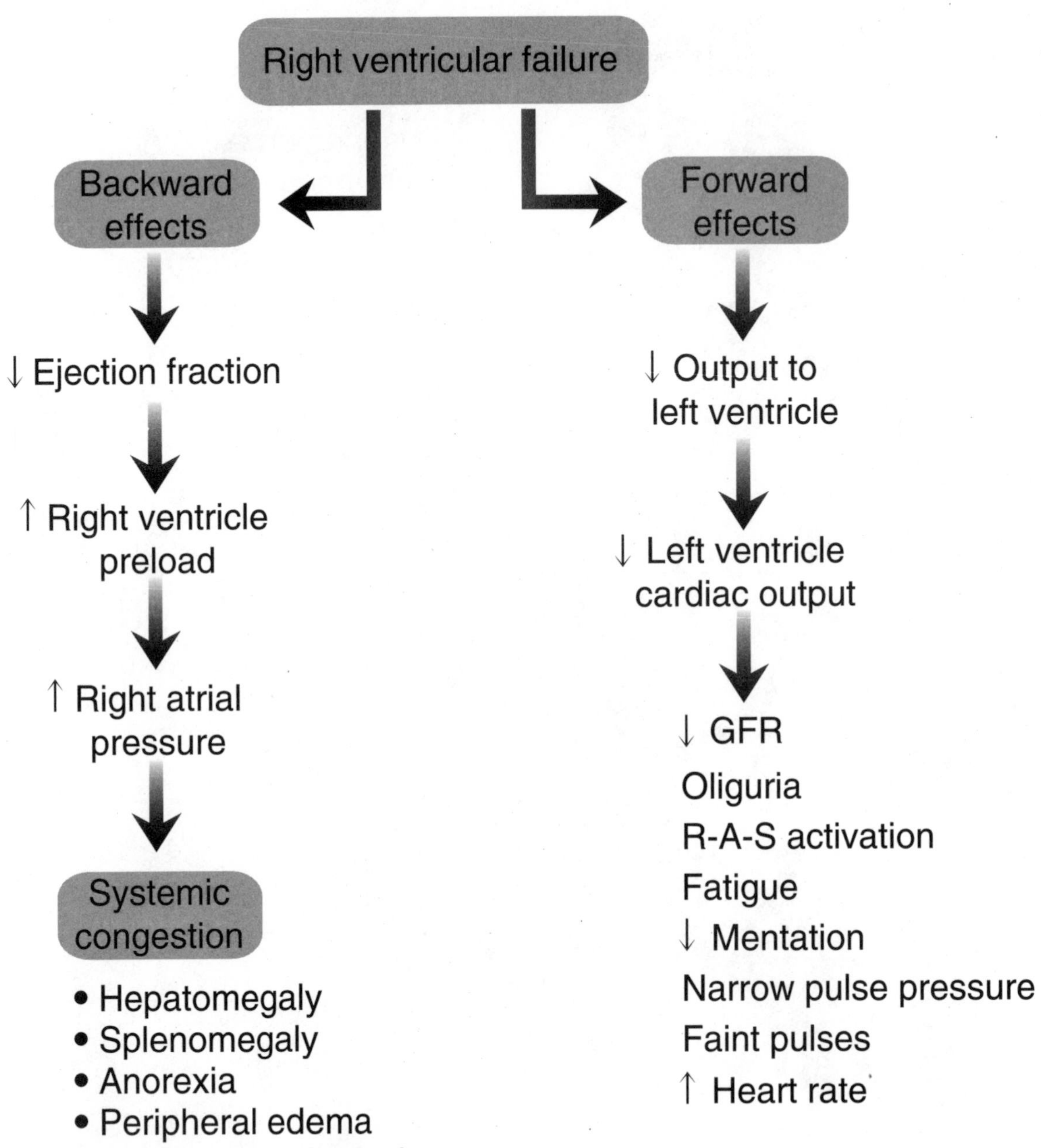


Pathophysiology of Right Heart Failure

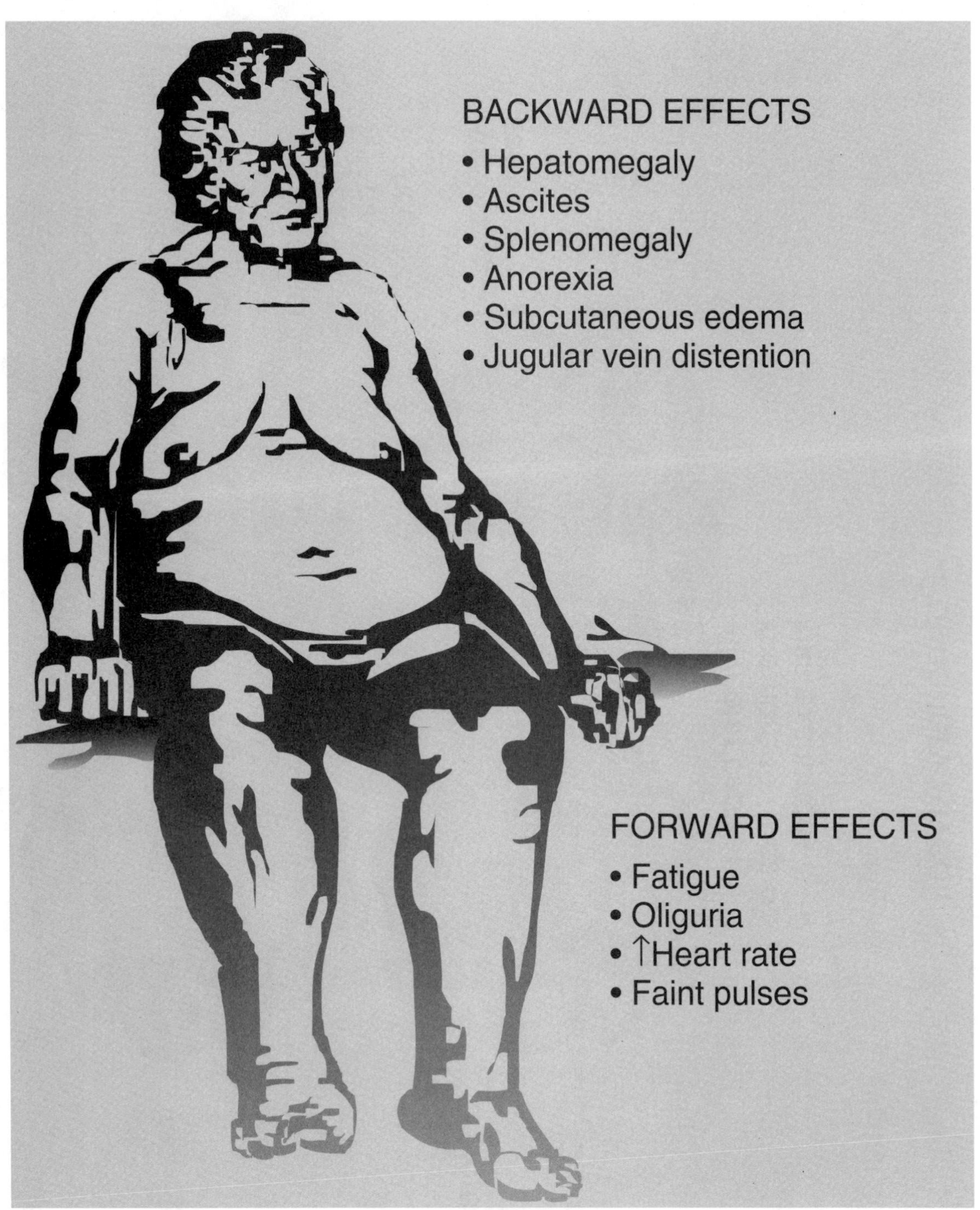


Manifestations of Right Heart Failure

Transparency #44

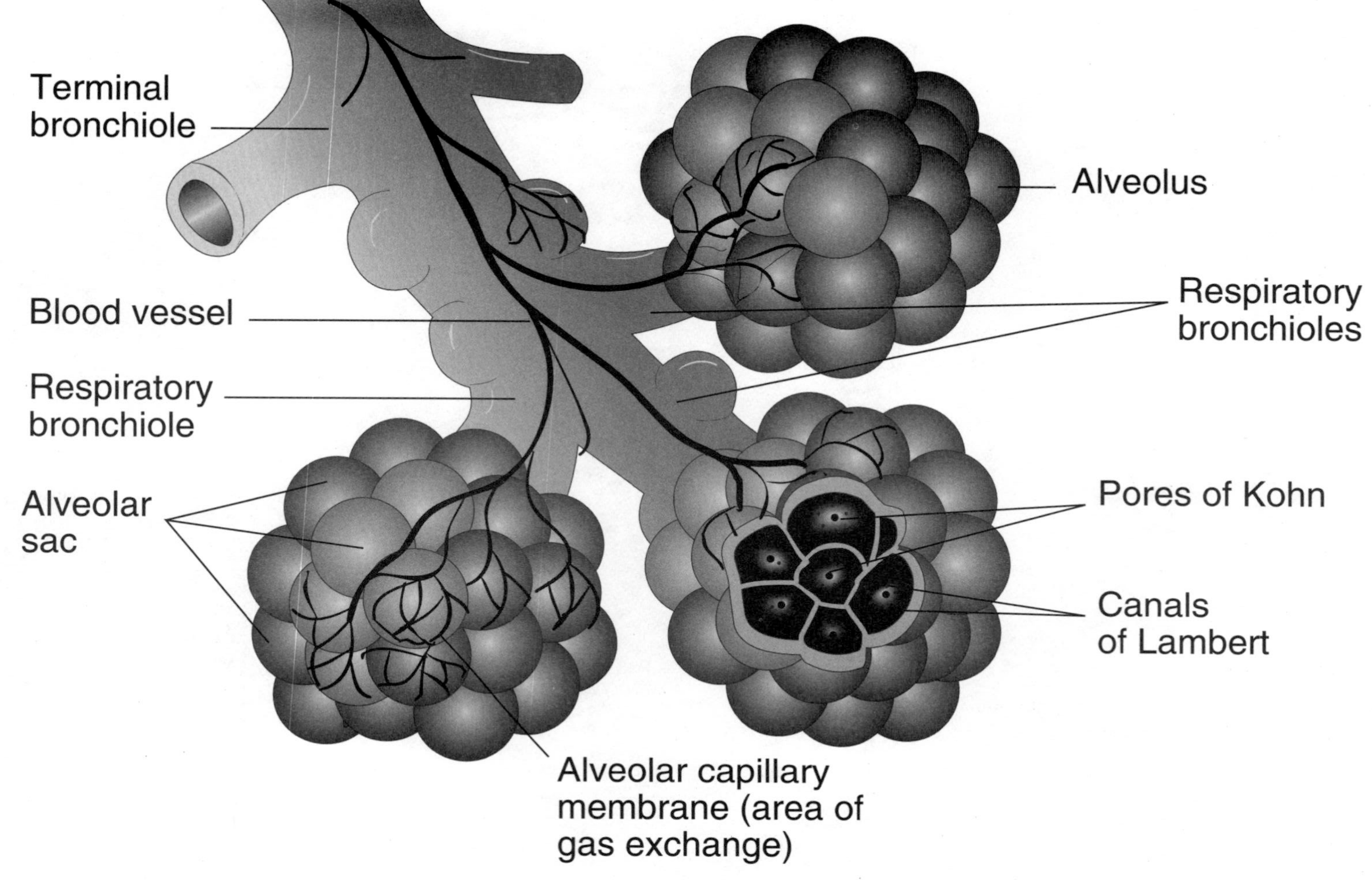


Pulmonary Alveoli

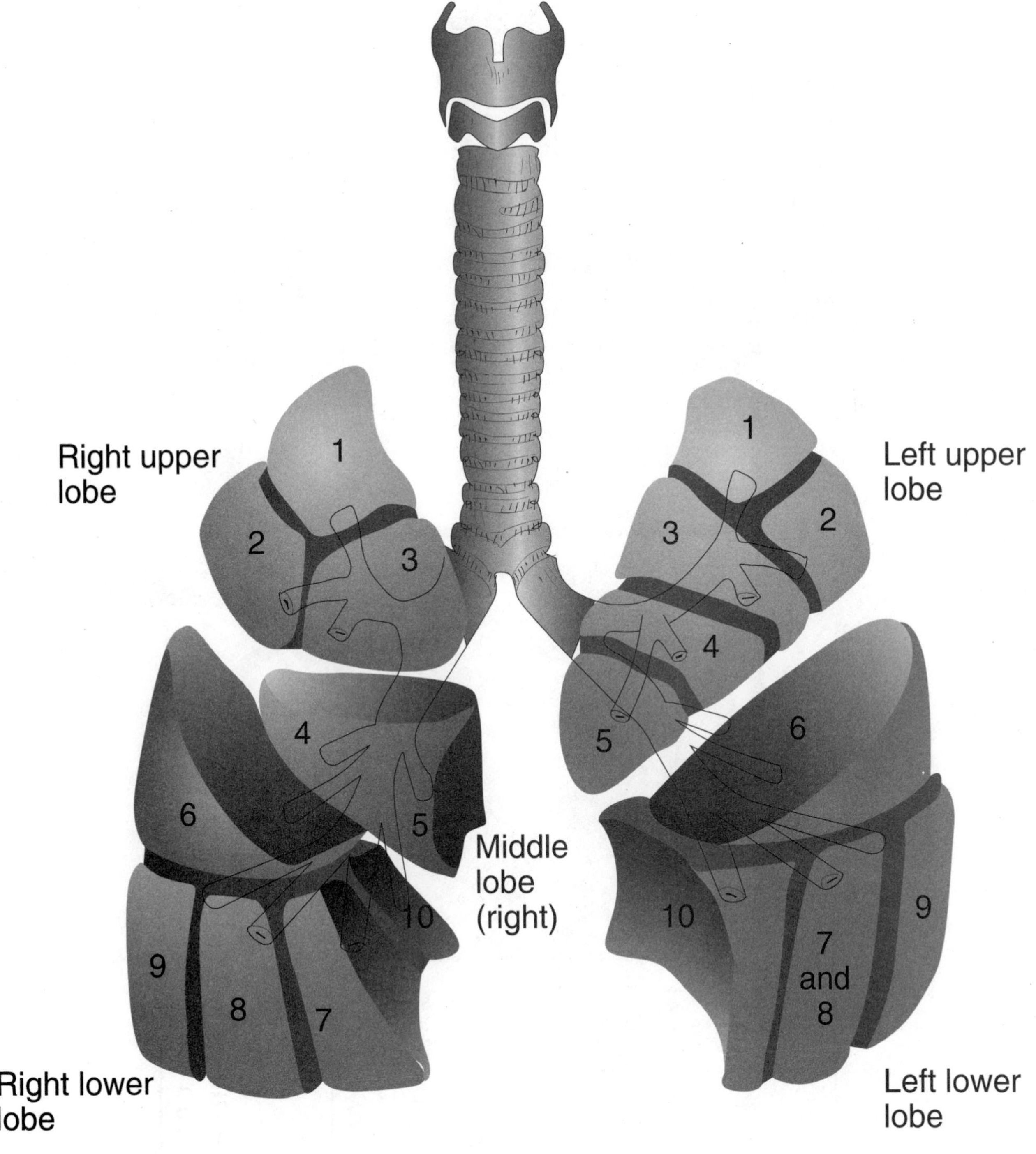


Lobes and Segments of the Lungs

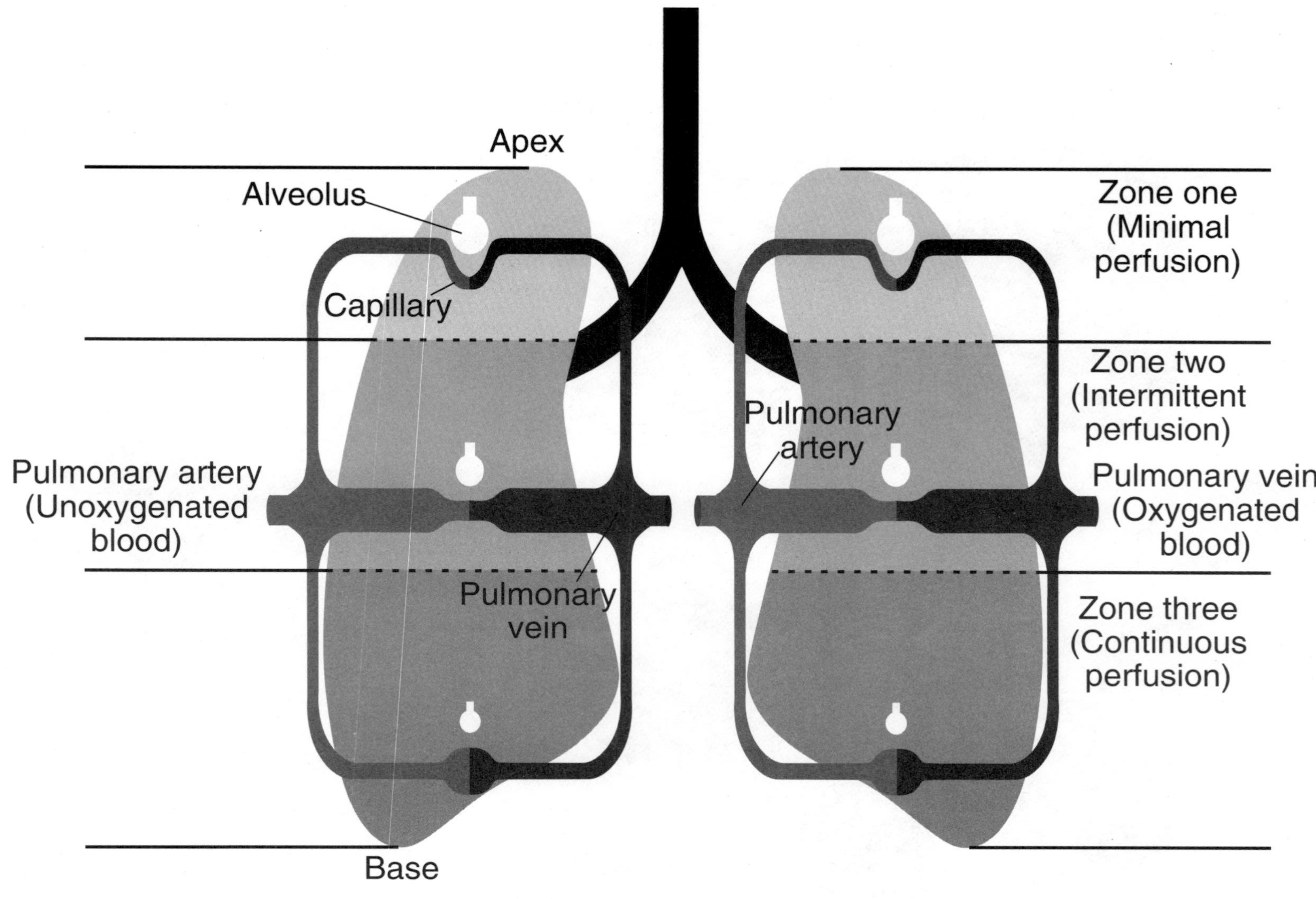


Functional Zones of the Lungs

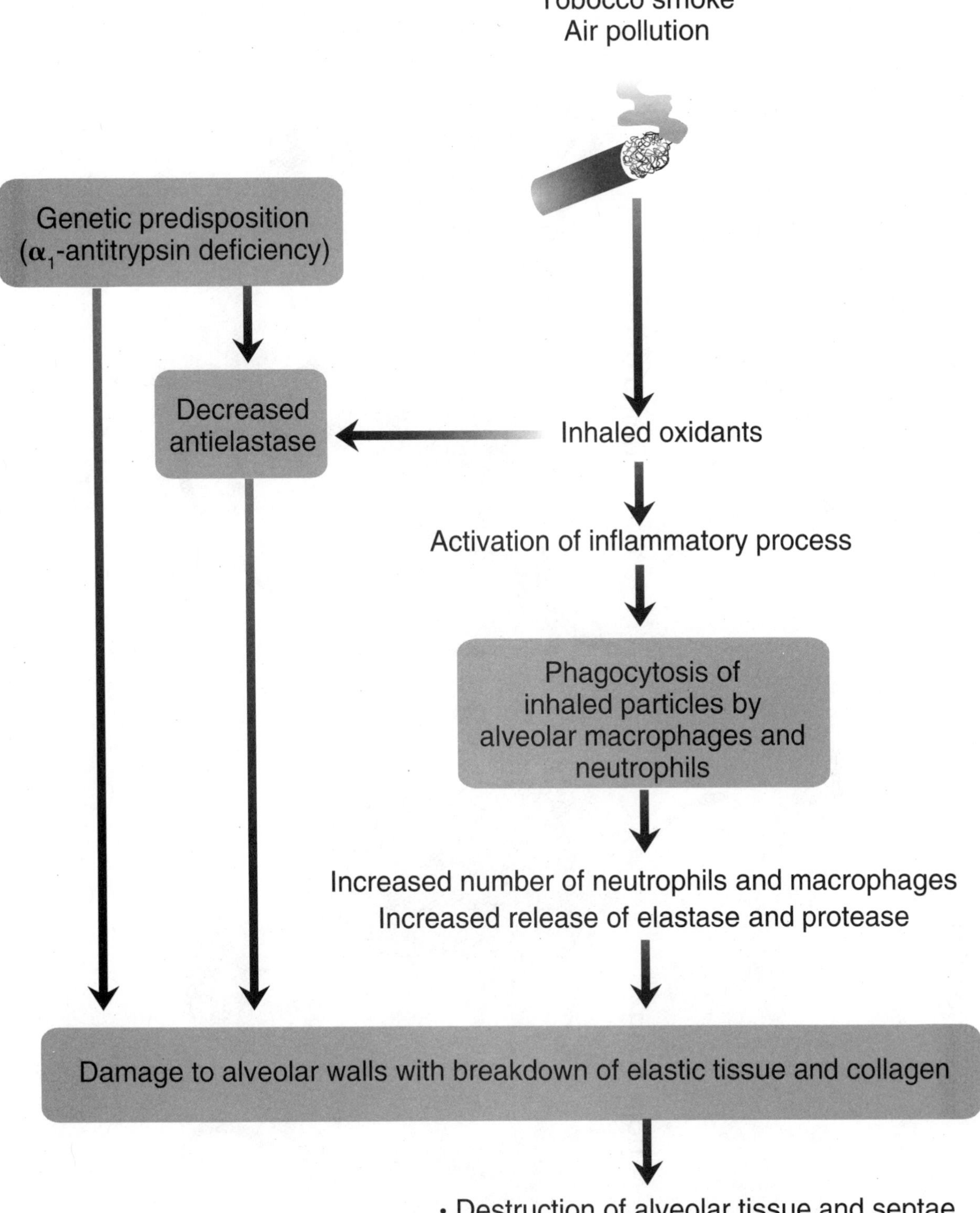


- Destruction of alveolar tissue and septae
- Increased mucus secretion
- Inflammation in the bronchioles
- Impaired airway clearance
- Loss of radial traction with collapse of bronchioles leading to air trapping

# Pathophysiology of Emphysema

Transparency #48

# Mechanism of Tension Pneumothorax

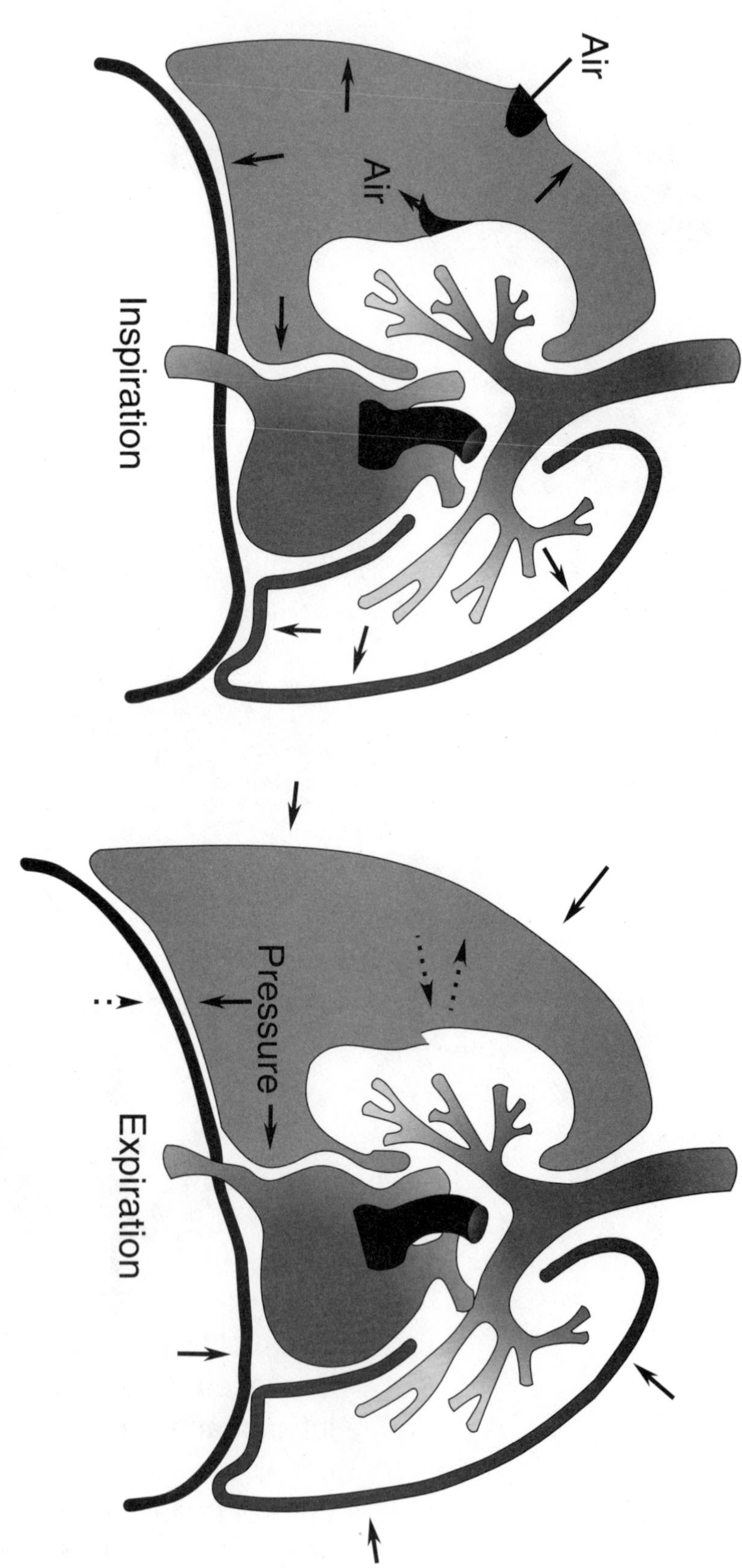

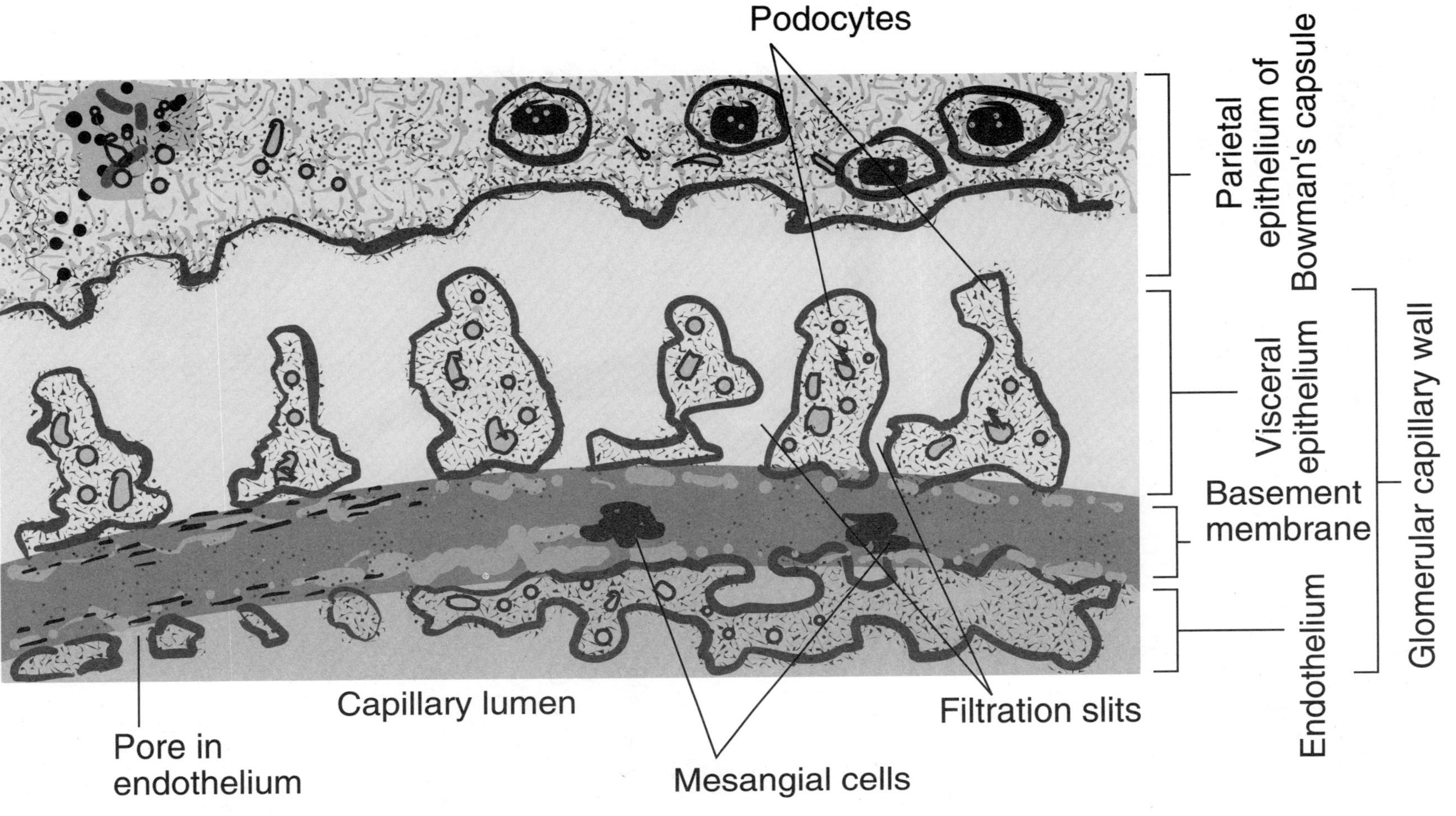


Microanatomy of Glomerular Membrane

Transparency #50

DISTAL TUBULE
5% GF reabsorbed
Reabsorption of $Na^+$(controlled by aldosterone), $Cl^-$ and $Ca^{++}$ (controlled by PTH), $HPO_4^-$ (controlled by PTH), $Mg^+$, $HCO_3^-$
Secretion of $K^+$,(controlled by aldosterone), $H^+$, $NH_3$

GLOMERULAR CAPILLARIES AND BOWMAN'S CAPSULE
Filtration of $H_2O$, electrolytes, creatinine, sugars, nitrogenous wastes (urea, uric acid), $HCO_3^-$, AA

PROXIMAL TUBULE
60%-70% GF reabsorbed
Reabsorption of $Na^+$, $Cl^-$, $K^+$, $Mg^+$, $Ca^{++}$, $HPO_4^-$, creatinine, AA, sugars, some nitrogenous wastes, $HCO_3^-$, $H_2O$
Secretion of $H^+$

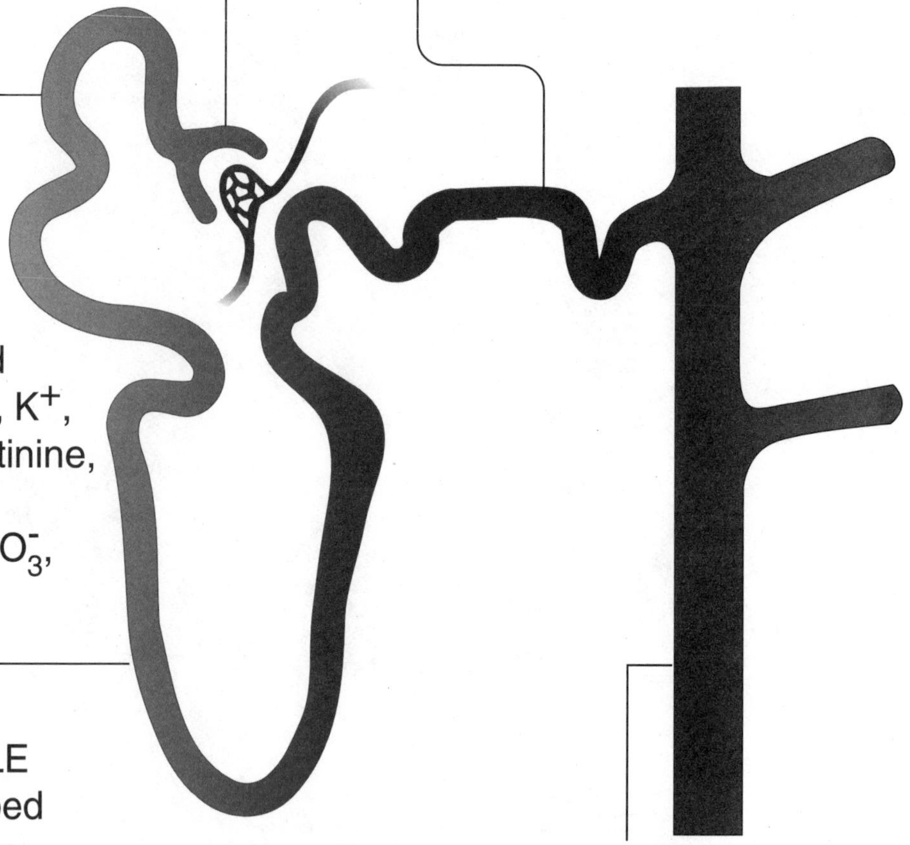

LOOP OF HENLE
5% GF reabsorbed
Descending loop:
Reabsorption of $H_2O$,
Secretion of urea
Ascending loop:
Reabsorption of $Cl^-$, $Na^+$, $K^+$, $Mg^+$, $Ca^{++}$

COLLECTING DUCT
19% GF reabsorbed
Reabsorption of $H_2O$ (controlled by ADH)
Reabsorption and secretion of urea, $Na^+$, $Cl^-$
Formation of titratable acids

Functional Anatomy of the Nephron

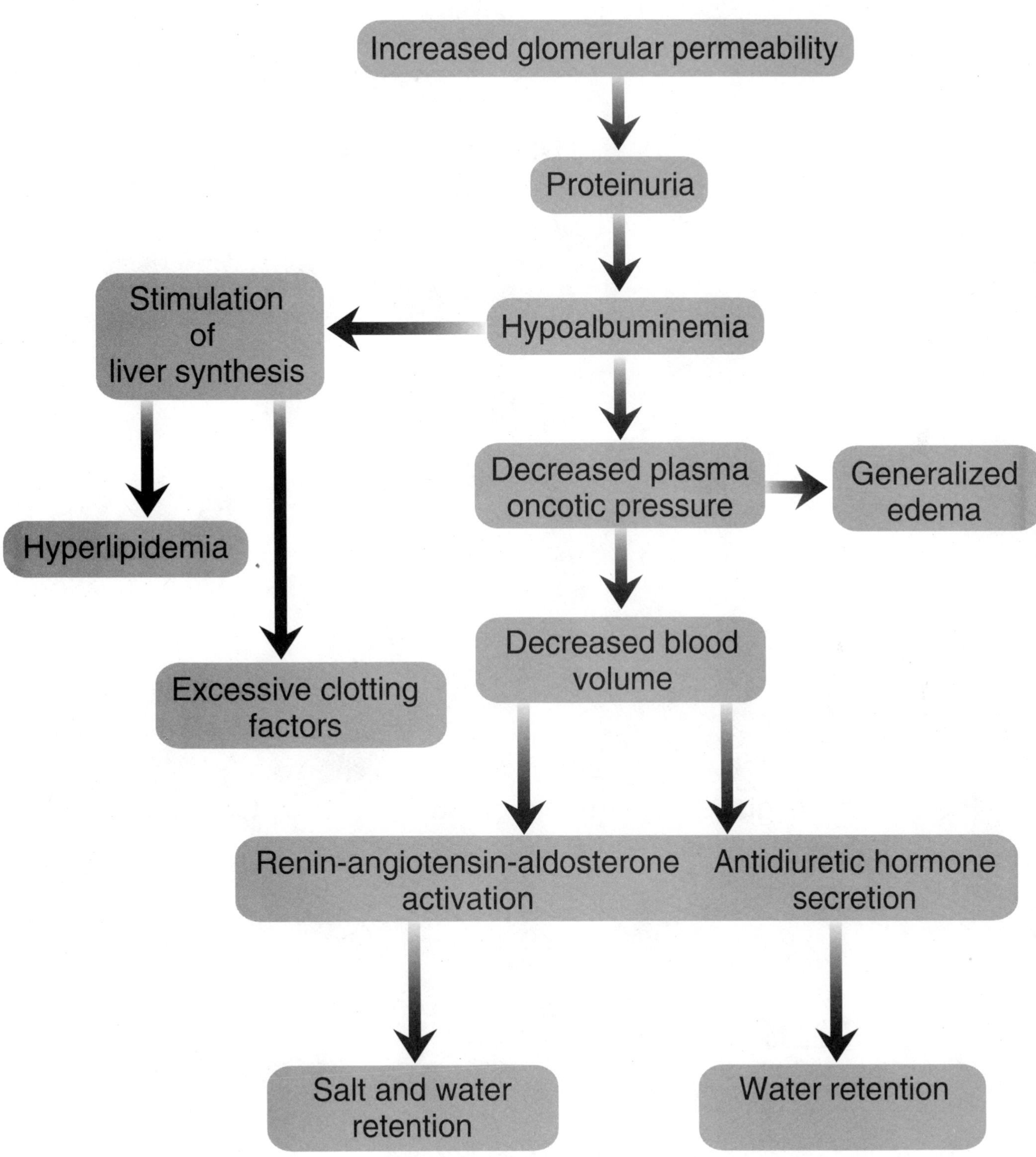


Nephrotic Syndrome

Transparency #52

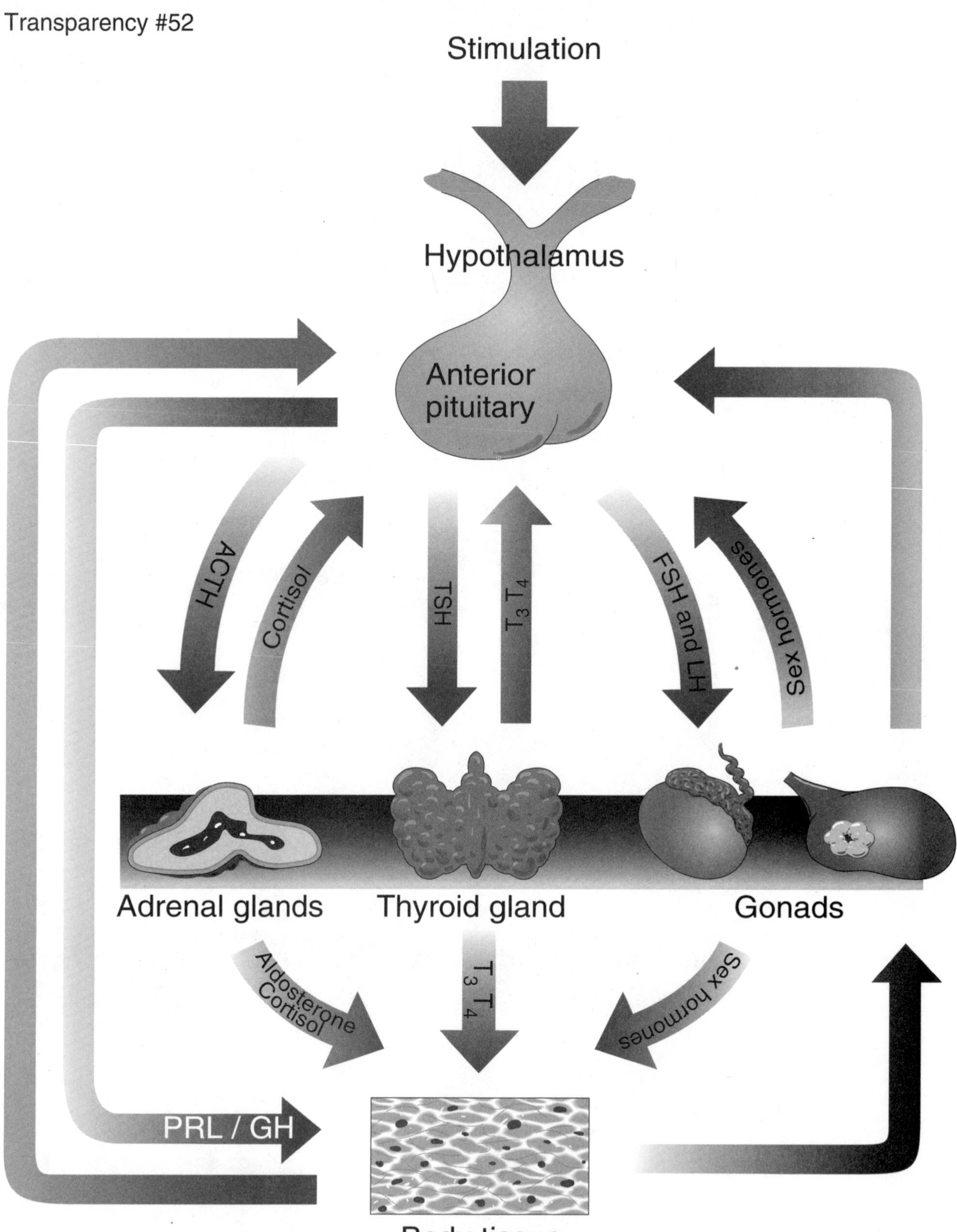


Major Pituitary Hormones, Target Tissues and Feedback Mechanisms

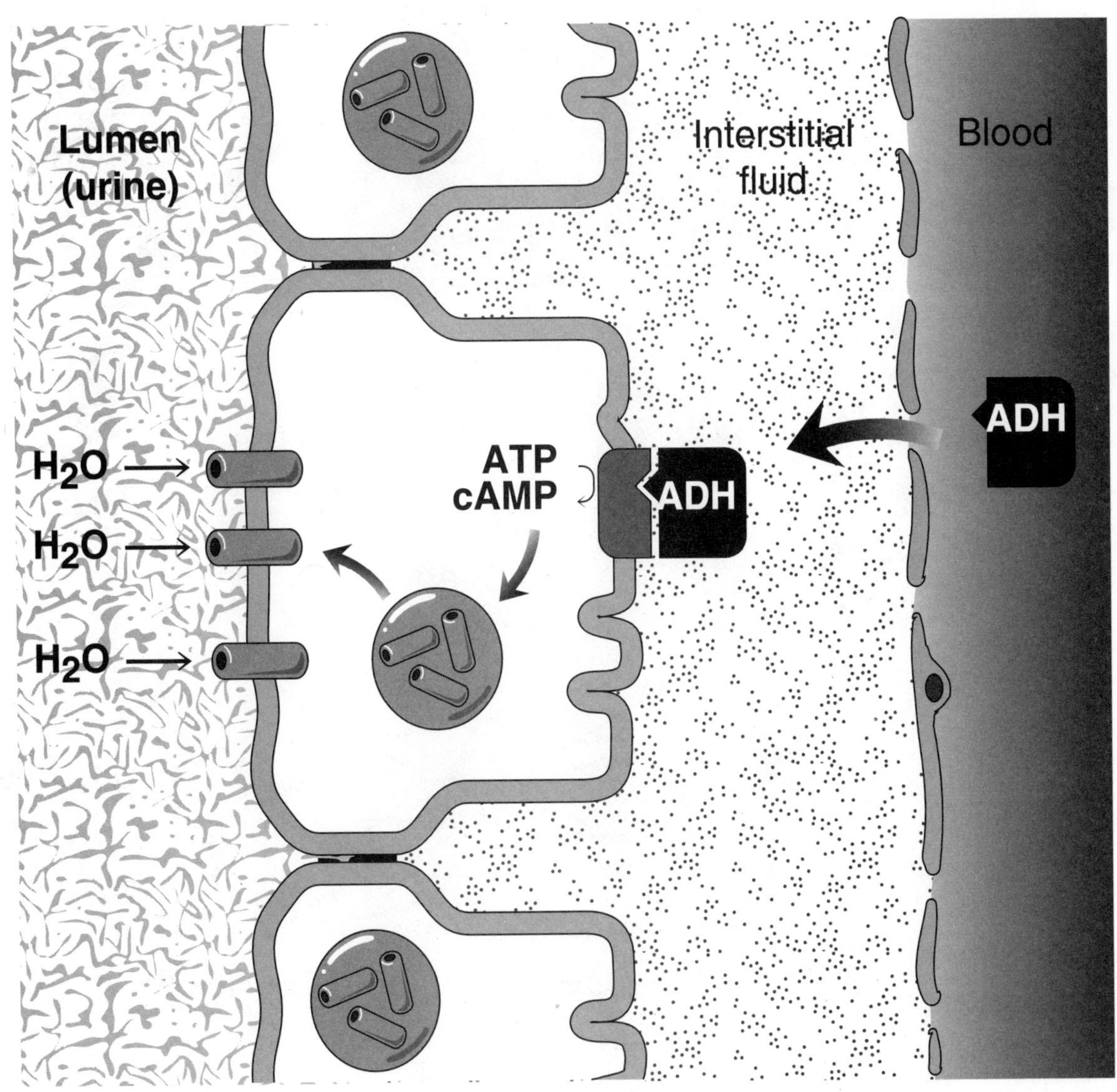


Mechanism of ADH Action on Renal Tubule Cells

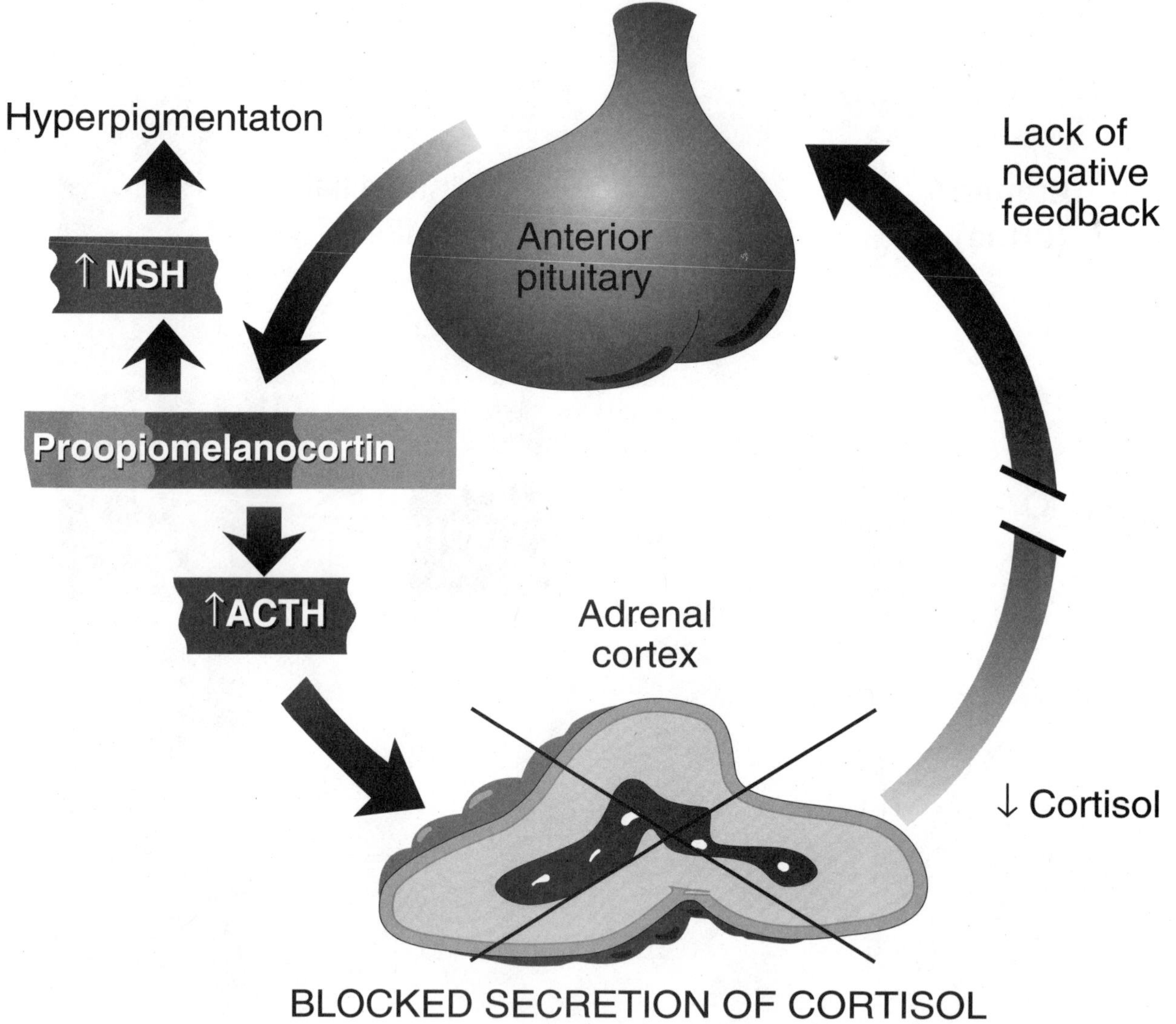


Negative Feedback in Primary Adrenocortical Insufficiency

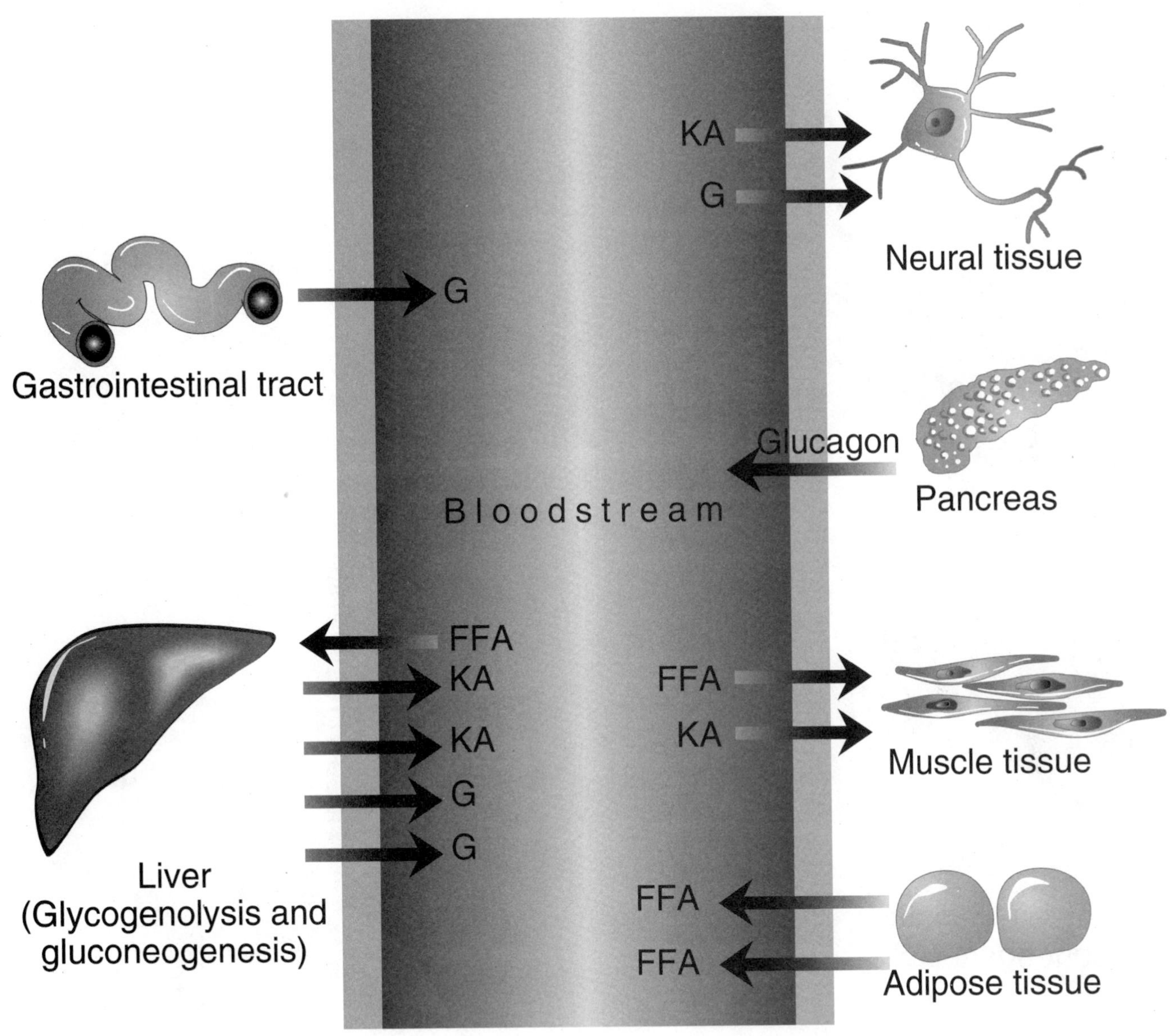


KEY:
G = glucose
FFA = free fatty acids
KA = Ketoacids

Metabolic Effects of IDDM

Transparency #56

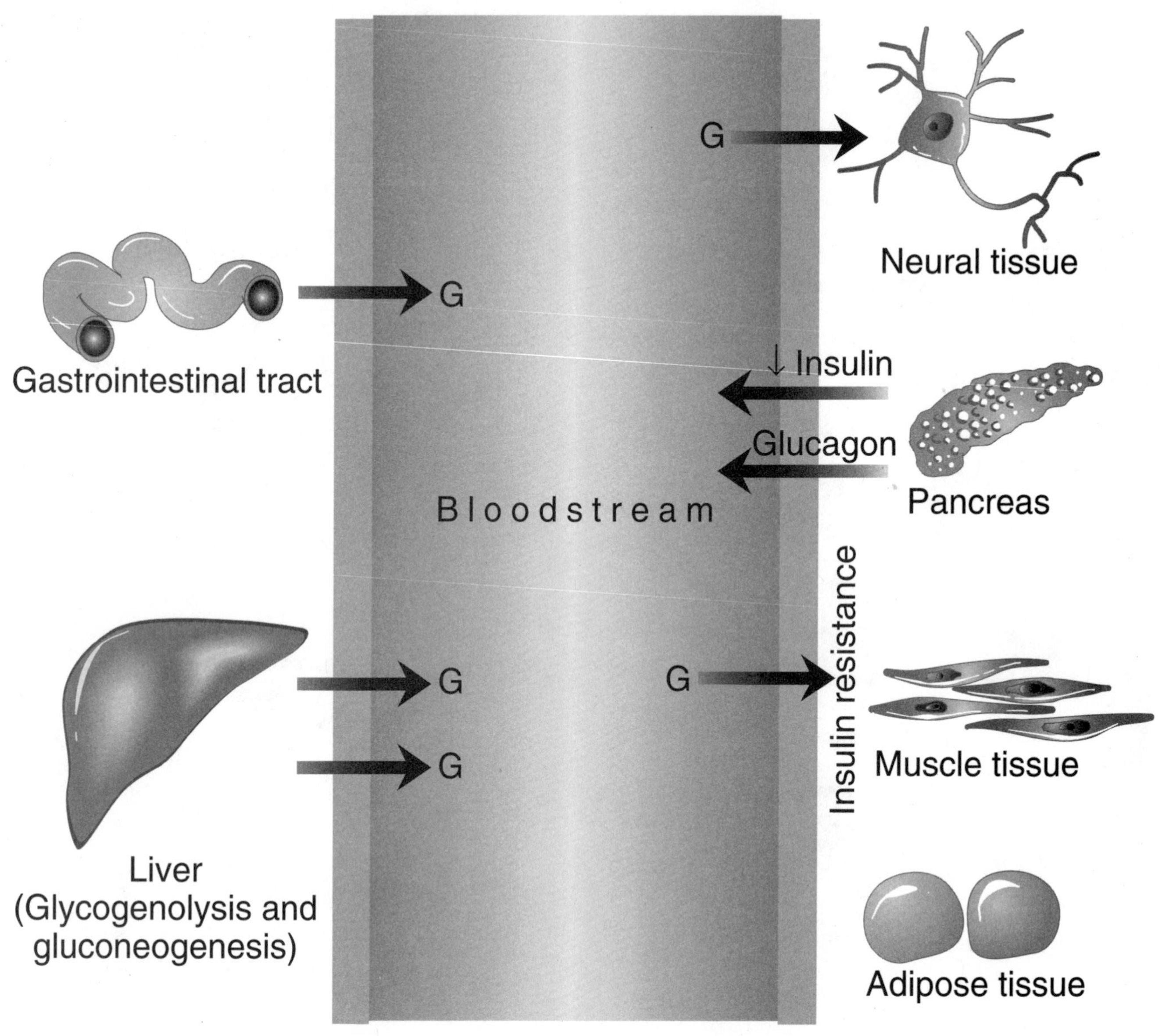


KEY:
G = glucose

Metabolic Effects of NIDDM

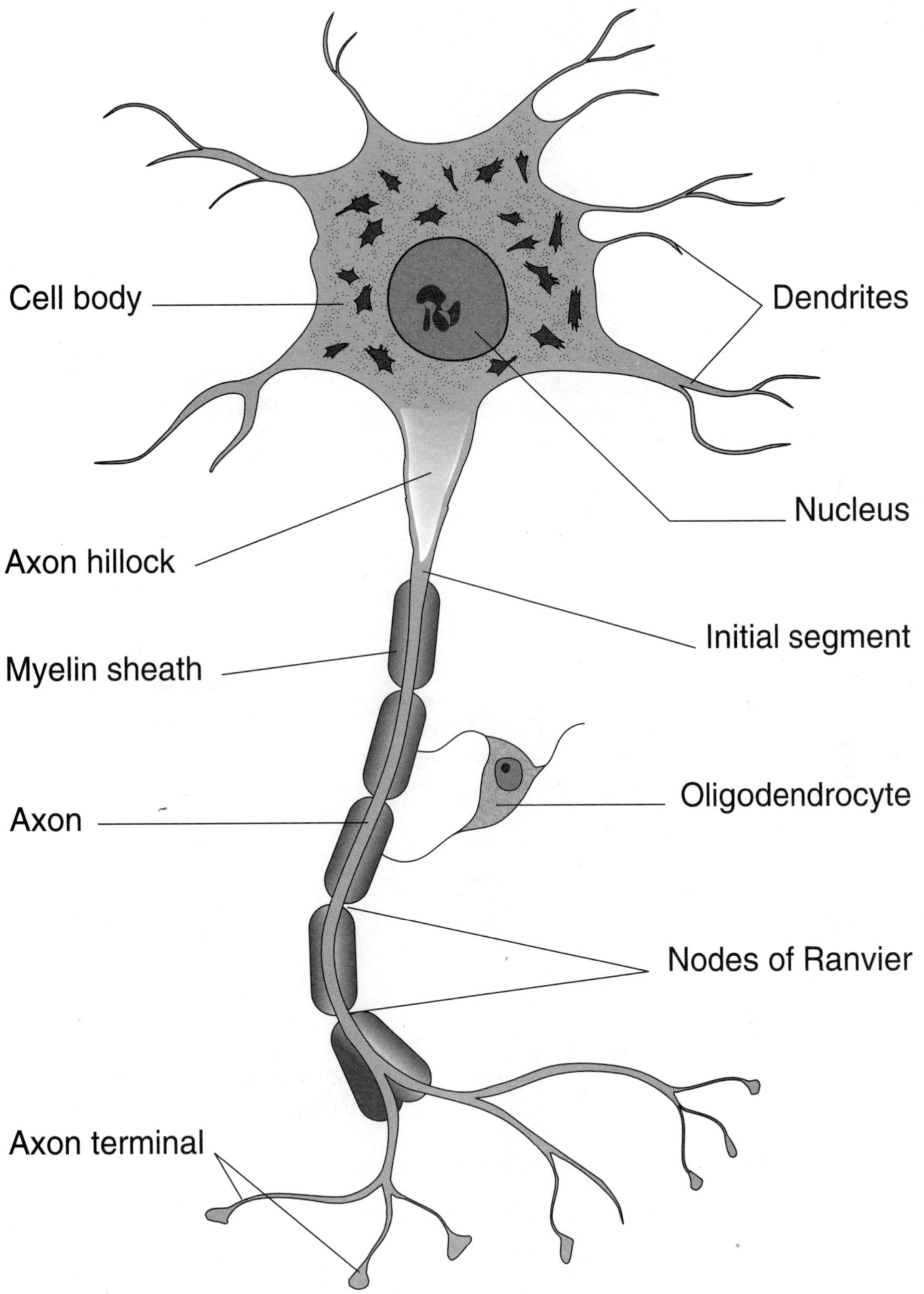


Anatomy of a Neuron

Transparency #58

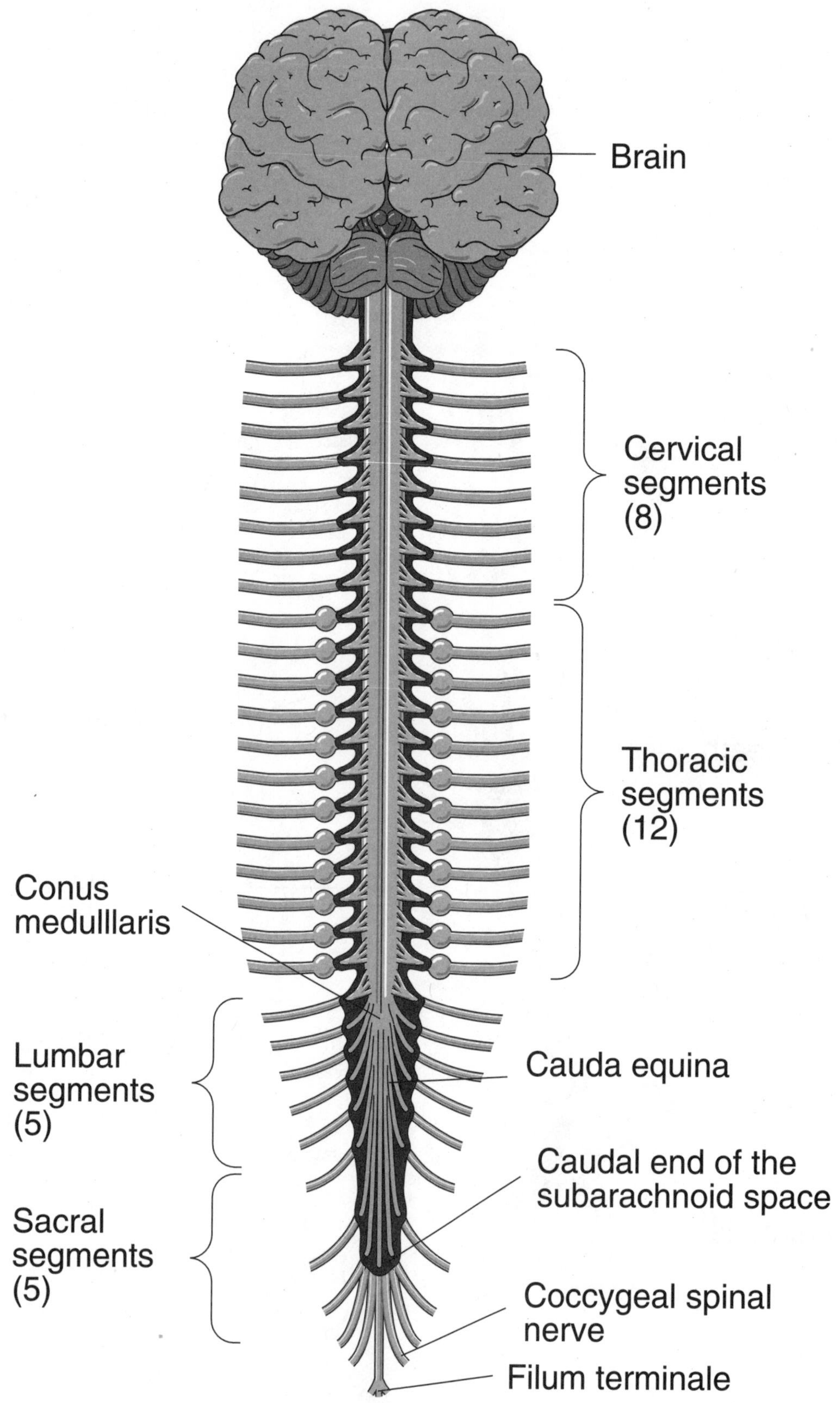


Spinal Nerves

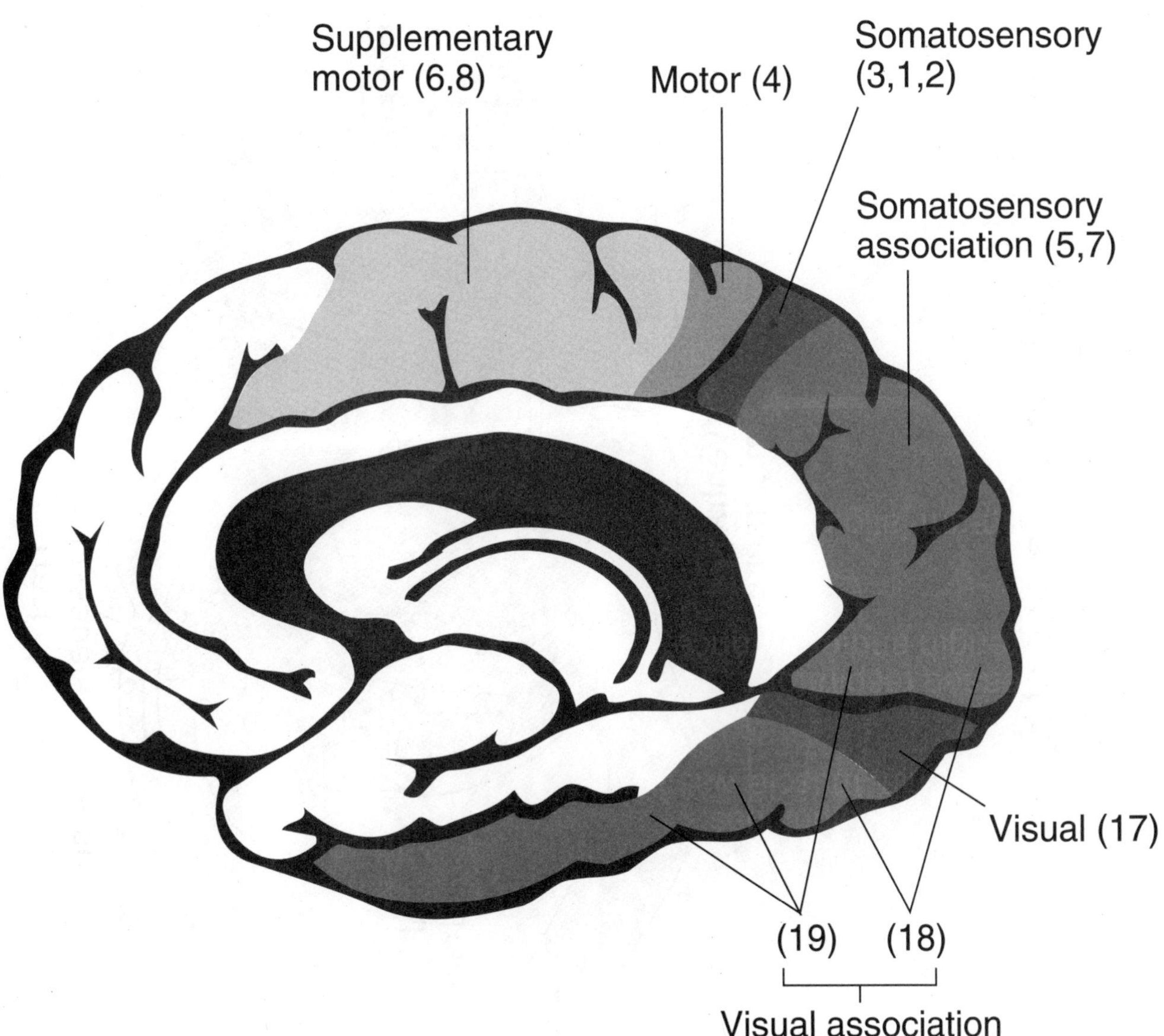


Functional Areas of Cerebral Cortex

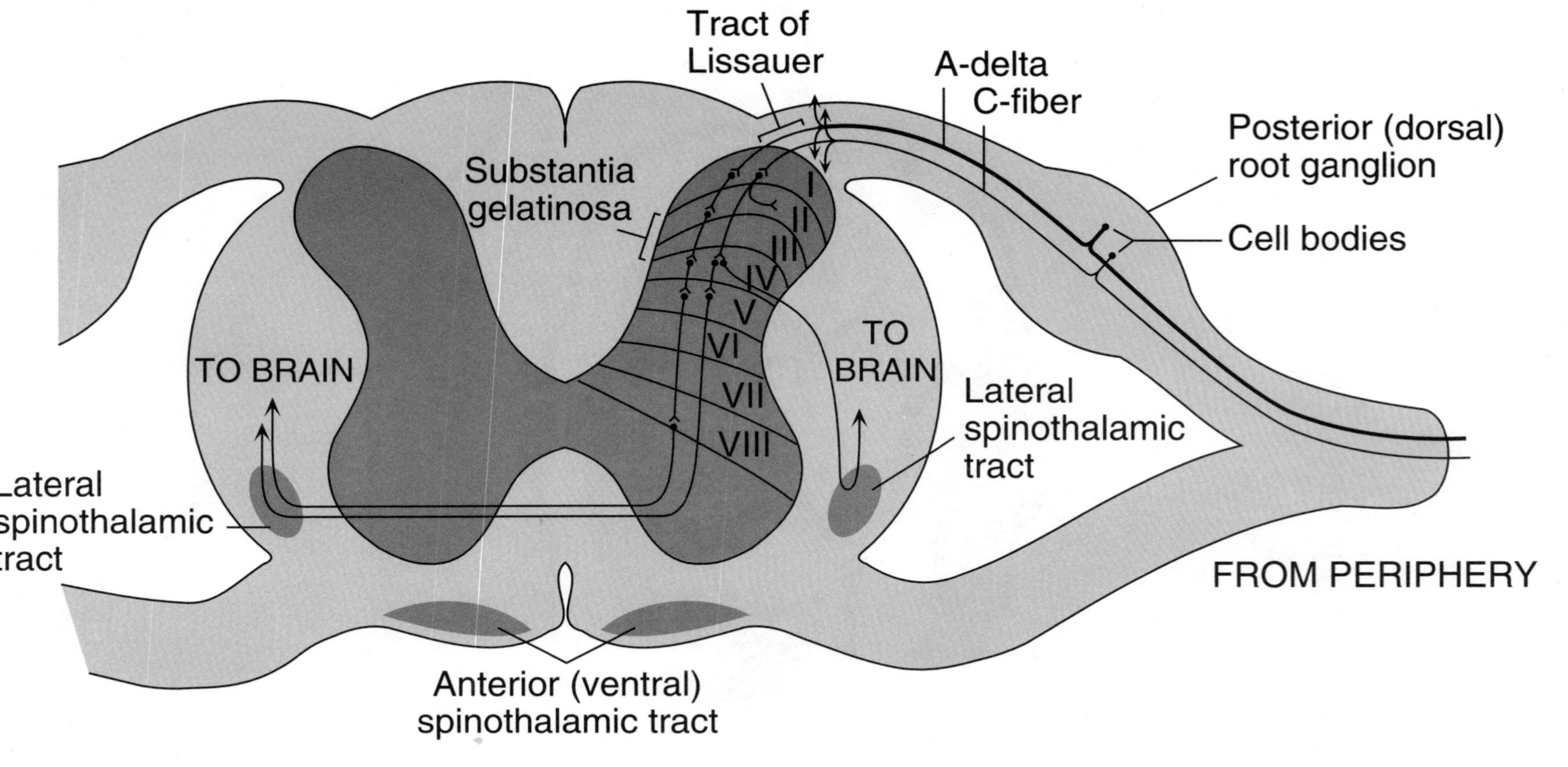


Transverse Section of Spinal Cord Showing Pain Pathways

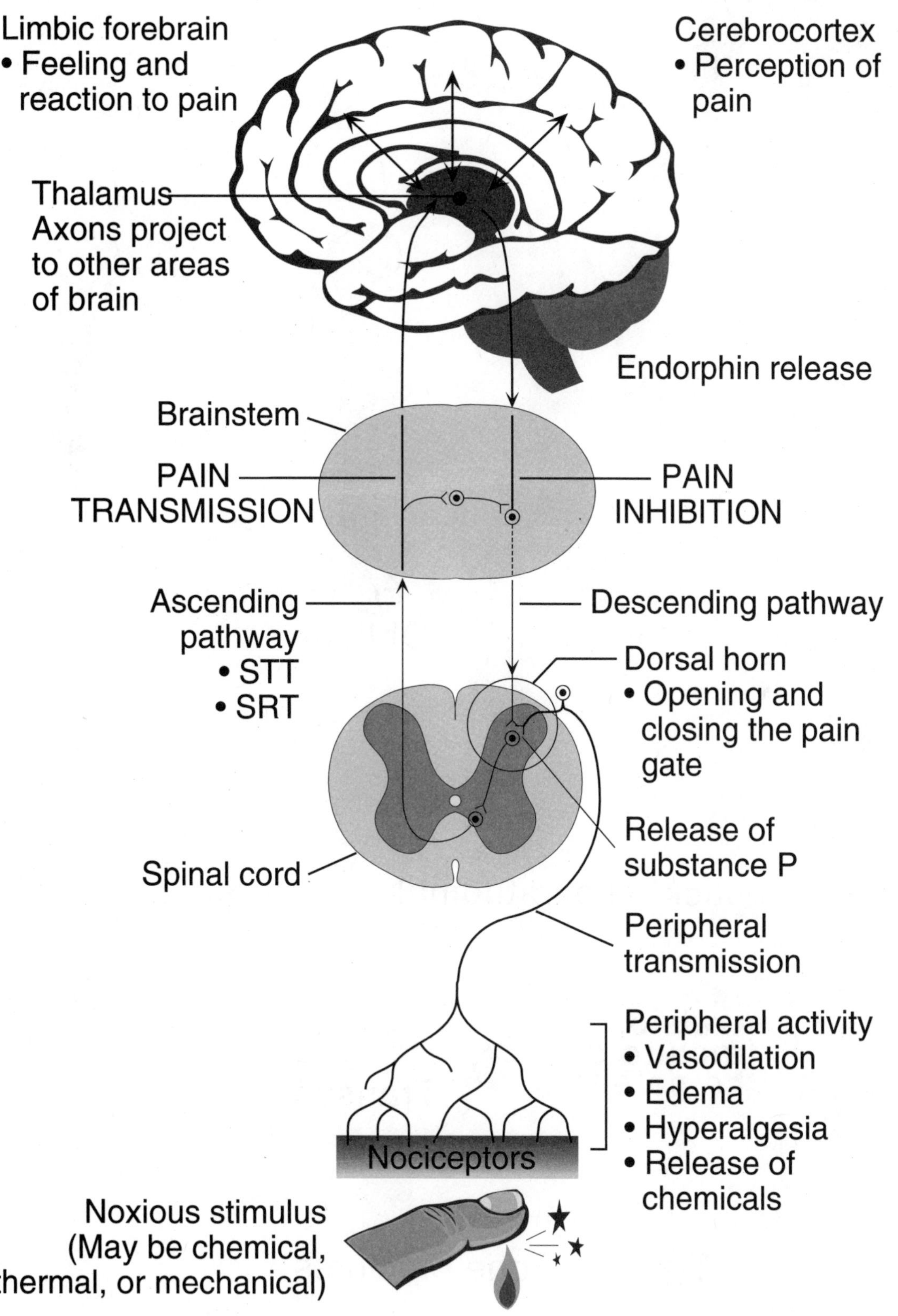


Mechanism of Pain Transmission and Inhibition

Transparency #62

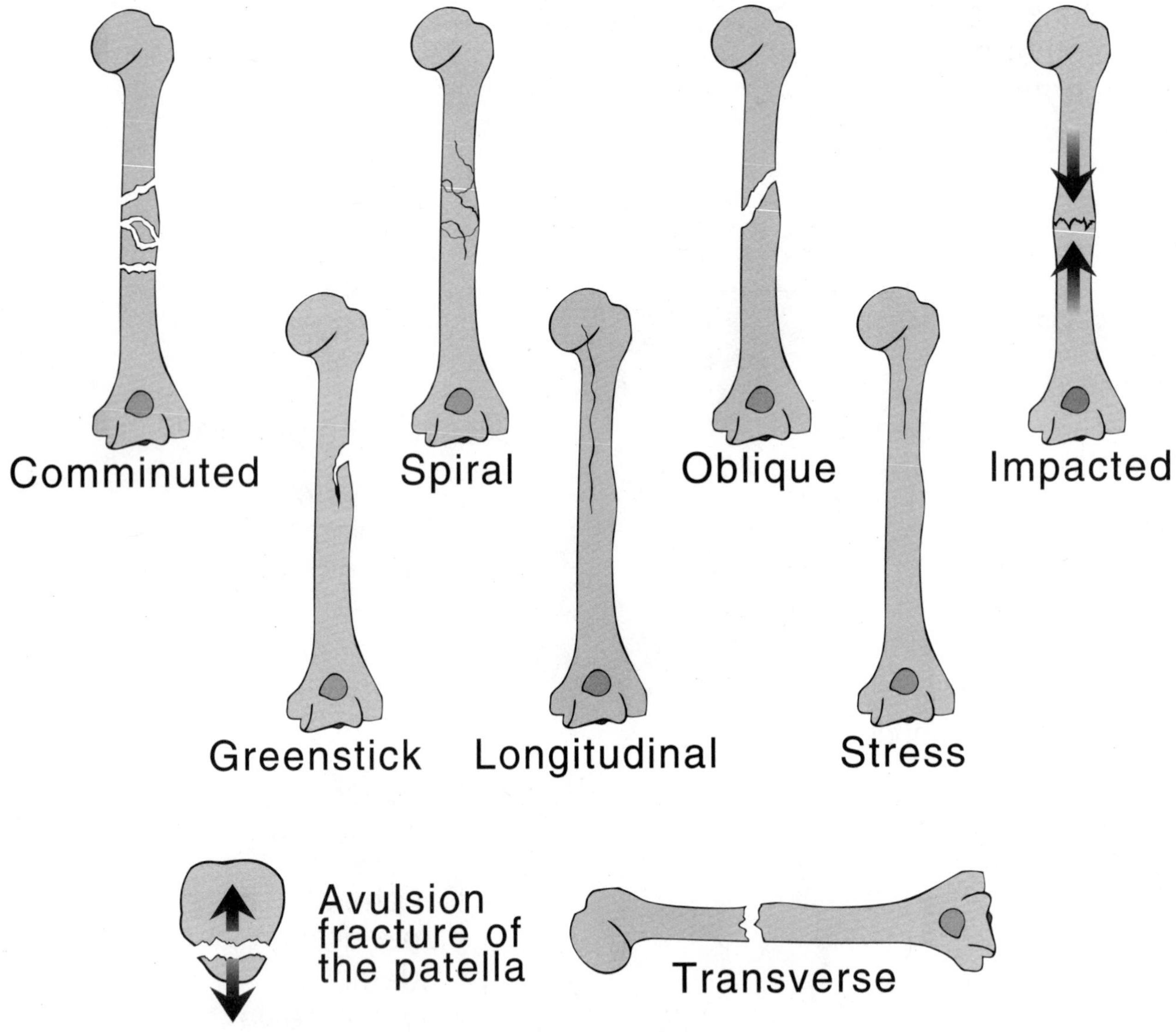

Comminuted
Spiral
Oblique
Impacted
Greenstick
Longitudinal
Stress
Avulsion fracture of the patella
Transverse

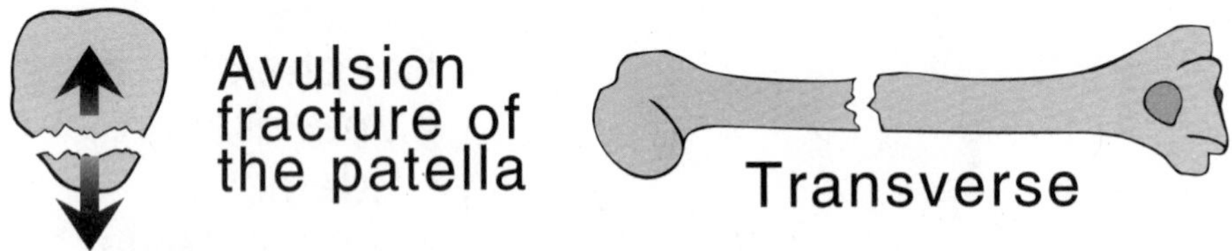

Types of Bone Fractures

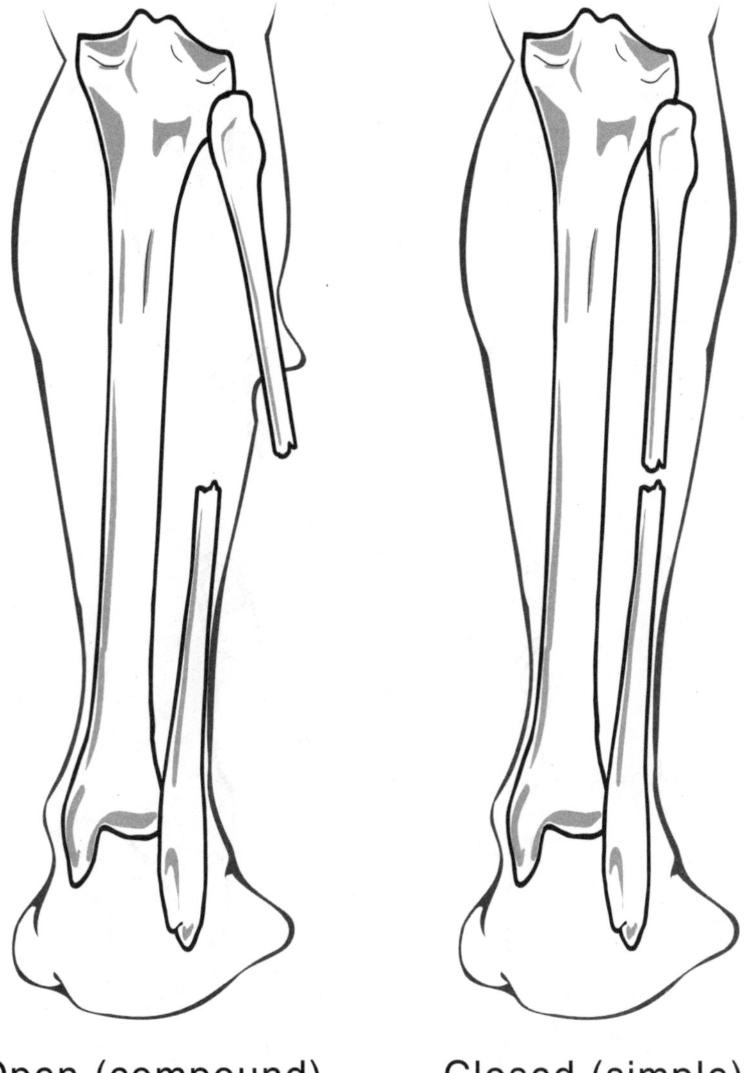


# Open and Closed Fractures

Transparency #64

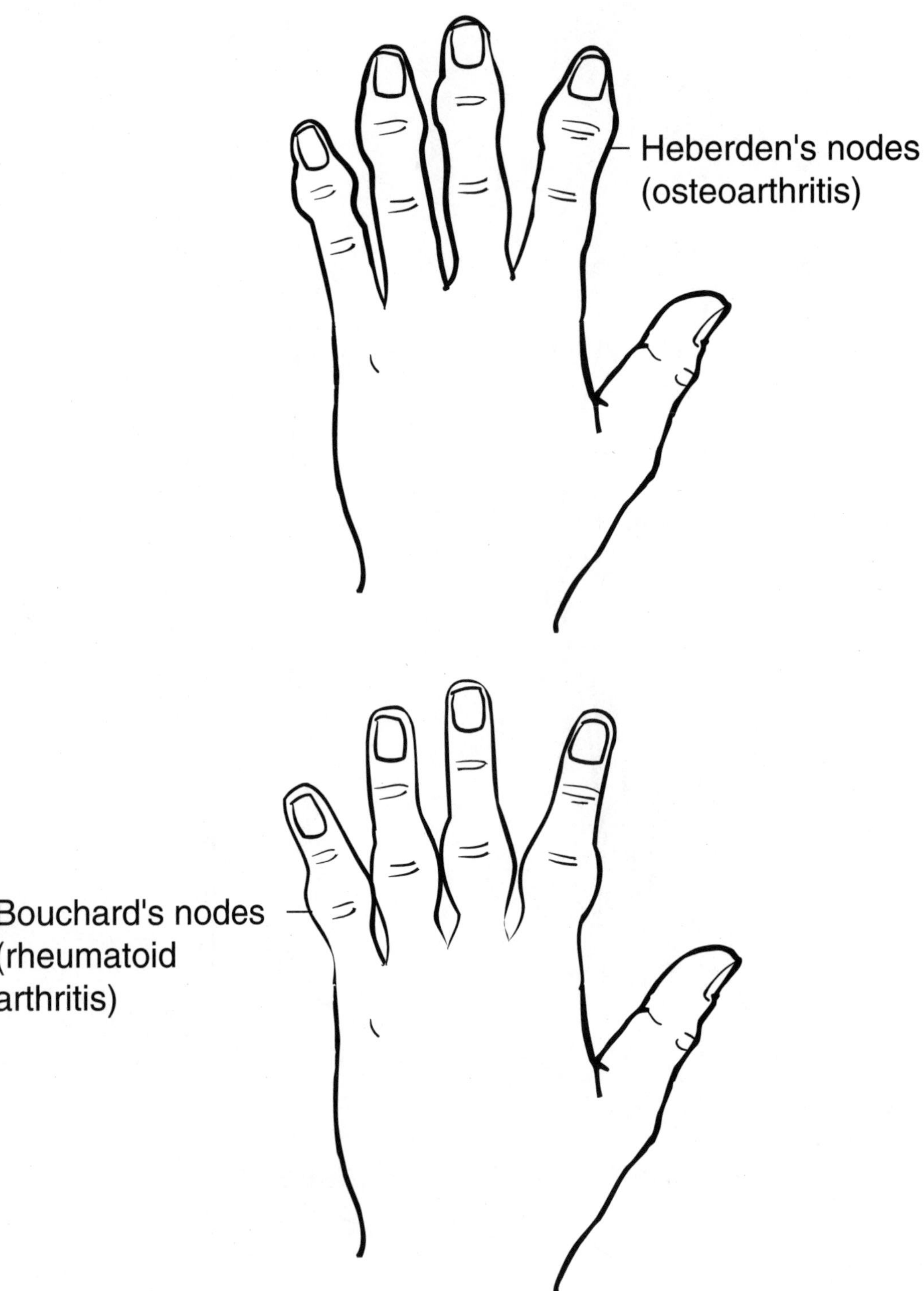


Affected Joints in Rheumatoid and Osteoarthritis

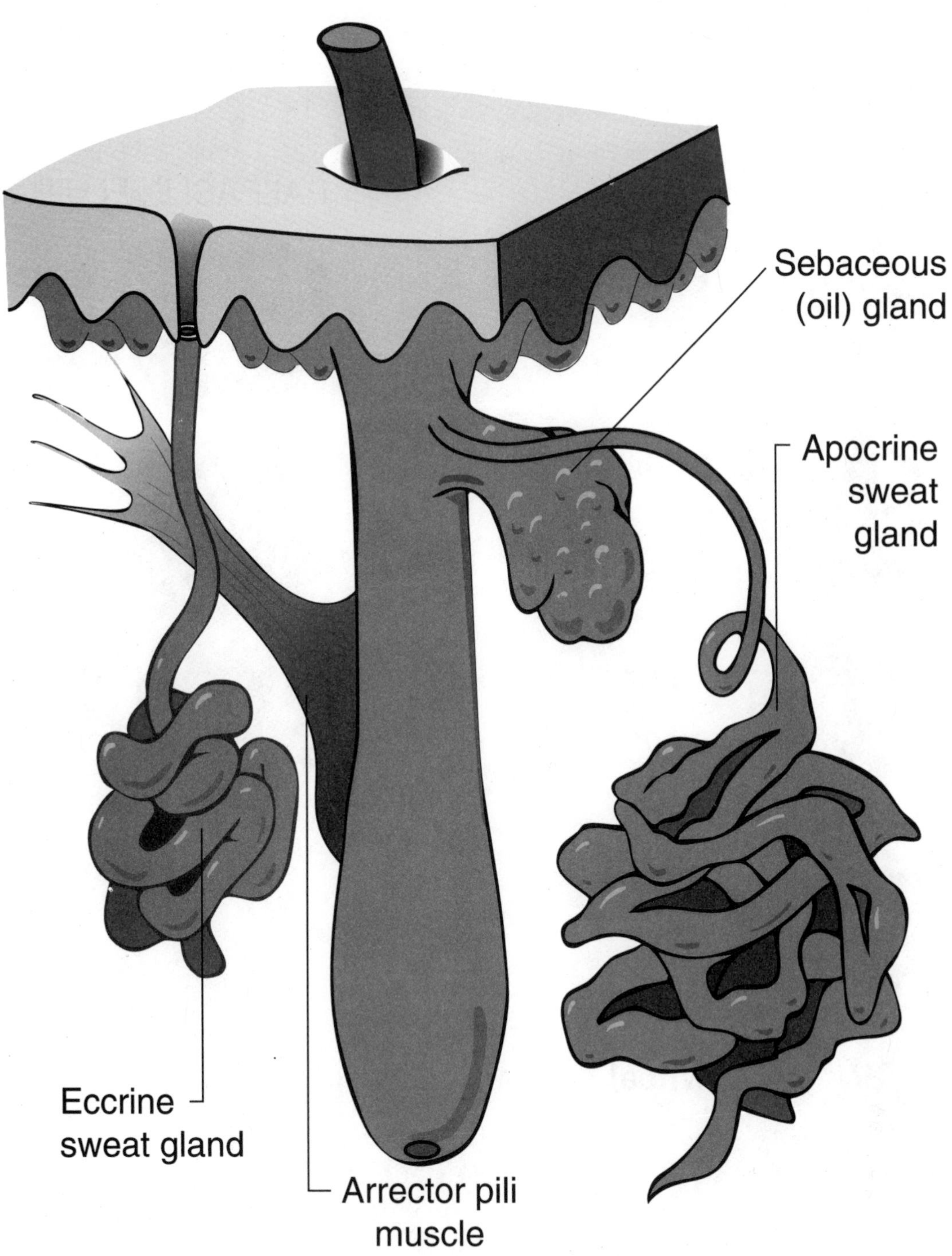


Accessory Structures of the Skin

Transparency #66

NONPALPABLE

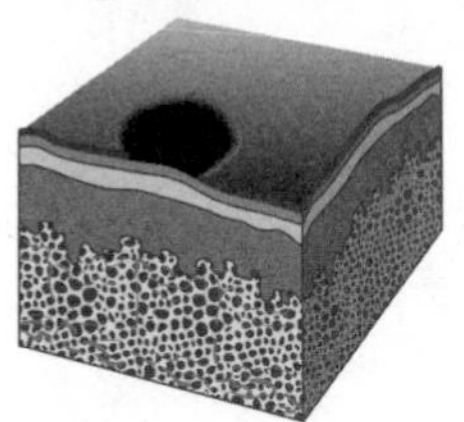

**Macule**

PALPABLE, SOLID

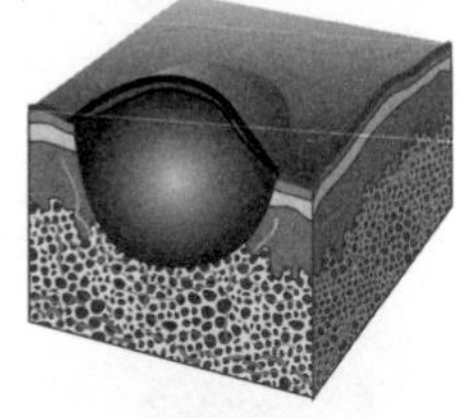

**Papule**

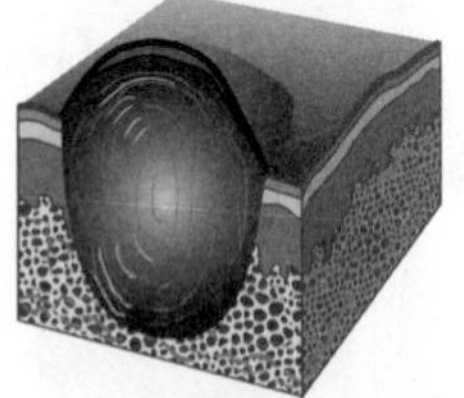

**Nodule**

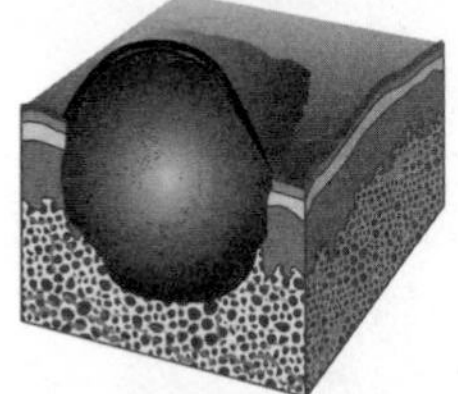

**Tumor**

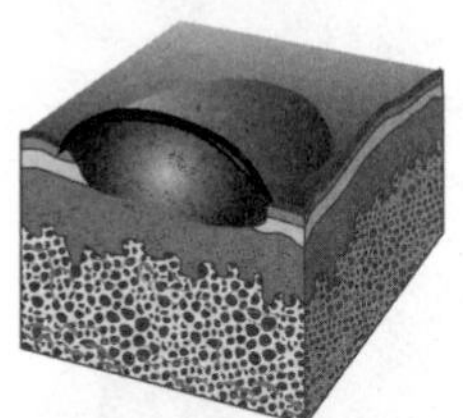

**Plaque**

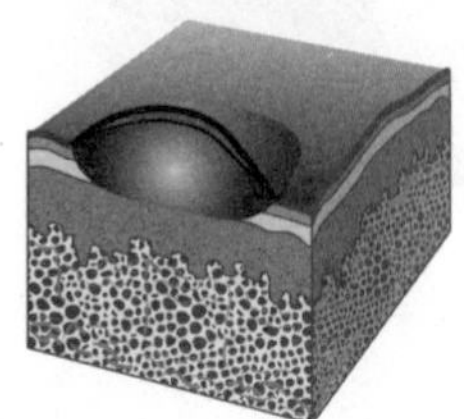

**Wheal**

PALPABLE, FLUID-FILLED

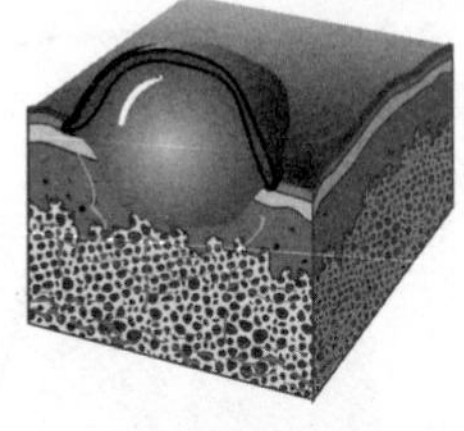

**Vesicle**

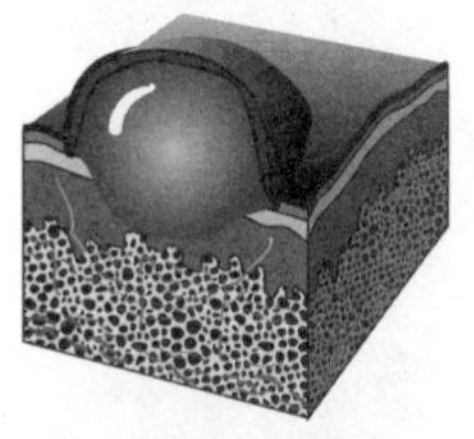

**Bulla**

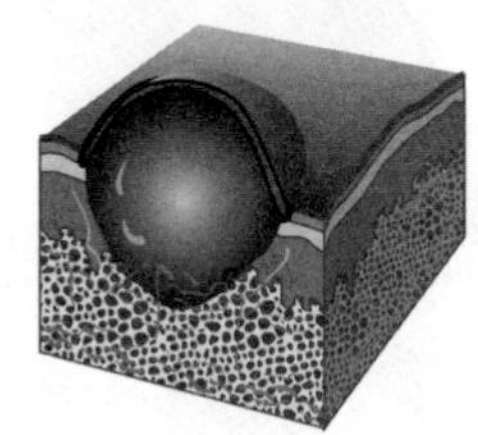

**Pustule**

Primary Skin Lesions

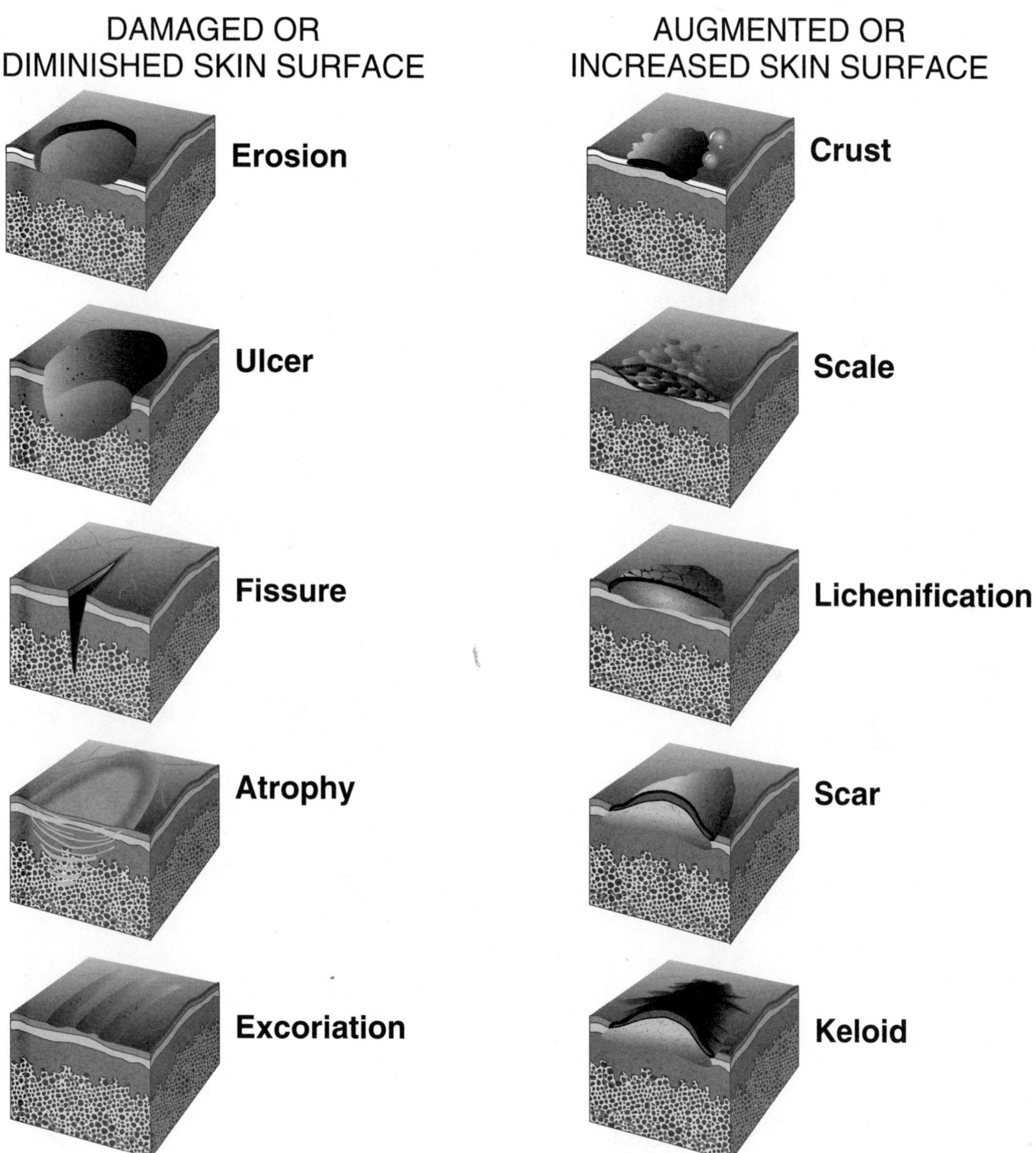


Secondary Skin Lesions

Transparency #68

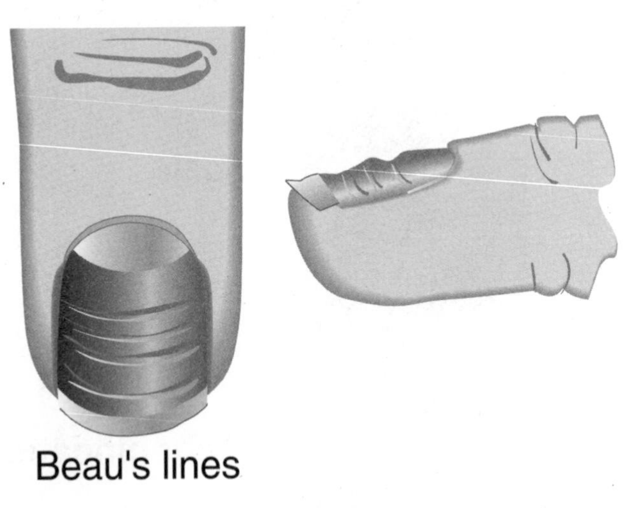

Beau's lines

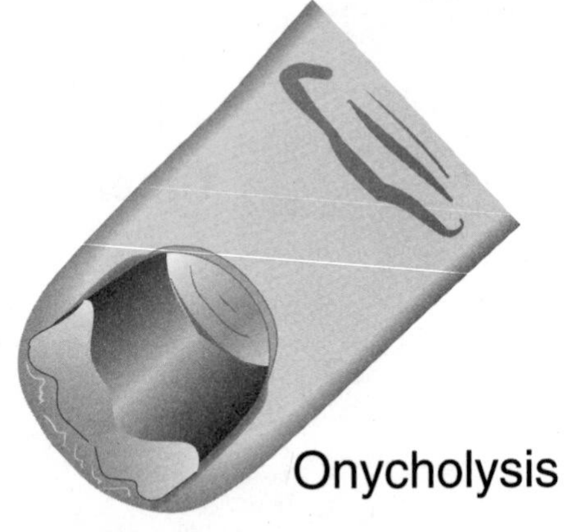

Onycholysis

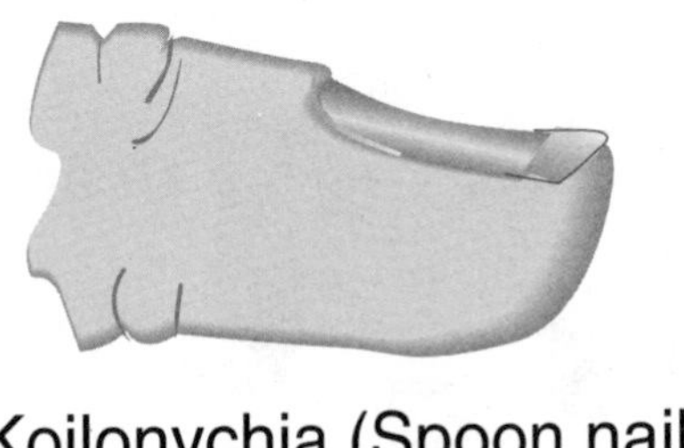

Koilonychia (Spoon nails)

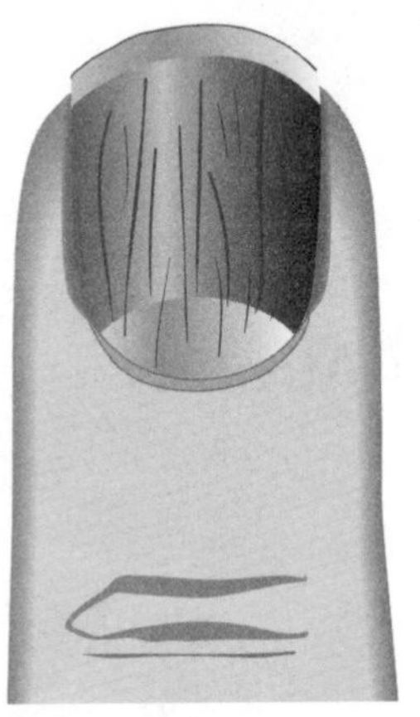

Splinter hemorrhages

## Fingernail Abnormalities

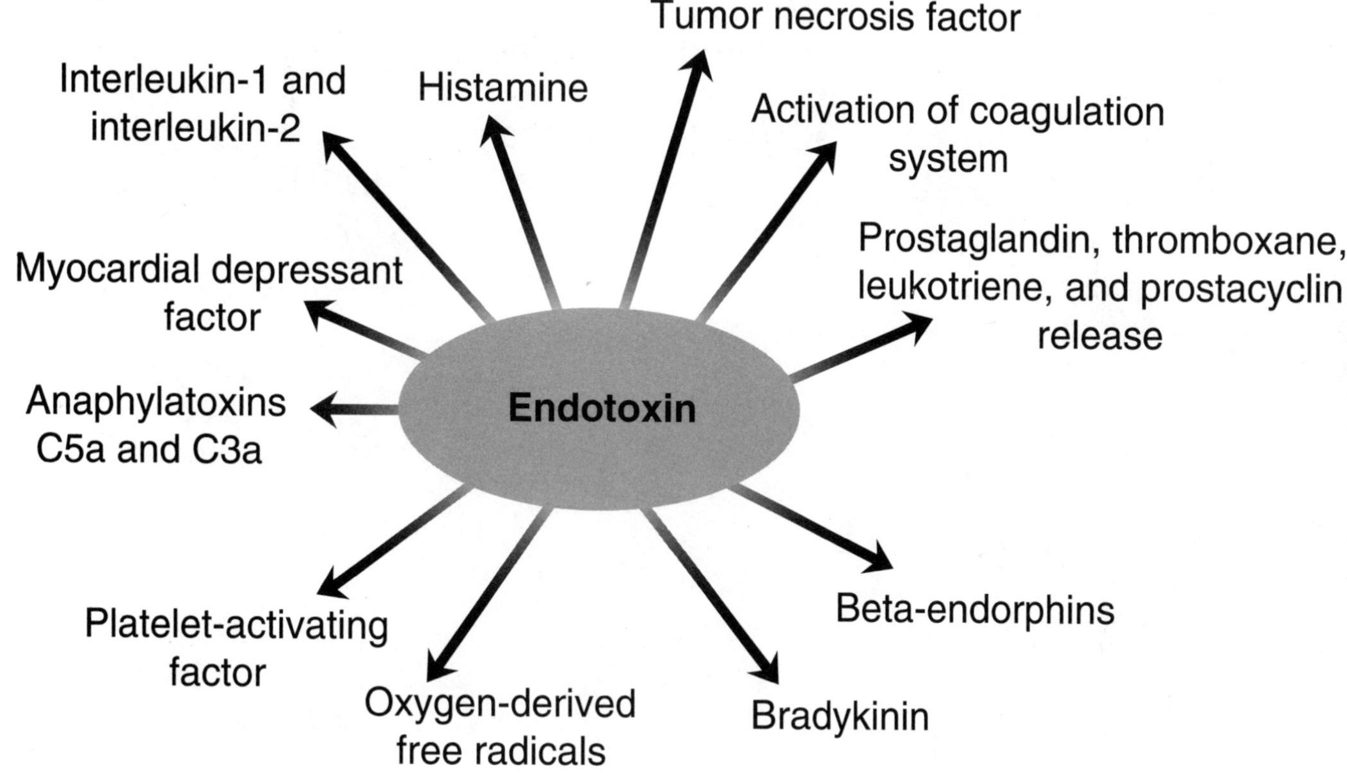


Mechanisms of Endotoxin Activity

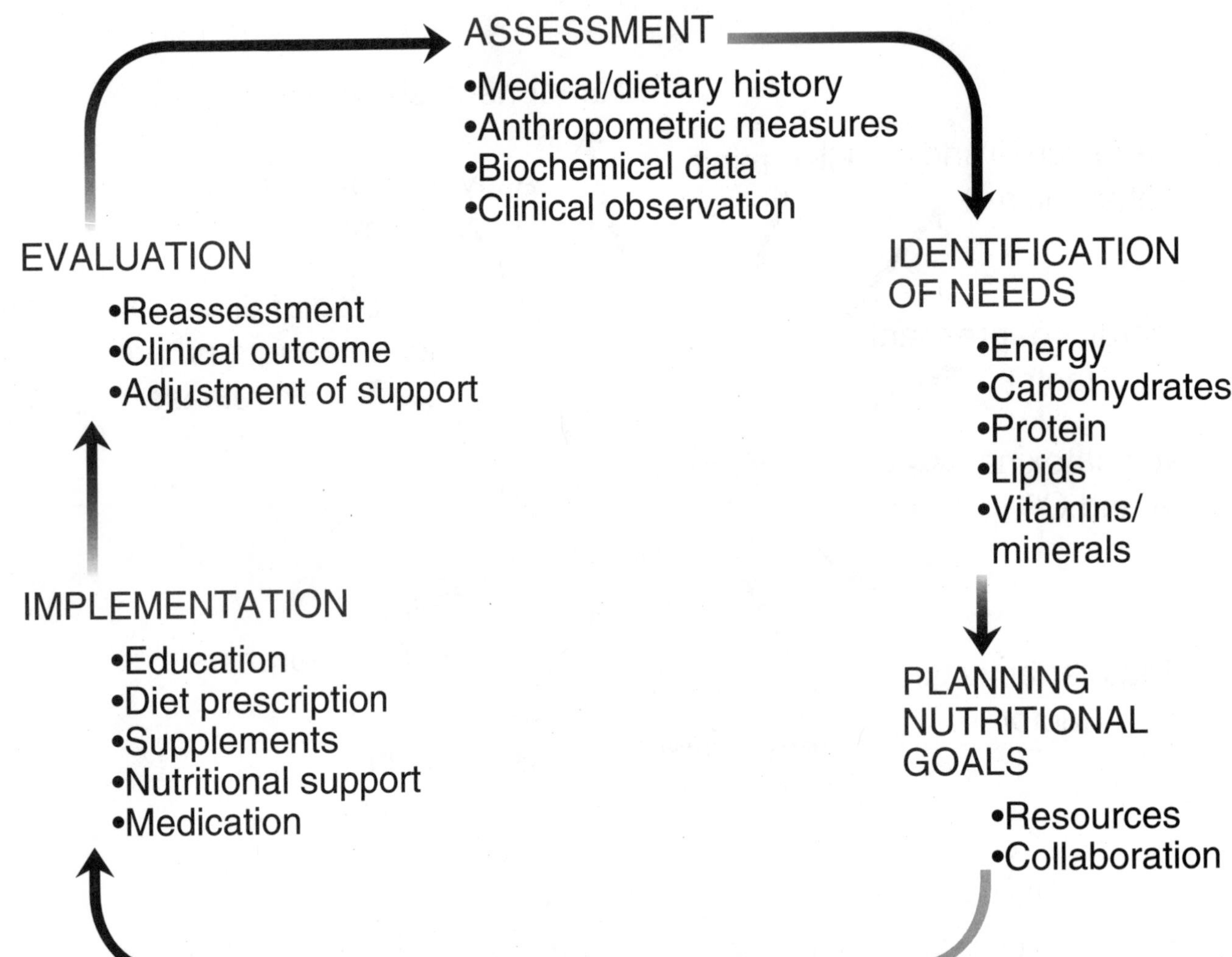


Nutritional Assessment and Intervention

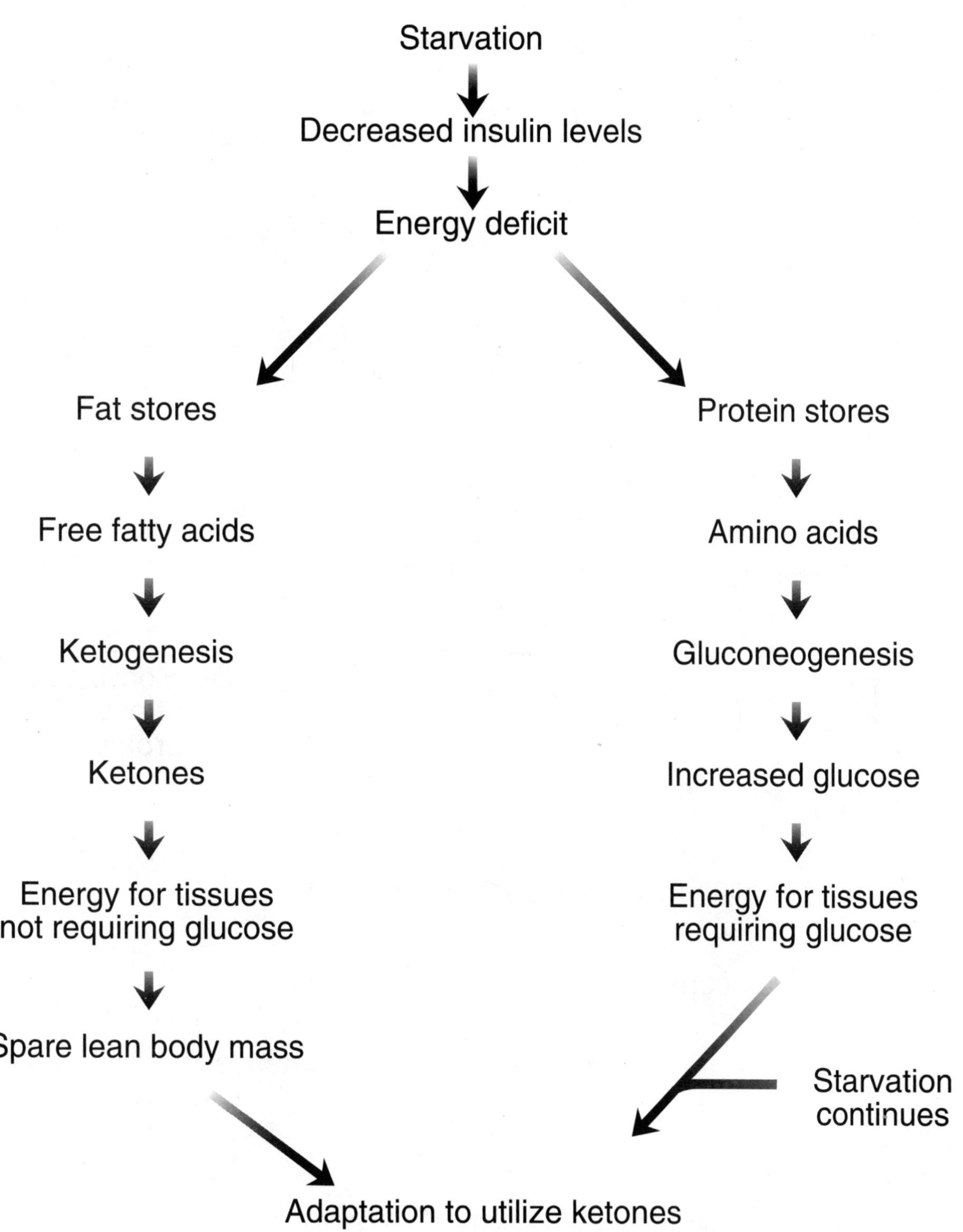


Catabolic Response to Starvation

Transparency #72

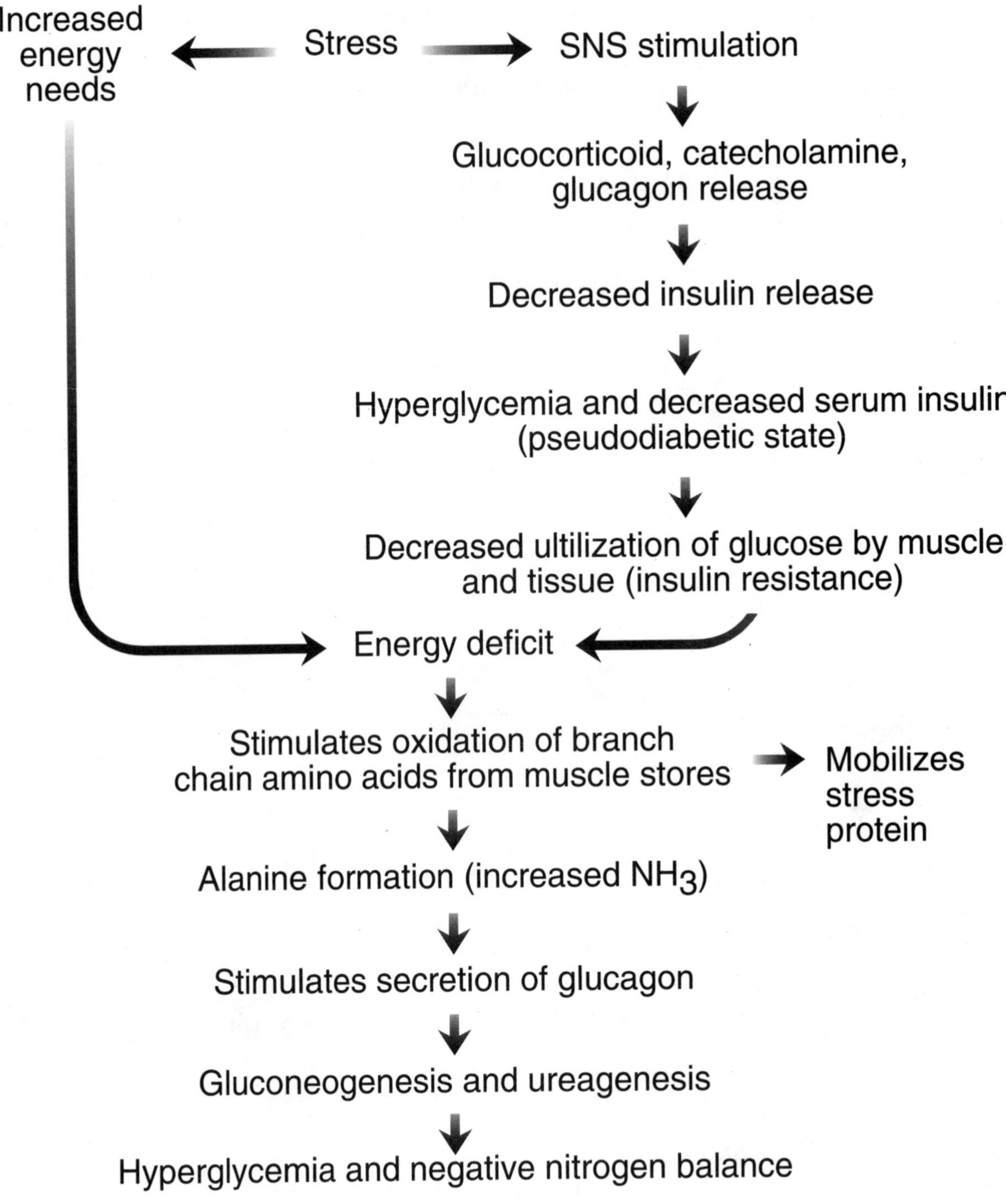


Immediate Catabolic Response to Stress

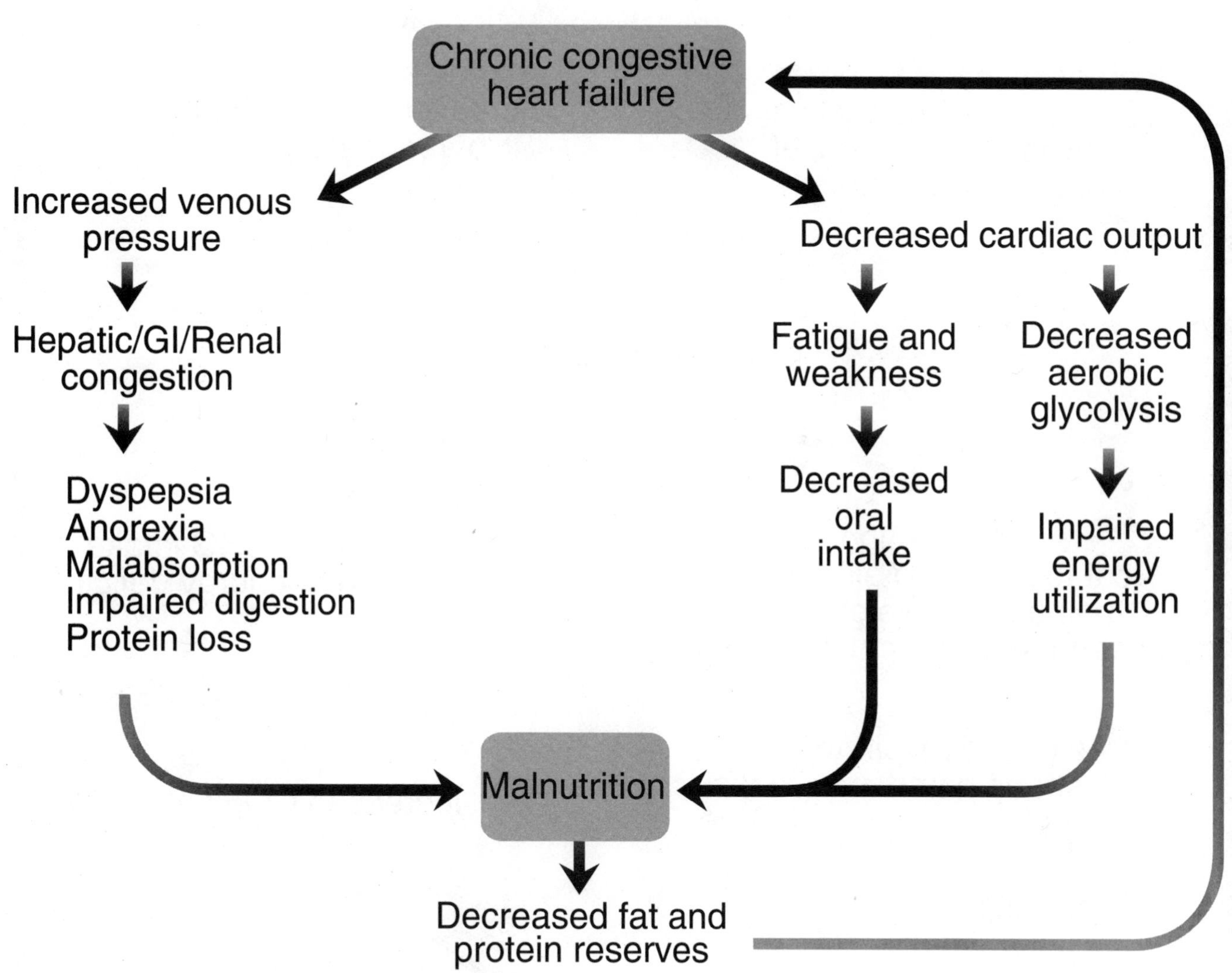


Malnutrition and CHF

Transparency #74

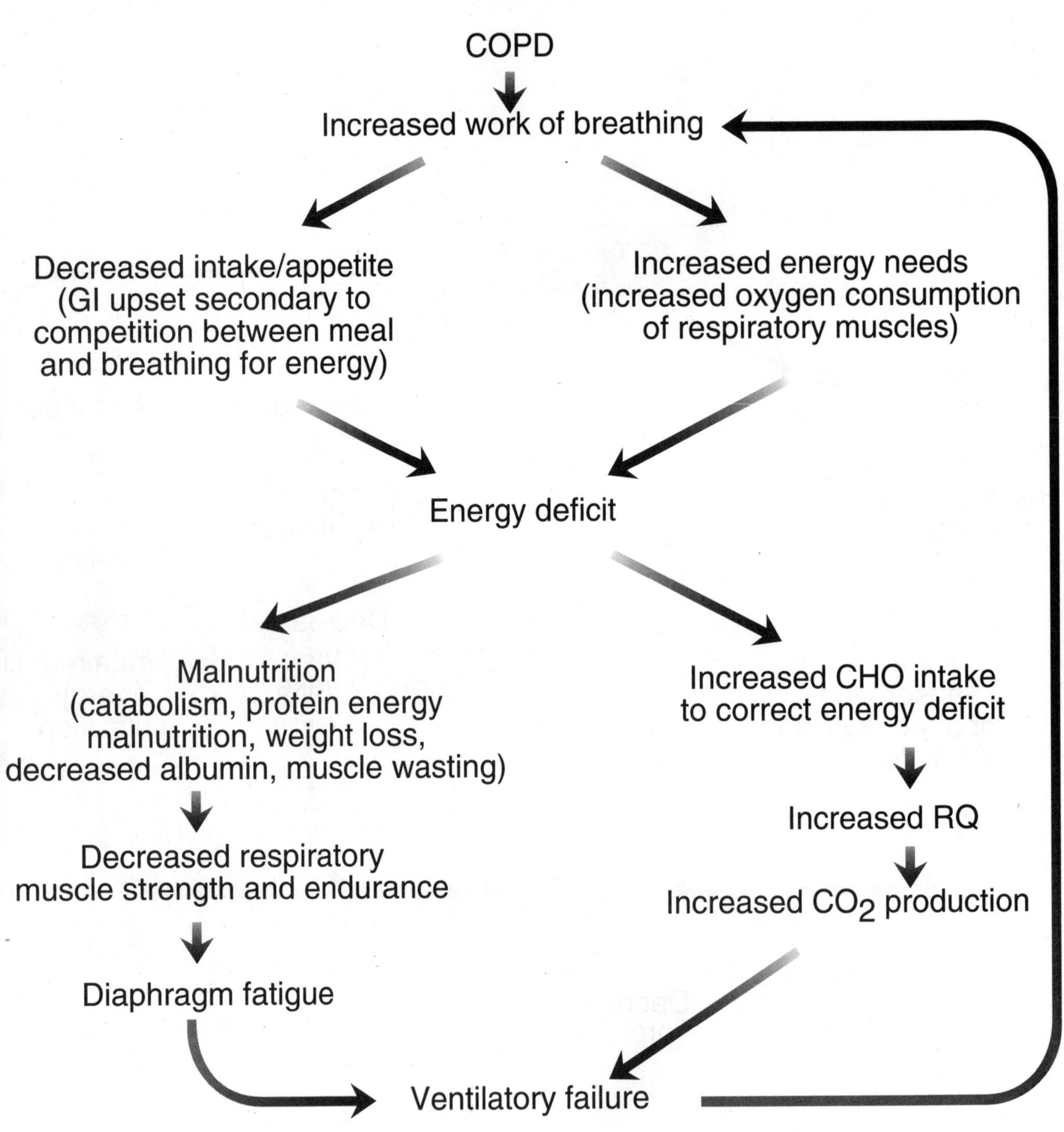


Malnutrition and COPD